Reading the Book of Nature

Habent sua fata libelli

Volume 41
of
Sixteenth Century Essays & Studies

Raymond A. Mentzer, General Editor

Composed by Thomas Jefferson University Press
at Truman State University, Kirksville, Missouri 63501
Cover Art and Title Page by Teresa Wheeler, TSU Designer
Manufactured by Edwards Brothers, Ann Arbor, Michigan
Body text is set in Galliard Old Style by Carter & Cone, 10/13

READING THE BOOK OF NATURE

THE OTHER SIDE OF THE SCIENTIFIC REVOLUTION

Allen G. Debus and
Michael T. Walton
EDITORS

This book has been brought to publication
with the generous support of
Truman State University, Kirksville, Missouri

Library of Congress Cataloging-in-Publication Data

Reading the book of nature : the other side of the Scientific Revolution /
Debus, Allen G., and Michael T. Walton, eds.
    p.   cm. — (Sixteenth century essays and studies : v. 41)
    "The present volume is composed of papers read at a series of sessions
centered on the history of renaissance and early modern science and med-
icine held in St. Louis at the Sixteenth Century Studies Conference 24–27
October 1996"–Pref.
    Includes bibliographical references and index.
    ISBN 0-940474-47-6 (alk. paper; casebound)
    ISBN 0-940474-48-4 (alk. paper; paperback)
    1. Medicine–History–16th century–Congresses. 2. Alchemy–History–
16th century–Congresses. 3. Science–History–16th century–Congresses.
I. Debus, Allen G. II. Walton, Michael Thomson, 1945– . III. Sixteenth
Century Studies Conference (1996, St. Louis, Mo.) IV. Series.
R146.R43 1997
509'.031–DC21   97–33101
                                             CIP

The paper in this publication meets or exceeds the minimum requirements of the
American National Standard—Permanence of Paper for Printed Library Materials,
ANSI Z39.48 (1984).

CONTENTS

PREFACE

THE PRESENT VOLUME IS COMPOSED OF PAPERS read at a series of sessions centered on the history of Renaissance and early modern science and medicine held in Saint Louis at the Sixteenth Century Studies Conference, October 24–27, 1996. These sessions were organized at the request of Robert V. Schnucker by Allen G. Debus and Michael T. Walton in part to bring together a group of scholars with similar interests from several disciplines and in part to present this work to the Sixteenth Century Studies Conference, which traditionally has had relatively few papers on science and medicine at its meetings.

The history of science has changed considerably over the course of the past few decades. Forty years ago the emphasis was on the Scientific Revolution of the sixteenth and seventeenth centuries, but interpreted largely on the development of the physics of motion and astronomy from the publication of the *De revolutionibus orbium* of Copernicus (1543) to the *Principia mathematica* of Isaac Newton (1687). To a large extent the historian's task was thought to be a positivistic enterprise in which earlier science was evaluated in relation to modern science. The work of Kepler, Galileo, and other predecessors to Newton was examined carefully to seek out the "modern" elements of their thought. There was far less interest in the biological sciences, with the exception of William Harvey because of his description of the circulation of the blood in the *De motu cordis* (1628). The background to his anatomical work was recognized in a series of great Paduan anatomists beginning with Andreas Vesalius (whose monumental *De fabrica* was also published in 1543) and leading to Hieronymus Fabricius, who taught Harvey as a student. Thus, as the development of classical mechanics was presented as a series of positive steps leading from Copernicus to Newton, the discovery of the circulation of the blood was presented as a "ladder of success" stretching from Vesalius to Harvey. In short, the Scientific Revolution was presented largely in terms of the mathematicized physical sciences, but with a nod to one development in the biological sciences. As for the history of medicine, there was relatively little interest expressed by historians of science. The founder of the discipline in this century, George Sarton, believed that the biological sciences stood far below the mathematical sciences, and he believed that medicine was lower still. Because he was convinced that medicine was a practical art, he was distressed by those medical historians who claimed that medicine is the real foundation of the other sciences. Indeed, he wrote that "the main misunderstandings concerning the history of science are due to historians of medicine who have the notion that medicine is the center of science."[1]

But what of other areas of interest to scholars interested in the Renaissance and early modern periods? The research of Lynn Thorndike, Paul Oskar Kristeller, Frances Yates, and Walter Pagel had pointed to the Neoplatonic revival and the prevalence of interest in natural magic, Hermeticism, and alchemy. Sarton felt that these subjects could largely be neglected. He wrote:

> The historian of science cannot devote much attention to the study of superstition and magic, that is, of unreason, because this does not help him very much to understand human progress. Magic is essentially unprogressive and conservative; science is essentially progressive; the former goes backward; the latter, forward. We cannot possibly deal with both movements at once except to indicate their constant strife, and even that is not very instructive, because that strife has hardly varied throughout the ages.[2]

In his very influential *The Origins of Modern Science 1300–1800* (1949) Herbert Butterfield wrote that historians who specialize in alchemy "seem to be under the wrath of God themselves; for like those who write on the Bacon-Shakespeare controversy or on Spanish politics, they seem to become tinctured with the kind of lunacy they set out to describe."[3] Even Marie Boas titled the chapter on the mystical natural philosophies of the Renaissance in her *The Scientific Renaissance 1450–1630* (1962) "Ravished by Magic."[4]

Only in the past thirty years has more attention been given to these subjects due mainly to the work of Dame Frances Yates and Walter Pagel. In particular Pagel's *Paracelsus: An Introduction to Philosophical Medicine in the Era of the Renaissance* (1958) proved to be an influential work for those interested in an alternative approach to the period of the Scientific Revolution. Many of the natural magicians and Paracelsians opposed ancient tradition and sought a new observational base for the understanding of nature. While it is true that theirs was not "modern" science, they certainly did contribute to modern

---

[1]George Sarton, *History of Science: Ancient Science through the Golden Age of Greece* (Cambridge: Harvard University Press, 1952), xi.

[2]George Sarton, *Introduction to the History of Science,* 3 vols. (Baltimore: Williams and Wilkins, 1927–1947), 1:19.

[3]Herbert Butterfield, *The Origins of Modern Science 1300–1800* (New York: Macmillan, 1952), 98.

[4]Marie Boas, *The Scientific Renaissance 1450–1630* (New York: Harper, 1962), 166–196.

science because of specific discoveries and concepts, and because of their debates both with the proponents of ancient tradition and with seventeenth-century mechanists. Indeed, they played a significant role in the methodological debates crucial to the rise of a new science. Here Paracelsus (1493–1541) may be seen as a major figure. A younger contemporary of Copernicus (1473–1543) and an older contemporary of Vesalius (1514–1564), Paracelsus produced an extensive corpus of writings touching on many topics, among them of special importance, the joining of chemistry and medicine. He rejected the ancient authors and relied on observational evidence, but he distrusted mathematics and sought truth in the macrocosm-microcosm analogy. The influence of Paracelsus extended to disciples over a period of more than a century. They developed a Chemical Philosophy that was fully as well known to their contemporaries as the Mechanical Philosophy, which is much better known to historians of science today. This Chemical Philosophy resulted in heated debates not only between the Paracelsian chemical physicians and the Galenists, but also between various sects of chemists and mechanists who sought to develop a mathematically based rather than a chemically based interpretation of nature. The complex nature of these various strands of chemical thought are evident in current research detailing the alchemical interests of Isaac Newton and Robert Boyle, who previously were thought to be exemplars only of the new mechanical science of the seventeenth century.

As we probe deeper into these texts we find also that their ramifications extend beyond the sciences into related cultural, political, and intellectual spheres. A large proportion of the Paracelsian authors were Protestant rather than Roman Catholic. As a result we find opposition based upon religious views—as well as opposition from the educational establishment that remained largely wedded to the ancients. Both in England and France political factions sought to support either the chemists or the ancients in a bid for control of medical organizations. Here and in other cases we can see a resulting debate on many levels.

The papers from this conference reflect current research in this area. Some of these papers center on specific technical aspects of Renaissance alchemy, chemistry, and Paracelsian thought, but others deal with the impact of this thought on other areas ranging from religious and political considerations to the role of alchemy in the methodology of the history of science. The volume begins appropriately with the beginning itself, a paper on the profound influence of the creation account in Genesis on sixteenth- and seventeenth-century scientists. Michael T. Walton's account opens with a Renaissance Jewish scholar, Ovadiah Sforno, whose commentary on the Pentateuch dealt with the creation of the earth and the elements while referring to chemical terminology. Although Sforno accepted many aspects of Aristotelian thought, the next author discussed, Paracelsus, challenged the Greek authors at every turn. For him the very basis of understanding should be a belief in God and the biblical account of creation which in practice could be evidenced in a proper union of medicine and chemistry. His was a "Mosaical" philosophy, and Walton follows this concept through the work of the Dane, Peter Severinus, the Englishman, R. Bostocke, and the German, Oswald Croll, all of whom sought a true Christian philosophy that in practice emphasized chemistry and medicine. Robert Fludd and Jean Baptiste van Helmont, two very different chemical philosophers, continued to base their philosophy on the creation account, and even Robert Boyle founded his concept of corpuscularian matter on the divine creation.

Like Walton, Jole Shackelford views the influence of the chemical philosophy over a long period, pointing to the sixteenth-century iatrochemist and Paracelsian, Peter Severinus, whose work was read widely and may be seen to have influenced Robert Boyle a century later. Shackelford centers his discussion on the *semina* or seeds of Severinus which were developed by him into a complete biological philosophy, one in which they were pictured as the principles from which bodies arise and to which they return. Again, there was a chemical basis for this since their nature was determined by stripping off their outer husk to reveal their inner virtue. This was to be accomplished by chemical means. Shackelford also points to the use of the term "mechanical" by Severinus when referring to chemical activity on a seminal level, thus noting the danger of using this term only in reference to an atomistic philosophy. The influence of Severinus' work was considerable and Shackelford notes the use of the *semina* by many authors, but pays special attention to the English scene concluding with Robert Boyle, whose corpuscular views and use of a "mechanical philosophy" are shown to have been influenced by Severinus.

From the persistent Paracelsian concepts that link the sixteenth- and seventeenth-century scientific and medical literature, Charles D. Gunnoe, Jr., turns to arguments used to counter this new medical and philosophical school. Here he rightly compares the religious reformation initiated by Martin Luther with the reformation in natural philosophy begun by Paracelsus. The rapid spread of Paracelsian thought after 1550 brought charges of heresy which culminated in the *Disputations on the New Medicine of Paracelsus* (1571–1573) of Thomas Erastus. Gunnoe takes up two points, Paracelsus' views on the creation, and his views on Adam's flesh and the resurrection. Erastus attacked Paracelsus first for teaching that matter was uncreated, a heretical viewpoint. No better was the Swiss reformer's belief in a threefold division of man (elemental, sidereal, and divine) which, for him, helped to explain the interrelation of the macrocosm and the microcosm. But for Erastus this meant that the resurrection would only be of the divine part of the body rather than the body in its entirety. Even worse was the fact that to save Mary from the original sin, Paracelsus taught that Mary was not descended from Adam, but from Abraham. From these examples it is clear that the religious implications of the Paracelsian corpus were fully as inflammatory to sixteenth-century scholars as were his views on natural magic, chemistry, and medicine.

Bruce Moran's paper deals with the debate between Andreas Libavius and Pierre Le Paulmier. The latter, a member of the Parisian Faculty of Medicine, had attacked Libavius as an alchemist and Paracelsian—this at a time when the medical school at Paris had rejected Paracelsian medicine and chemistry, insisting on reliance on Hippocratic and Galenic texts. Accordingly the Parisian physicians rejected the work of their colleague Le Paulmier, who had advocated use for chemistry in medicine that seemed to reflect alchemy. This he had called *Galenochymia*. As for Libavius, he had attacked Paracelsus himself, but at the same time he had called for practical chemical preparations. At times he had accepted alchemical procedures and he seems to have accepted some accounts of the philosophers' stone. Although Libavius may have been unique in his own definition of the proper use of chemistry and pharmacy in medical practice, his insistence on the proper use of words and clear language indeed sets him apart from many other chemical authors in this period. In short, the debate between Libavius and Le Paulmier warns us that we cannot read the texts of this period with preconceived notions of what key words mean. Rather, it is essential that we try to understand what those words meant to their authors.

With William R. Newman we turn to a group of papers related to English authors. Newman emphasizes the work of Francis Bacon, who had been neglected by historians of science for many years, but has recently been named as a major figure in ending the Aristotelian belief that art and nature "were distinct and inviolable realms which could not interact." In this way Bacon is presented in the work of Daston, Dear, and Pérez-Ramon as key players in the establishment of the new science. Newman demolishes this view through the citation of medieval alchemical texts that reject the belief that art and nature were distinct. These alchemists were both Aristotelian in their views on natural philosophy and proponents of observational and experimental studies. In short, it was not necessary to attack Aristotle to erase the division of art and nature since these alchemists saw no such dividing line. There seems little doubt that it is essential to reassess the alchemical background to the Scientific Revolution.

Stephen McKnight next discusses the role of antiquity in Francis Bacon's *New Atlantis*. McKnight first notes Bacon's belief in the need to halt the intellectual decline that had occurred since Adam's Fall and the need to begin true advancement of knowledge. He refers to the work of Charles Whitney and Charles Webster and to Bacon's view that science and technology are essential for the establishment of the religious millennium. But at the same time proper reading of the ancient fables became fundamental for Bacon's program. Here we see the significance of the *De sapientia veterum*. Although Bacon's repeated references to the real meaning of ancient myths may be found throughout his writings, comparison between the *New Atlantis* and the references of Plato to Atlantis indicate that Solomon's House, often looked upon solely as an inspiration for the Royal Society, may also be seen as an attempt to restore the truths of the ancient magi. The desired instauration of Bacon then requires both recovery of the original divine knowledge given to Adam and recovery of the pristine religion. His emphasis on religious purity and the recovery of the original knowledge points to Bacon less as revolutionary figure in the establishment of the new science than as scholar seeking return to the true *prisca theologia*.

Nicholas H. Clulee's paper is on "John Dee and the Paracelsians." The topic is a significant one because although Dee did not publish on any Paracelsian topics, he had close to one hundred editions of works by Paracelsus in his library plus many other works by contemporary Paracelsians. It was Dee's *Monas Hieroglyphica* (1564) that was looked upon as an alchemical text, and continental authors—including Libavius—rejected this work of Dee's along with that of avowed Paracelsians. Clulee points out that Gerhard Dorn's *Chymisticum Artificium Naturae* (1568) includes Dee's symbol of the monas on its title page, surely an indication of the interest of an important Paracelsian in Dee's work. But there is ample evidence that Dee's *Monas Hieroglyphica* was of interest to other authors who may be classed as Paracelsians. And if today we are most likely to turn to Dee's "Mathematical Praeface" to the English translation of Euclid (1570), his interest in navigation, or to any number of his other interests, there is little doubt that in the late-sixteenth and the seventeenth centuries he was most widely known for his alchemical work expressed in the *Monas Hieroglyphica*.

Ana Maria Alfonso-Goldfarb turns her attention to John Wilkins' *Mathematical Magick* (1648). Wilkins has been considered one of the more important forerunners of the mechanical philosophy. While one would not wish to reject this view in its entirety, it is less than correct if one takes into account all of his work. Certainly this is true of the *Mathematical Magick*, one of his most celebrated publications. Here the second book is titled "Daedalus: Or Mechanical Motions." Included is a discussion of perpetual motion, and, of more interest, a description of the eternal lamps that had been found in ancient tombs still shining. This led Wilkins to a consideration of alchemy, which he did not discredit. Indeed, he returned to the problem of perpetual motion at this point suggesting that it might finally be achieved through chemical means. As he proceeded, Wilkins cited authors ranging from Aristotle to Francis Bacon as well as books on natural magic penned by Johannes Wecker and J. B. della Porta and the account of the lamp supposedly in the secret cave of the Rosicrucians. Wilkins' discussion ultimately leads to an attempt to identify the wick and the oil used in such lamps and he suggests that perhaps asbestos and an oil prepared from asbestos or gold might be the answer. This conclusion is to be found in a "little chymical discourse to prove that *Urim* and *Thummin* is to be made by art," an unexpected conclusion from one of the better known "new philosophers."

In his paper Allen G. Debus illustrates the fate of Spanish science in the Scientific Revolution through the reaction to the Paracelsian texts. In the late sixteenth century when chemistry was leading to heated debates throughout Europe in the established medical faculties, Philip II, fearing the spread of Protestantism in the Iberian peninsula, closed the borders of Spain to foreign books and even forbade Spanish students to study in any but a handful of theologically orthodox foreign universities. The result was that very little of the new science was available in Spain after 1560. This is particularly true of alchemical and Paracelsian works which were widely known and discussed in other parts of Europe. The few references to Paracelsus for the most part were highly critical and his work was placed on the Spanish *Index* of prohibited books for their theological implications. It is only after the death of Philip IV (1665) that this changed. His natural son, Don Juan of Austria, was instrumental in lifting the ban on foreign books, and shortly thereafter we find a flood of new ideas being discussed. It is then that we see the work of Paracelsus being introduced along with that of Copernicus, Harvey, Bacon, Descartes, and others. Debates that had been common in Paris and London earlier in the century now were repeated in Madrid and Seville. In fact, the question of the acceptance or rejection of chemistry in medicine remained a serious and unresolved topic throughout the first half of the eighteenth century. It would seem then that Philip II's closing of the border to foreign ideas, although meant to protect Roman Catholicism, had the additional effect of retarding

Spain's participation in the pan-European scientific debate during the critical period of the development of modern science.

From Spain we move to Denmark for the locale of Martha Baldwin's paper. Simon Paulli's catalog of native Danish plants (1648) became the basis for the defense of Danish medicines (1666) made by Thomas Bartholin, who called for the revival of Danish folk medicines. This is a theme frequently presented by Paracelsians and normally associated with them rather than with Galenists, such as Bartholin. Indeed, today he is generally remembered primarily as one of the most gifted of the seventeenth-century anatomists. However, Bartholin had revised his views on the traditional Galenicals in the mid-1660s arguing that diseases should be cured with medicines from their country of origin and that Danish diseases were best treated with homegrown remedies. His plea included praise for his country and for all things Danish. He attacked foreign foods and praised the simple diet of Danish farmers. Even strong Danish beers were to be preferred over French wines which brought about diseases of the kidneys and joints. Along with other imported substances coffee and tobacco were to be condemned and associated with eastern depravity. Baldwin pictures this call for reliance on simple homegrown remedies at least in part as an attack on the Danish empirics and pharmacists, a not uncommon move among seventeenth-century physicians who sought control over their profession.

The final group of papers deals with French authors. Lawrence M. Principe writes of Gaston "Claveus" DuClo (b. 1530), an influential French alchemist who has been largely ignored by historians. Even his name appeared in different forms during the course of the seventeenth century. And yet, he was cited favorably both by Stahl and Boyle while his work was attacked at length by Andreas Libavius. Principe finds the significance of DuClo's alchemical works in his attempts to present alchemical theory clearly. DuClo was well schooled in Aristotelian philosophy and his presentation reflects the scholastic method as he deals with matter theory and the problem of mixtures. Still, there is ample evidence to show that he was well aware of the corpus of alchemical texts. For him transmutation involved mixture of sophic mercury with an aurific seed and he presented a series of examples of transmutation to the reader. Principe notes that in contrast to other alchemists of the period, DuClo ignored the medical chemistry of the Paracelsians and rejected the vitalism so common to this group of authors. Rather, Principe sees here a "purely physical, rational, and coherent system of transmutational alchemy," devoid of the mysticism and obscurantism of other authors.

Thomas Willard turns to another French alchemist, Jean D'Espagnet, who was a magistrate and mathematician as well as a literary figure and an alchemist. He is best known for his *Enchiridion Physicae Restitutae* and *Arcanum Philosophiae Hermeticae Opus* (1623). Published together, the former was a general guide to cosmology, and the latter, a guide to alchemy. He spoke favorably of the possibility of many worlds and the beauty of Copernican space. Still, he accepted the macrocosm-microcosm analogy. In the *Arcanum* D'Espagnet compared the creation with the work of the alchemist. Similarly, he accepted sympathetic action and believed both in soul in matter and in the *anima mundi*. Willard goes on to show the importance of the influence of the pseudo-Lullian texts, and the work of Sendivogius and Paracelsus on D'Espagnet. In short, we have here an author perhaps no less influential than DuClo, but one whose approach is far different, pointing once again to the wide spectrum we find in alchemical authors.

A third French figure is presented in the paper by Kathleen Wellman, who turns to Théophraste Renaudot (1584–1653), a chemical physician and a bureaucrat patronized by Cardinal Richelieu in his attempt to control the medical profession. Renaudot established a system of free medical consultations as well as a low-interest-loan program for the poor and an employment and housing agency. At his Bureau d'adresse he began a series of conferences held weekly between 1633 and 1642. These conferences covered a wide range of subjects and are of interest to us here primarily because the subject matter centered so often on scientific, medical, and occult topics. The discussions were recorded and published. In printed form they represent perhaps the earliest account of a scientific gathering. Unfortunately, the opinions are presented anonymously and we are unable to identify the speakers. In this paper, Wellman centers her remarks on the occult topics discussed at the Bureau d'Adresse. She summarizes the discussion on talismans as an example and then goes on to deal with the frequent need of the participants to define their terms, to present evidence on the subject being discussed, and to explain the significance of the topic for an understanding of nature. Sorcery and black magic are not ignored while the work of Paracelsus is the subject of heated debate, although the subject of chemical medicines is generally approved. The conferences were open to everyone and clearly the recorded discussions are of importance for all areas of seventeenth-century science.

Ursula Klein distinguishes the chemical textbooks of the seventeenth century from the work of the more mystical Paracelsians. Taking as her example the *Traicté de la Chymie* (1660) of Nicaise Le Febvre, she proceeds to indicate the differences between this French author and Paracelsian tradition. The complex nature of the Paracelsian principles is noted and compared with the work of Le Febvre who—like many other textbook authors—used a five principle rather than a three principle system. His system was based in part on the results of distillations. The Paracelsians and Le Febvre agreed that all natural mixes "undergo natural destruction or putrefaction." Thus, separation by fire is a natural process, one that is only hastened by the operator. And yet, fire could also alter substances in the preparation of essences, elixirs, tinctures, and extracts by changing the procedure. In this case Le Febvre believed that the artist could correct nature, a necessity resulting from the world flood that had mixed the elements of water and earth. In spite of the similarities between Paracelsian tradition and the text of Le Febvre, Klein insists that the latter made a distinction between artificial and natural mixes, the former being created only by nature, the latter being only mechanical or artificial mixtures.

With the final paper we leave the chemical, alchemical, and Paracelsian themes that dominated these sessions. Vera Cecília Machline turns her attention to the French physician Laurent Joubert (1529–1582), who sought medical value in laughter. She turns to traditional accounts in the medieval medical literature recommending laughter and mirth, which was joined with a stern warning that intemperate joy and laughter might affect the heart and cause death. Such concern was to be found in the sixteenth-century works of both Girolamo Fracastoro and François Valeriole. For Joubert laughter provided a healthy mean between joy and sadness. Still, this "laughter of the mean" was to be distinguished from the more dangerous laughter stemming from humoral imbalance and illness. The *Traité du ris* (1560) testifies to the Renaissance interest in the physiology of laughter and its medical consequences.

If the present volume presents us with a lesson, it is perhaps that we must judge the work of earlier authors in its entirety as Walter Pagel insisted more than fifty years ago. The work of recent decades has established the fact that giants such as Boyle and Newton were deeply interested in alchemy and religion. We cannot judge them solely by their so-called positive contributions to our science since they were influenced by a much broader spectrum of thought. But we must also go beyond the work of the individuals of the period to examine the development of modern science in its totality. We must surely go beyond the progressions leading to classical mechanics and the circulation of the blood to study the debates of the chemists and the Paracelsians with the followers of both the ancients and the mechanists. And beyond this we must relate these views to the medical, religious, and even the political maelstrom of the period. Only after we have done this will we begin to truly understand the origins not only of our science, but of the modern world. ▨

Michael T. Walton

GENESIS AND CHEMISTRY IN THE SIXTEENTH CENTURY

ALTHOUGH CATHOLICS, PROTESTANTS, AND JEWS often disagreed on the interpretation of Holy Writ, all accepted the Genesis account of the creation as part of God's communication to man and therefore true. In particular, the first chapter of Genesis formed a bridge between theology and the natural world. In the King James Version,[1] the first ten verses of this chapter are translated:

> In the beginning God created the heaven and the earth. And the earth was without form, and void; and the darkness was upon the face of the deep. And the Spirit of God moved upon the face of the waters. And God said, Let there be light: and there was light. And God saw the light, that it was good: and God divided the light from the darkness. And God called the light Day, and the darkness he called Night. And the evening and the morning were the first day.
>
> And God said, Let there be a firmament in the midst of the waters, and let it divide the waters from the waters. And God made the firmament, and divided the waters which were under the firmament from the waters which were above the firmament: and it was so. And God called the firmament Heaven. And the evening and the morning were the second day.
>
> And God said, Let the waters under the heaven be gathered together unto one place, and let the dry land appear: and it was so. And God called the dry land Earth; and the gathering together of the waters called he Seas: and God saw that it was good.

[1] Unless there is a specific reason to give the Hebrew, the biblical text will be given in the King James Version's English.

1

Natural philosophers were fond of pointing out that God had given his children two books: the Bible and the book of nature. As the word of God, Genesis both stimulated thought about the book of nature and measured the adequacy of theories about the functioning of nature. Because chemistry, like Genesis, dealt with the basic components and processes of God's creation, chemical theory was dependent for its acceptance not only on its conformity with observation, but also on its agreement with God's written revealed truth. Indeed, natural phenomena were only intelligible because they reflected the pattern of the divine mind that could be glimpsed in Genesis.

Scholars who adhered to older Aristotelian ideas of matter and chemical processes, no less than advocates of the new chemical philosophy, worked in an intellectual milieu that stressed the light of Mosaical-Christian truth over the purely intellectually derived teachings of pagan philosophy. Certainly, most chemists accepted the four elements, but elemental theory was modified and adapted to new interpretations of observations and demands of theology. Scholars like Ficino, Pico, Reuchlin, Agrippa, and Postel, who reinterpreted and harmonized classical, Jewish, and Christian traditions, provided a model for those who wanted a more correct Mosaical reading of nature.[2] Both traditional Platonic-Aristotelians, like Rabbi Ovadiah Sforno, and the revolutionary

---

[2]The conflict between pagan philosophy and Christian truth arose with the advent of gentile Christianity. Saint Jerome's dream trial in which the heavenly tribunal declared him a Ciceronian rather than a Christian became an archetype of the tension between the two worldviews. Numenius and Saint Augustine suggested a solution which posited that Pythagoras and Plato knew and adapted Hebrew wisdom. Plato became Moses Atticus. Marsilio Ficino and Pico della Mirandola gave the Renaissance explication *par excellence* of the harmony between Greek and Christian (Hebrew) thought. Ficino's Platonic-Mosaical philosophy was developed in his *Theologica Platonica* and his commentaries on Plato's works, *Omnia Opera Platonis*, especially in his commentary on the *Timaeus* where he equates Plato's *caos* with Moses' "without form and void." Ficino was not as consumed with Hebraic thought and tradition as was his friend Pico; see Ficino, *De vita libri tres*, book 2 (1489). In his *Heptaplus*, a commentary on the seven days of creation, Pico linked the Cabalistic notion of creation by emanation to both Genesis and Greek philosophy. Later, Heinrich Cornelius Agrippa firmly tied traditional elemental doctrines to the Neoplatonic-Cabalistic universe of Ficino and Pico. In his *De occulta philosophia* (Cologne, 1533), Agrippa taught that the four elements exist in both the celestial and sublunary spheres (book 1, chap. 10), but that based on Genesis, we know that only earth and water actually bring forth a living soul (book 1, chap. 6). The element of fire, seen in the light of the sun and symbolized by the fire on the altar of the Temple, is the mother of all elements, because it can purify all. To elemental doctrine, Agrippa tied Cabalistic alphabetical and numerological notions, believing they gave man the key to understanding both celestial virtues and matter (book 2). Agrippa was a friend of Trithemius. Trithemius was Paracelsus' teacher. Agrippa, like Ficino and Pico, helped create the intellectual context that gave birth to Paracelsianism and aided in its acceptance.

Paracelsus and his successors, sought to illuminate Moses with chemistry and chemistry with Moses.

*   *   *

The work of Ovadiah Sforno (1470–1550), teacher of Johannes Reuchlin and friend of Cardinal Egidio Grimani, illustrates the application of traditional Platonic-Aristotelian ideas of matter to Genesis. His study of philosophy, mathematics, and medicine in Rome allowed him to compare and harmonize Jewish teachings with the Platonic-Aristotelian worldview. Sforno accepted western astronomy, physics, and elemental theory as they existed in the Christian world. He also followed medieval Jewish philosophers, especially Maimonides, in rejecting the eternity of the world in favor of the revealed truth of divine creation. His ability to weave the strands of the various intellectual traditions is seen in his commentary on the Pentateuch, a classic of rabbinic thought that remains a standard text in the orthodox Jewish curriculum.[3]

Sforno composed his commentary with the stated purpose of strengthening his co-religionists who found their secular learning and life at variance with Jewish tradition. He believed that a correct understanding of the Pentateuch would help those who "question the importance of our holy Torah...for they do not understand it properly."[4] The commentary rests firmly in the rabbinic tradition with its appreciation that nature declares God's glory. Religiously, Sforno, as a "Maimonidean" rationalist, apparently was little influenced by the then controversial *Zohar* or other works in the Cabalistic tradition, and his death in 1550 preceded the dissemination of the Paracelsian corpus. His commentary relied on a traditional Aristotelian understanding of the elements and chemical properties to describe the creation of the earth and the "sublunar" region. In his discussion of the separation of the elemental waters and the appearance of dry land, Sforno referred to the four elements, distillation (a process alchemists often associated with creation), and the physics of elements moving to their natural place:

---

[3]Ovadiah Sforno was born at Cesena, Italy, about 1470, but spent most of his adult life in Rome and Bologna. He was Jewishly educated by his father and older brother. He studied secular subjects in Rome and became a practicing physician. The extent of his Latin skill is revealed in his translation of his own *Or Amim* [Light of the Gentiles] (1537) published two years before his death as *Lumen Gentium* (Bologna, 1548). During his lifetime, much of Sforno's reputation rested on this work, in which he analyzed the points of convergence and divergence between Jewish tradition and the Platonic-Aristotelian worldview.

[4]Introduction to Sforno's commentary on the Pentateuch in *Mikra'ot Gedolot* (New York: Abraham Isaac Pridman, n.d.), (my translation).

and the spirit (or wind) of Elohim hovered above the surface of the waters" [Gen. 1:2]: the movers of the celestial spheres are called the spirit or wind, as it is said "He makes His angels, wind" [Psalms 104:4]: [These wind angels] moved the dark air over the surface of the waters which surrounded the foundation of the earth. And thus the midst of the waters near the celestial sphere were heated through movement and became the element of fire ....

And there was an expanse [firmament] in the midst of the water" [Gen. 1:6]: thus it was that the nature of the elemental waters became like a wheel turning, dividing one part from another, such that the upper part of the waters, near the air, returned to the nature of vapor. And thus they are raised to the level of elemental air. This elemental air becomes a place for the portion of water which became vapor. It greatly expands into a larger area than it first occupied [forming an expanse or firmament].[5]

As is apparent, Sforno viewed the words of Moses in terms of traditional ideas of matter and physics. The Master of the Universe created the elements from the vast churning abyss. After creation, the elements functioned according to the dictates of natural philosophy. The world is intelligible in Aristotelian terms, but it is always under God's control and is absolutely the product of his creative impulse. Nature is correctly understood only when the processes of the natural world are viewed from a Mosaical perspective.

*   *   *

Theophrastus Bombastus von Hohenheim, called Philippus Aureolus Paracelsus, stands in marked contrast to Sforno. Paracelsus reveled in challenging tradition and mocking university learning. He immersed himself in the revelatory insights of Cabala in radical Neoplatonism. His works, and those attributed to him, called for the overthrow of the old pagan medicine and for the creation of a new medicine and chemistry based on observation of nature.[6] Like Sforno, however, Paracelsus decreed that all knowledge gained from that observation would have, of necessity, to comport with God's revealed word. What the word of God meant was subject to Paracelsus's peculiar magical, spiritualist religion. The idiosyncratic nature of his religious ideas was a major impediment to the acceptance of his philosophy. Thomas Erastus' criticism of Paracelsus' impiety and magic, along with Johannes Oporinus' claim that Paracelsus rejected both the pope and Luther, placed Paracelsus outside of any

---

[5] Sforno's commentary on Gen. 1:6 in *Mikra'ot Gedolot*, 13–14 (my translation).

[6] The genuineness of any work attributed to Paracelsus is immaterial for the purpose of this study. Works believed to be by the master constituted the source of Paracelsianism. What that tradition said about Genesis is my focus.

religious orthodoxy.[7] Yet his religious heresy and his medical and chemical theories were intertwined with his desire to make chemistry and medicine truly Christian by freeing them from their pagan roots. The book of nature, man [the microcosm], and the book of Scripture, Paracelsus taught, had all been imperfectly understood before him. The great exegetes had missed the kernel and stuck only to the rind.[8] He would expose the kernel for all to see.

In opposition to the Peripatetic philosophy, Paracelsus rooted his thought in the belief in God and in the biblical account of creation. The author of *Three Books of Philosophy to the Athenians* (Erastus and others believed him to be Paracelsus) "corrected" the Athenian Aristotle.[9] The *Three Books*, a commentary on the creation, taught that in the beginning, God created all things from the Great Mystery by means of the process of separation. By separation, the elements broke out of the Great Mystery: fire became the heaven; air occupied the space where there was no substance; water moved to the center; and earth coagulated into dry land.[10]

The theme of creation recurs in Paracelsus' writings, using different terms than in his *Three Books,* but always relating his perceptions to the Genesis text. In the *Meteorology*, for example, Paracelsus stated that "God began creation with the heavens, or chaos, the ethereal realm which is above the other elements."[11] In Paracelsus' constant coping with creation and its relationship to matter and process in the created world, Paracelsianism is most Mosaical. It is here, too, that we see that Paracelsianism found a Cabalistic interpretation of Genesis. Paracelsus and the works attributed to him adhered to the hidden tradition revealed to Moses rather than the vulgar philosophy of the plain text of Genesis. Paracelsus claimed that he had been called by God to "blott out false works…through the light of nature."[12]

---

[7]Charles D. Gunnoe, Jr., "Thomas Erastus and His Circle of Anti-Paracelsians," in *Analecta Paracelsica*, ed. Joachim Telle (Stuttgart: Franz Steiner Verlag, 1994), 147–148, covers the Erastian challenge to Paracelsianism and cites most earlier work. He also reproduces the essential parts of Oporinus' letter on Paracelsus.

[8]Oporinus' letter, in Gunnoe, "Thomas Erastus," 148.

[9]Paracelsus, *Philosophiae ad Atheniensis libri tres*, translated into English by H. Pinnel as *Philosophy Reformed* (London, 1657) and by Arthur Edward Waite, *The Hermetic and Alchemical Writings of Aureolus Philippus Theophrastus Bombast, of Hohenheim, called Paracelsus the Great…translated into English*, 2 vols. Vol. 1 *Hermetic Chemistry;* Vol. 2, *Hermetic Medicine and Hermetic Philosophy* (1894; reprint, Berkeley, Calif.: Shambala, 1976); hereafter cited *Writings of Paracelsus.*

[10]*Writings of Paracelsus*, 2: 249. See Walter Pagel, "The Prime Matter of Paracelsus," *Ambix* 9 (1961): 117–135.

[11]Paracelsus, *Meteorologicae*, in *Philosophiae magnae* (Cologne, 1567), 35 (my translation).

[12]*Tincture of Philosophy*, in *Writings of Paracelsus*, 1:19–20.

Paracelsus saw the Great Mystery very much as others saw the 'boundless' of philosophy or the *ein soph* of the *Zohar*. From the Great Mystery came the elements, but, as Genesis teaches, water is the mother, seed, and root of all minerals.[13] All elements are necessary and have their place, but only water is the mother. What could be more profound? What could be more at variance with the uncreated elements of Aristotle? What could be more Mosaical? From the foundation of a true understanding of creation, cabalistically and chemically interpreted, correct knowledge could proceed.

Paracelsus' "inspired," but unsystematic, thought presented many problems, both chemically and theologically. His doctrines challenged university knowledge. His newly minted terms for his ideas sounded strange. His religious discourse and comments on the Bible were unorthodox. His thought was "cabalistic" at best. However, the fact that his theories and odd terminology allowed chemical and medical problems to be viewed in a new light did much to recommend his ideas to those dissatisfied with accepted medical practice. His cabalistic approach to chemistry and the study of nature fit the intellectual disposition of many. His interpretations of nature were at root religious, and it is appropriate that the seemingly miraculous nature of his cures converted dedicated, if not fanatical, followers.[14]

The potential of Paracelsianism was seen and embraced by Peter Severinus, who systematized the doctrines of the master. In his *Idea medicinae philosophicae* (1571), Severinus not only presented Paracelsianism in an orderly manner but he also explained its recondite terminology.[15] Although he avoided intricate theology, Severinus helped establish Paracelsus as a *Christian* philosopher by describing him as a disciple of the Mosaical philosophy.[16] By this he meant that Paracelsus rejected Aristotle and taught doctrines in harmony with Scripture. In his discussion of the elements, Severinus refers to the Paracelsian separation of the four elements from the "primary receptacle." This separation was cast in very literal biblical language.

> On these four [elements], by nature incorporeal, unorganized, void, the Creator established light and number, the seeds of all things. [This was done] completely incomprehensibly by power of his word and spirit which hovered over the water.[17]

[13]*The Economy of Minerals*, in *Writings of Paracelsus*, 1:92.

[14]See *Analecta Paracelsica* for discussions of many early Paracelsians.

[15]Jole Shackelford, *Paracelsianism in Denmark and Norway in the 16th and 17th Centuries* (Ph.D. diss., University of Wisconsin, 1989). This excellent source on the work of Severinus demonstrates that Erastus drew heavily on Severinus for his understanding of Paracelsian ideas.

[16]Peter Severinus, *Idea medicinae philosophicae* (Basel, 1571), 41.

[17]Ibid., 40–41 (my translation).

Severinus' spin on Paracelsus was in the direction of the literal reading of Genesis and in orthodox Christianity. Many Christian adepts had come to believe that there was a need for a new Christian philosophy of nature, and that the need could be met by studying the thought of the German prophet Paracelsus. Many others who read his works did not accept Paracelsus' heretical religious outlook. For example, in Erastus' critique of the new medicine, Paracelsus was pictured as an impious magician, not a Mosaical philosopher. But the undeniable religiosity of Paracelsianism, when modified to appear more orthodox, proved able to withstand the criticisms of Erastus and to establish itself as a Christian alternative to pagan natural philosophy.

The "reformed" nature of Paracelsianism provided the context for the first extended reference in England to Paracelsus. Robert Bostock, in his *Difference between the Auncient Phisicke…and the Latter Phisicke* (London, 1585), argued for a restored, true Christian, i.e. Paracelsian, science and medicine to replace the medicine received from pagans and practiced by the medical establishment.[18] Bostock believed that God had revealed the true healing art in biblical times. Adam "was endowed with singular knowledge, wisdom, and light of nature." Abraham also "did see and perceive, the invisible things of God…." In a like manner, Moses and then Hermes Trismegistus were possessors of the true wisdom.[19] The Greeks had received the divine teachings about nature from the Hebrews and other adepts, but in an imperfect, corrupt form. This corrupt knowledge was passed on by the Greeks and formed the basis of "modern" chemistry and medicine. Like the church, medicine and chemistry needed reformation by a return to the divine original.

> Theophrastus Paracelsus was not the inventor of this arte, but the restorer therof to his puritie. [He was] no more than Wicklife, Luther, Oecola[m]-padius, Swinglius, [or] Calvin…when they…disclosed, opened and expelled the Clowdes of the Romish religion…[which] had darkened the trueth worde of God.[20]

So Bostocke taught that the restoration of chemistry and medicine for the healing of men's bodies was analogous to the restoration of religion for the healing of men's souls. A kind of medical Lollard, Bostocke sought a return to a true Christian medicine restored by the divinely ordained Paracelsus, a medical Luther, whose salvatory writings Bostocke would open to the people in English.

[18]Allen G. Debus, "An Elizabethan History of Medical Chemistry," *Annals of Science* 18 (1962): 5, reproduces and analyzes part of Bostocke's text.

[19]Ibid., 5–7, examine sig. F of Bostock's text.

[20]Debus, "Elizabethan History of Medical Chemistry," 25–26.

On the continent, the German chemist Oswald Croll was also attracted to the religiosity of Paracelsianism. In his *Admonitory preface* (1609), Croll equated Paracelsus' ideas of illumination with birth by the Holy Spirit.[21] True medicine was learned "from God alone." A physician should be "born out of the light of Grace and Nature of the inward invisible man...." True philosophy is grounded in Christ and teaches that God made all from first matter which is "a kind of ineffigiate confused essence" called the mother of the world.[22] Again with Croll, as with Bostocke and Severinus, Paracelsus' philosophy was accepted as the true philosophy because it was grounded in nature and agreed with Genesis.

*   *   *

In addition to chemists who read Genesis more or less in light of Paracelsus' doctrines, the late sixteenth and early seventeenth centuries produced several chemists, such as Robert Fludd and Joan Baptist van Helmont, who read nature and Genesis with a detailed knowledge of technical Cabala and a more critical chemical perspective. Robert Fludd scrutinized Genesis with a knowledge of and devotion to Cabala far beyond that of Paracelsus. In his *Mundi historia* (1621), Fludd set forth doctrines of divine emanation, sephirotic action, and alphabetic creation,[23] all Cabalistic concepts, which he later fully integrated with chemistry in his *Mosaicall Philosophy*.[24]

In the *Mosaicall Philosophy,* Fludd sought to elucidate and apply the knowledge he had gained from his studies of Genesis, Cabala, and chemistry. He taught that, with the aid of alchemy and Cabala, an adept could explore the connection between the heavenly and earthly realms. Fludd began his description of the cosmos with a commentary on Genesis. The world was created by the "Eternal spirit of wisdom: or the *Ruach Elohim*" who "doth

---

[21]"Praefatio Admonitoria" in *Basilica chemica* (Frankfurt, 1609). The preface was translated into English, *The Admonitory Preface of Oswald Crollie*, trans. H. Pinnel (London, 1657).

[22]Ibid., English ed., 22, 58.

[23]Robert Fludd, *De praeternaturi utriusque mundi historia* (Frankfurt, 1621). The *Mundi historia*, like the *Zohar,* compares the tetragrammaton to the parts of the human body and uses the Zoharic names for the sephiroth. As in the early Cabalistic work *Sefer Yezirah, The Book of Formation*, Fludd teaches that all was created from earth (*aleph* [א]), fire (*shin* [ש]), and water (*mem* [מ]).

[24]The Latin edition of the *Mosaical Philosophy* was published in 1638, the year after Fludd's death. The English edition, published in London in 1659, was apparently also prepared by Fludd. The term "Mosaical philosophy" was not original to Fludd, but was a code phrase for the new Christian philosophy which would supplant the ancient pagan philosophy taught in universities. The title was similar to Kort Aslaksson's *Physica et ethica Mosaica* (Hanover, 1613); see Jole Shackelford, "Rosicrucianism in Early 17th Century Denmark," *Bulletin of the History of Medicine*, 70, (1996): 188–191.

operate by his Angelicall Organs of a Contrary fortitude, in the Catholic Element of the lower waters." The contrary actions were condensation and rarefaction. The "potent angell" Michael governed the angelical organs of the *Ruach Elohim* and its subservient forces, the four winds. The sun, by "celestial Alchemy, or spagyrick vertue of the divine illumination," divided the waters into upper and lower parts. The upper waters, the home of good angels, "were obedient unto bright Divinity, and were converted into a fiery nature" whereas the lower waters, Satan's habitat, "being fecall, gross, impure, and therefore more rebellious unto light," were converted into an elementary nature subject to change.[25]

Fludd demonstrated the sun's role in the rarefaction of creation by pointing to the weather glass. In sunlight the water in the glass expands, but in darkness, which is the cold north influence of the elementary world, the water contracts. Between the upper waters and the lower waters existed the third part of the universe, the firmament. The firmament was the mediator between the dwelling place of the *Ruach Elohim* and the fecal world.[26]

Above the firmament, all stood in the changeless similitude of God, while in the world below the action of contraries led to change. As an example of the existence of opposite actions in the elementary world, Fludd cited the heart's systole (contraction), darkness, and diastole (dilatation), light.[27]

One of the central aspects of Fludd's commentary on the creation was his use of distillation. He pictured the divine emanation as an alchemist using beams of light to separate the primordial waters into their constituent parts. The finest material rose, leaving the debris of gross matter in the elementary world. In distillation, putrefaction, and generation, Fludd believed that he had glimpsed the processes used by God in the creation.[28] His chemical and Cabalistic explanation of Genesis was the basis of the true and complete

---

[25]Fludd, *Mosaicall Philosophy,* 192–193.

[26]Ibid., 193–194. As in Sforno above and Helmont below, many biblical commentators are concerned with the nature of the firmament and how it divides the waters.

[27]Ibid., 193–194. The contraction and dilation mirror, the *tzimtzum* or contracting of the divine light before the bright light, filled the then empty space to form the world as described in the *Zohar.* Fludd's universe was not only Cabalistic but also Hermetic in that it made use of ideas found in the *Pimander.* In his unpublished *Philosophicall Key* (1618), Fludd wrote of a creation by a Demogorgon which worked by means of two intermediaries, chaos and eternity, an elucidation of Moses' account in Genesis. See Allen G. Debus, *Robert Fludd and His Philosophicall Key* (New York: Science History Publications, 1977), 77.

[28]Debus, *Philosophicall Key,* 34.

Mosaical philosophy, not an abbreviated gloss, such as that provided by less diligent students of nature and Scripture.

*   *   *

Jean Baptiste van Helmont's criticism of Paracelsus and the new chemistry, and Baptista's attempt to place chemical study on a more certain base, have been well chronicled by Walter Pagel.[29] His criticism notwithstanding, Helmont was himself perhaps the archetypal Cabalistic chemist. He was profoundly committed to obtaining a true knowledge of nature by means of observation and divine illumination. Knowledgeable in rabbinic and Cabalistic thought, Helmont was committed to the truth of Scripture. The creation account in Genesis, therefore, provided essential data for his chemical thinking. His understanding of creation and chemistry was informed by observation, Scripture, and, ultimately, the mystical illumination, called *Binsicam*, divine kiss, by the rabbis.[30] The search for such illumination was a dangerous, but indispensable, step to discovering the underlying truth of nature.

Helmont expressed his divinely inspired insights in a chemical commentary on Genesis. Although mystical, his thoughts are not the imaginative, vague, Neoplatonic-Cabalistic conceptions of Paracelsus, nor do they correspond to Fludd's detailed amalgamation of alchemical and Cabalistic doctrines. Helmont's experiments and specific discoveries shaped his view of Genesis, and, from the details of his discussion, it is clear that the biblical text predisposed him to formulate certain experiments and to develop his chemical theories. The essence of his reading of Genesis is found in his discussion of the *Gas of Water*.[31]

> Gas and Blas are new terms introduced by me which were unknown to the ancients [the German translation defines *Gas* as a subtle water vapor or spirit and *Blas* as a wind or movement from heavenly bodies]. Gas and Blas are among the first physical necessities; therefore, these new concepts must be amplified and expanded. First it must be shown how Gas is produced from water, that it is different from [the products produced by] heating water until vapor rises. To understand how this happens, one must learn the anatomy of water; therefore, I will repeat that the most glorious God in the beginning

---

[29]Walter Pagel, *Joan Baptista van Helmont: Reformer of Science and Medicine* (London: Cambridge University Press, 1982).

[30]Jean Baptiste van Helmont, *Ortus medicinae* (Amsterdam, 1652), 24. Pagel, *Helmont*, 24, discusses the divine kiss.

[31]Jean Baptiste van Helmont, *Aufgang der Artzney-Kuenst* (Sultzbach, 1683), 109. The *Aufgang* is an interpretive translation of the *Ortus*. The passage in the *Ortus* begins on page 59. The translation is mine, based on both texts. The "Dutch" text referred to is in the German translation.

created the heavens and the earth and the abyss of waters. The abyss began at the vault of the heavens [the Dutch reads "at the far end of the dwelling place of the souls"] and ends above the globe of the earth. Nothing is written about the creation of air, which is also a body and was made into an element. Only after the six days of creation, and there was a place [for it] to fill, was there air. Thus "heaven" means air and the matter of the heavens is air, something not known before [I discovered it]. [The Dutch reads "and after the beginning, the air was with the water together in one body and known by one name, heaven"]. The Eternal created the eternal firmament and separated the water which ought to remain below from the water which ought to remain above. Now this firmament was not a cataract or passive division of the waters, but by the power of its operation, the very principle of separation. Just as the sun is not a dividing wall between day and night but is rather itself the source of division, the heavens or air is the source of division between the waters.[32]

After a chemical discussion of creation and a demonstration of the origin of air, Helmont continued by describing "Gas," his discovery, and what he meant by it and related terms.

Now I will turn to the history of *Halitus* under which term both steam and Gas can be meant. It is nothing more than the examination of what is in air. By Gas, I do not understand the dry, oily body the ancients called exhalation but rather another watery, vaporlike [body] which in the past was associated with the substance of meteors. I consider [Gas] the body [corpus] of water, containing the elements in it and the spirit of Mercury, a liquid, most simple, a tasteless, simple salt of water. It contains in itself a uniform, homogenous, simple and inseparable sulphur.[33]

In Helmont's chemical system, primordial air and water were similar in composition. Air, or heaven, was created to separate the waters above from the waters below. Air, like water, contained the elements necessary for creation, because it contained gas. Gas, the watery salt of air, contained the elements. Helmont's discovery of gas was not simply justified by Genesis, but, in part, grew out of his chemical reading of the text. Primordial water contained the elements, especially the subtle vapor—gas. These elements are now distributed in both air and water, from whence creation continues.

Helmont's famous tree experiment proved that creation from water was ongoing. In five years, he grew a tree which eventually weighed 169 pounds. The soil in which it grew diminished by only two ounces. Helmont, therefore, concluded that water supplied the vastly greater part of the tree's matter. Both

[32]Helmont, *Ortus medicinae*, 59–60; *Aufgang der Atzney-Kuenst*, 109.
[33]Helmont, *Ortus medicinae*, 60; *Aufgang der Artzney-Kuenst*, 110.

the experiment and Genesis proved the primacy of water in creation past and present.

> Therefore, coal gas, which I do not dare light but in an open vessel, likewise with its burning makes pure water. Seeds, indeed, are the property of concretion which abide in Gas...when it returns to [its] original water. That all plants arise immediately and substantially from the element of water alone I learned from the [tree] experiment.[34]

In Helmont's work, Genesis suggested experiments and helped in the interpretation of the work. This distinguishes him from other chemical theorists who used Genesis to explicate their chemical theories or to connect theory to Scripture. With an eye to Genesis, Helmont discovered the properties of water, air, gas, and the elements in the laboratory. The divine kiss enabled the diligent observer to be inspired by nature and Holy Writ. Helmont's insights and their basis, Genesis, became important with the mosaification of atomism and the rise of corpuscularian chemistry.

*　　　*　　　*

The development of early modern atomism is a complex story that exceeds the bounds of the present essay.[35] It is, however, important for my purposes to note that atomism had to be divorced from the pagan atheists Epicurus and Lucretius, and married to Moses before being considered as an acceptable theory of matter. In order to mosaify atomism, both Daniel Sennert and Pierre Gassendi cited Strabo's *Geography*, which identified the Phoenician, Moscus, as the source of Greek atomism.[36] The Phoenicians were related to and influenced by the Hebrews. Natural philosophers of the seventeenth century recognized the possibility that Moscus was actually Moses.[37] Gassendi taught that atoms were the first matter of creation, coming forth from the *tohu,* or abyss, by God's fiat.[38] The non-Greek origin of atomism was important to Robert Boyle. In his *Sceptical Chemist* (1680), he placed the origin of Phoenician atomism in the Hebrews. Further, Boyle concluded, as had Helmont, that water was the "primitive and universal matter."[39] He wrote,

---

[34]Helmont, *Ortus medicinae*, 88.

[35]Danton B. Sailor, "Moses and Atomism," *Journal of the History of Ideas* 25 (1964): 3–16.

[36]Ibid., 6–7.

[37]Ibid., 6–12.

[38]Walter Charleton, *Physiologia Epicuro-Gasseno-Charltoniana* (London, 1654), 87.

[39]Robert Boyle, *Sceptical Chymist,* Everyman's Library, Science, no. 559 (London: J. M. Dent, 1911), 71.

by perusing the beginning of Genesis, where the waters seem to be mentioned as the material cause, not only of sublunary compound bodies, but of all those that make up the universe; whose component parts did orderly, as it were, emerge out of that vast abysse, by the operation of the Spirit of God, who is said to have been moving Himself, as hatching females do (as the original, *Merahephet*, is said to import, and it seems to signifie in one of the two other places, wherein alone I have met with it in the Hebrew Bible) upon the face of the waters; which being, as may be supposed, divinely impregnated with the seeds of all things, were by that productive incubation qualified to produce them.[40]

Boyle acknowledged the similarity of his ideas to Helmont's, but argued that his own work was distinguished by its experimental rigor. In discussing the tree experiment and his own hydroponic endeavors, Boyle presented more detailed data proving that water is prime matter.

And though it appears not that Helmont had the curiosity to make any analysis of this plant, yet what I lately told you I did to one of the vegetables I nourished with water only, will I suppose keep you from doubting that if he had distilled this tree, it would have afforded him the like distinct substances as another vegetable of the same kind. I need not subjoyne that I had it also in my thoughts to try how experiments to the same purpose with those I related to you would succeed in other bodies than vegetables, because importunate avocations having hitherto hindered me from putting my design in practice, I can yet speak but conjecturally of the success: but the best is, that the experiments already made and mentioned as you need not the assistance of new ones, to verifie as much as my present task makes it concern me to prove by experiments of this nature.[41]

Of course, common water is not primordial water and only retains some of the creative virtues or seeds. Still,

we find that our common water (which indeed is often impregnated with a variety of seminal principles and rudiments) being long kept…will putrifie and stink…according to the nature of the seeds that were lurking in it.[42]

Boyle's discussion of water with its active seeds is Helmontian in a mosaic-corpuscularian garment. Boyle, like Paracelsus, Fludd, and Helmont, accepted

[40]Boyle, *Sceptical Chymist*, 71–72.
[41]Boyle, *Sceptical Chymist*, 68. See also C. Webster, "Water as the Ultimate Principle of Nature: The Background to Boyle's Sceptical Chymist," *Ambix* 13 (1966): 96–107, and Michael T. Walton, "Boyle and Newton on the Transmutation of Water and Air, from the Root of Helmont's Tree," *Ambix* 27 (1980): 11–18.
[42]Boyle, *Sceptical Chymist*, 73.

the water of Genesis as prime matter, for in the beginning, and to a lesser degree at the present, water was a mixture of corpuscles that could be combined to produce all things.

Boyle added experimental rigor to his corpuscular chemistry, which recognized water as prime matter. Yet, although he refers to Genesis and even relies on his knowledge of Hebrew to define the verb *merahephet*, Boyle regarded the study of nature as something to be distinguished from the study of Scripture. To that end, he broke off his Genesis commentary with the words, "[b]ut you, I presume, expect that I should discourse on this matter like a naturalist, not a philologer."[43]

Boyle's critical "naturalist" insight, in addition to revealing Genesis's influence on his theory of matter, illustrates a trend to treat chemistry apart from Scripture that grew in popularity from the mid-seventeenth century. By Boyle's day, chemistry was Mosaical; it needed little scriptural justification. It was assumed that nature declared God's glory and that a new, successful Christian philosophy of nature would roll forth to prove it. By the final third of the seventeenth century, the pagan philosophers had been christianized and the biblical text vindicated. To be sure, natural philosophers like Boyle were committed to Holy Writ; they did not, however, need to invoke it in the same way as had previous virtuosi to prove the validity of their science. Reasoning from experiment eventually became a sufficient basis upon which to read the book of nature.

[43]Ibid., 72.

14

Jole Shackelford

SEEDS WITH A MECHANICAL PURPOSE

SEVERINUS' SEMINA AND SEVENTEENTH-CENTURY MATTER THEORY

THE APPARENTLY ANTITHETICAL RELATIONSHIP between mechanical philosophy and occult philosophy once led scholars of seventeenth-century science to suppose that a decisive shift away from occult philosophy occurred in the Scientific Revolution of the seventeenth century, and that a more rigorously experimental and mechanical philosophy emerged triumphant and defined the foundations of modern science. But in light of studies published over the last thirty years, this view is no longer tenable. In England, for example, where atomism and Cartesianism were forged into a mechanical, corpuscular philosophy during Newton's lifetime, occult philosophical traditions continued to flourish, as recent work on Robert Boyle and his contemporaries has demonstrated.[1] Boyle himself was influenced by the chemical philosophy of Jean Baptiste van Helmont, and vestiges of Helmontian agencies persisted in a decidedly vitalist corner of Boyle's corpuscular hypothesis, which is in most other respects a model of mechanical philosophy. Indeed, the transition that Boyle apparently made from entertaining Helmontian chemical ideas to expressing chemistry in terms of the mechanical operations of material corpuscles has been treated as a microcosmic study of the abandonment of occult

[1] The most recent contributions on this topic include John Henry, "Occult Qualities and the Experimental Philosophy: Active Principles in Pre-Newtonian Matter Theory," *History of Science* 24 (1986): 335–381; Antonio Clericuzio, "A Redefinition of Boyle's Chemistry and Corpuscular Philosophy," *Annals of Science* 47 (1990): 561–589; idem, "Robert Boyle and the English Helmontians," in *Alchemy Revisited; Proceedings of the International Conference on the History of Alchemy at the University of Groningen, 17–19 April 1989*, ed. Z. R. W. M. von Martels (Leiden: E.J. Brill, 1990, 192–199).

15

philosophy in the older historiography of the Scientific Revolution. As a result, Boyle's matter theory and its relation to alchemical, atomic, mechanistic, and Paracelsian antecedents has become a testing ground for arguments over continuity and change in seventeenth-century science, consideration of which will necessarily be a part of the reconstruction of a new overview of scientific change in early modern Europe.

Recent work by Antonio Clericuzio and John Henry has strengthened the efforts of Walter Pagel, Allen Debus, Charles Webster, Nina Rattner Gelbart, and others to place Boyle in a Helmontian tradition and therefore to argue for continuity between sixteenth-century Paracelsian thought and the new science of the seventeenth century. Clericuzio has even traced key elements of this vitalism, namely the operation of seminal principles on inert matter (water) to form bodies, back to ideas developed by the sixteenth-century Danish Paracelsian physician and philosopher Petrus Severinus.[2] This aspect of Paracelsian metaphysics, at least, continued to fill a philosophical need well over a century after its decisive formulation by Severinus and found its way into the theories of matter and causation expounded by prominent English mechanical philosophers. The nature of Severinus' theory of the generation of bodies, its assimilation into the nascent corpuscular theory, and what this can tell us about the meanings of mechanical philosophy in midcentury England, is the subject of the present study.[3]

Antonio Clericuzio's claim that Helmont was heavily influenced by Severinus' ideas agrees with my own observations on the similarity of their

[2]Clericuzio, "Redefinition of Boyle's Chemistry," 583, claims that Severinus was one of Boyle's sources. Also, Clericuzio, "From to Boyle: A Study of the Transmission of Helmontian Chemical and Medical Theories in Seventeenth-Century England," *British Journal for the History of Science* 26 (1993): 303–334, 310: "A central aspect of van Helmont's natural philosophy was his theory of seminal principles (itself a development of Severinus' ideas), which was to play an important role in the iatrochemistry of the second half of the seventeenth century." Also Clericuzio, "Redefinition of Boyle's Chemistry," 583, notes that Boyle's views on seminal principles were based on works of chemical authors like Severinus, Etienne de Clave, and Helmont. The last two, however, were familiar with Severinus' ideas. Clericuzio's work in this and other recent papers has fleshed out the skeletal suggestion made by Charles Webster, *From Paracelsus to Newton: Magic and the Making of Modern Science* (New York: Cambridge University Press, 1982), 69, that Gassendian atomism, as it was received in England, carried with it important elements of Paracelsian doctrine.

[3]Severinus and his ideas are treated in Walter Pagel, *The Smiling Spleen: Paracelsianism in Storm and Stress* (Basel: S. Karger AG, 1984); Eyvind Bastholm and Hans Skov, *Petrus Severinus og hans Idea medicinae philosophicae* (Odense: Odense Universitetsforlag, 1979); Allen G. Debus, *The Chemical Philosophy: Paracelsian Science and Medicine in the Sixteenth and Seventeenth Centuries*, 2 vols. (New York: Science History Publications, 1977); and at length in Jole Shackelford, "Paracelsianism in Denmark and Norway in the 16th and 17th Centuries" (Ph.D. diss., University of Wisconsin, 1989).

theories of generation and corruption. Nevertheless, I will argue here that while Helmont was an important intermediary for the dissemination of Severinus' ideas in England, English natural philosophers were in fact reading and commenting on the Dane's work before Helmont's studies were known and that Severinus' ideas may therefore have reached Boyle's contemporaries directly or through intermediaries other than Helmont, forming part of an interpretive matrix in which Helmontian theory was understood. Moreover, the chronology of Helmont's writing suggests that he may have learned about Severinus' work while in England and that Helmont's published medical works, which only much later influenced Boyle and his contemporaries, therefore represent, in part, a repackaging and reimportation of Severinus' ideas. I will show that the theory of seminal principles, upon which Severinus built an entire biological philosophy, was widely known and contributed to the general body of speculation about matter theory in seventeenth-century England and elsewhere in Europe. Then I will propose that Severinus' concepts were enduring because they were framed in such a way as to make them amenable to theorists like Boyle, who desired to shape a natural philosophy around mechanical precepts, yet found the austere requirements of Cartesian matter theory insufficient for explaining organic phenomena. The ironic result is that metaphysical concepts elaborated by Severinus from Paracelsian, Hippocratic, and Neoplatonic sources, which ascribed the generation of bodies to immaterial forms and invisible agents, continued to offer explanatory power for the corpuscular mechanists of late-seventeenth-century English chemistry.

Finally, I will argue that the formulation of Severinus' ideas and the terminology he employed may not have been interpreted by mid-seventeenth-century readers as alien to mechanical interpretations and offer this as evidence that the conceptual distance between his Paracelsian vision and the mechanical philosophy of Gassendi, Walter Charleton, and Boyle may not have been as great as has been supposed by modern historians who have opposed "occult" to "mechanical"—at least not at the lowest level of organic processes.[4] John Henry has already made a case for the survival of occult qual-

---

[4]Take as an example of the standard dichotomy between Paracelsian and mechanical philosophy recent statements by Margaret Osler, "The Intellectual Sources of Robert Boyle's Philosophy of Nature: Gassendi's Voluntarism and Boyle's Physico-Theological Project," 178–198 in Richard Kroll, Richard Ashcraft, Perez Zagorin, eds., *Philosophy, Science, and Religion in England 1640–1700* (New York: Cambridge University Press, 1992), 183: "Mechanical philosophers, influenced by Descartes and Gassendi, advocated a mechanical analogy to explicate the phenomena of nature. Followers of Paracelsus espoused a chemical philosophy, which endeavored to account for natural phenomena in terms of a more or less occult, holistic, chemical metaphor." And, "The bulk of his [Boyle's] scientific writings have a dual thrust: to provide empirical and experimental support for

ities in late-seventeenth-century natural philosophy, specifically in pre-Newtonian mechanical philosophy, if "mechanical" is not restricted to the Cartesian sense.[5] Here I wish to persuade that a reverse process might also have existed; namely, that seminal principles, taken into corpuscular, "mechanical" philosophy from their origins in Paracelsian, "occult" philosophy, may not have appeared to be radically different from other mechanical ideas espoused by Boyle's contemporaries. I am suggesting that the very idea of "mechanical" may have been much more nuanced in seventeenth-century discourse than the clockwork metaphor implies and that a careful scrutiny of how such terms are used in the Latin and vernacular literatures is called for in order to ferret out their range of meanings. The historical link between "mechanical" agents in Severinus' biological theory and the mechanical philosophy of Boyle and his contemporaries underscores the complex evolution of matter theory in the seventeenth century, which must be recognized in any effort to revive or revise a grand narrative about the emergence of modern science in a seventeenth-century Scientific Revolution.[6]

---

his corpuscularianism and to render chemistry as respectable as her sister sciences, astronomy, mechanics, and optics, which had been so successfully wedded to mechanical principles. This latter task was complex and difficult because of the occult alchemical and Paracelsian associations that chemical thinking had acquired historically."

[5]Henry, "Occult Qualities," 344: "The mechanical philosophy, as it was presented by English natural philosophers, had a strong tradition of active principles"; ibid., 366: "The use of occult qualities or unexplained active principles in matter...was always a major feature of the mechanical philosophy in England." Anthony Clericuzio, "From Van Helmont to Boyle," 334, no. 172, claims that Henry "failed to recognize the importance of chemistry in Pre-Newtonian theories of matter," implying that he also failed to recognize that these occult qualities, which Clericuzio insists are really active corpuscles, were vested in the work of the chemists. However, Henry clearly placed those ideas in the context of the chemical philosophy of Paracelsus, Severinus, and Helmont; e.g. Clericuzio, "From Van Helmont to Boyle," 343: "Powers' concept of an active spirit...is in fact influenced by Paracelsian doctrines"; and ibid., 340: "The major source for Charleton's ideas in the *Physiologia* was, of course, Pierre Gassendi, whose matter theory was strongly influenced by the Paracelsian Petrus Severinus, and managed to reconcile materialism and vitalism."

[6]Modern historians have argued that mechanical philosophy, considered an essential component of the emergence of a new experimental science in Restoration England, was grounded in various factors, including (1) a wholesale rejection of occult philosophy and Aristotelian (occult) substantial forms, (2) the increasing role of mechanical instruments in the practice of science, with a concomitant influence of what has been described as the mechanics' philosophy (i.e. mathematics) on mechanical philosophy, (3) the importance of distinguishing the omnipotence of the Creator from atheist or pantheist positions that natural (or divine) law is unchangeably imprinted in the material world, and (4) the need to reassert social hierarchy in the Restoration. To these I would add the possibility that the forms that matter theory took in the late sixteenth and early seventeenth centuries already embodied social and political views that may have affected how the mechanical philosophers selectively adopted concepts from a large menu of Cartesian, atomist, Aristotelian, and chemical philosophies.

THE DOCTRINE OF SEMINA

The idea that diseases can be caused by "seeds" (*semina morborum*) had been entertained in the medical literature since Galen, but underwent division and elaboration in the sixteenth century. On the one hand, Girolamo Fracastoro spoke of *semina* (seeds), or usually *seminaria* (seedbeds), in addition to *fomites* as material causes of diseases. Lucretius had used the term *semina* to mean material atoms, and we can suppose that Fracastoro's use of the term also owed something to the ancient atomist, whose work was again read and discussed in the sixteenth century.[7] On the other hand, for Paracelsus the idea of seed was more closely connected with the general process of the generation of bodies—all bodies—and also with the original generation, as it is described in Genesis.[8] This latter use of *semina* had a long history behind it, too, but in theology. Paracelsus' *semina* were descendants of the seminal reasons of Neoplatonic philosophy (*rationes seminales*; *logoi spermatikoi*), which were implanted in nature at creation as reifications of God's ideas. Saint Augustine gave seminal reasons an explicit place in Christian creation theory, which was repeated and elaborated in the Hexameral literature down through the ages and was a familiar concept in sixteenth-century natural philosophy.[9] Paracelsus' concept of *semina*, with this theological interpretation, was taken up by Petrus Severinus, who made it a central component of his *Idea medicinæ philosophicæ* (1571)—Ideal of Philosophical Medicine—which proved to be enormously influential as an explanation of Paracelsian theory.[10]

[7]For a discussion of Fracastoro's use of these terms and how they affected sixteenth-century medical literature, see Vivian Nutton, "The Reception of Fracastoro's Theory of Contagion: The Seed That Fell among Thorns?" *Osiris*, 2d series, vol. 6 (1990): 196–234.

[8]See Paracelsus, *Labyrinthus medicorum errantium*, in *Theophrastus von Hohenheim genannt Paracelsus, Sämtliche Werke*, I. abt., ed. Karl Sudhoff, vol. 11 (Munich and Berlin: R. Oldenbourg, 1928), 187: "Nun wisset erstlich, von solcher kunst die ding zu verstehen, das got alle ding beschaffen hat, aus nichts etwas. Das etwas ist ein sam, der sam gibt das end seiner praedestination und seines officii." ["Now God created all things; He created something out of nothing. That something is a seed, which contains within itself its apparent end, its determination, its office, its task." Trans. Nicholas Goodrick-Clarke, *Paracelsus: Essential Readings* (Wellingborough: Crucible, 1990), 102.]

[9]On Augustine's *rationes seminales* theory see Michael J. McKeough, *The Meaning of Rationes Seminales in St. Augustine* (Washington: Catholic University of America, 1926); Christopher J. O'Toole, *The Philosophy of Creation in the Writings of St. Augustine* (Washington: Catholic University of America, 1944); and Jules M. Brady, "St. Augustine's Theory of Seminal Reasons," *New Scholasticism* 38 (1964): 141–158. On Henry of Langenstein's use of *rationes seminales* to explain causation, see Nicholas H. Steneck, *Science and Creation in the Middle Ages: Henry of Langenstein on Genesis* (Notre Dame: University of Notre Dame Press, 1976), 34, 95, 99, 109.

[10]Petrus Severinus, *Idea medicinæ philosophicæ fundamenta continens totius doctrinæ Paracelsicæ, Hippocraticæ et Galenicæ* (Basel: Henric Petri, 1571). In Pagel's judgment, "most of Severinus' biological ideas have influenced the subsequent generations of Paracelsists. This is particularly evident in the adoption of his concept of semina and their substitution for the elements of ancient lineage and tradition"; see, Pagel, *Smiling Spleen*, 22.

Severinus regarded *semina* as the fundamental immaterial principles from which bodies arise (generation) and to which they return (corruption).[11] They posession within them the knowledge, the ideal plan or blueprint, that is used for constructiong specific bodies from elementary matter by means of chemical separations. This knowledge (*scientia*) is also a body's predestination, which determines its functin and guides its return to an incorporeal, seminal existence at the predetermined time—unless there is an interventioon by a supervening form. since the seeds are dimensionless (incorporeal) and invisible, yet implanted in the elemental matter, they cannot be directly perceived and must be understood from observation of their effects, which are manifest in the chemical properties, life cycles, and periodicities exhibited by individual things. The true nature of seeds can also be determined by chemically stripping off the accidental properties from individuals, the "husks" that hide their true essences. This follows logically: since *semina* operate chemically, through separation, it makes sense that they and their operations can be studied by chemical means.[12] Severinus attributed this idea to Hippocrates, who used the concept of separation to explain the organic development of seeds, but Severinus specifically directed the reader to Paracelsus' *Philosophy to the Athenians*.[13]

For Severinus, *semina* served as links between the ideal and material natures. As forms bound to elemental *matrices* (wombs), they partook of both natures, for which reason Severinus said that people who variously called them corporeal and incorporeal were correct in both judgments.[14] This dual

[11]Severinus defines generation and corruption as a flowing forth and reflux of the seed; see, e.g., *Idea medicinæ*, 89: "Quid igitur est Generatio & Corruptio? Sunt fluxus & refluxus seminum, quæ dum fluunt augentur, minuuntur vero dum refluunt" [What then are generation and corruption? They are the flowing and reflowing of seeds, which when they flow out are increased, and when they flow back they are diminished] (my translation).

[12]The chemist imitates the creator by wielding his knowledge of the creative process. On Paracelsian separation ("scheidung") see Massimo L. Bianchi, "The Visible and the Invisible from Alchemy to Paracelsus." In *Alchemy and Chemistry in the 16th and 17th Centuries*, ed. Piyo Rattansi and Antonio Clericuzio (Dordrecht: Kluwer, 1994), 17–50.

[13]Severinus, *Idea medicinæ*, 86.

[14]In brief, *semina* guide the process by which bodies are generated from spirit. This is a reification in which form, soul, or spirit emanates from material being. This function conveys a unique ontological status to *semina*. Occupying the no-man's-land between the intelligible, ideal world and the sensible world of bodies, *semina* must partake of both. They must be essentially formal, dimensionless, and without quality, but able to dress themselves in matter and take on qualities, quantity, and dimension as they evolve into bodies. The basic idea that *semina* link the ideal and material worlds is found in Paracelsus, *Philosophia sagax*; see Walter Pagel, "Paracelsus and the Neoplatonic and Gnostic Tradition," *Ambix* 8 (1960): 136. Paracelsus presented a case for invisible, corporeal principles uniting with matter to clothe themselves in bodies in *De podagricis*; see Bianchi, "Visible and the Invisible," 26. Ultimately the roots of this fuzzy distinction between formal and material goes back to Plotinus, who taught that both incorporeal and corporeal beings were constituted from one principle that was both form and matter; see P. O. Kristeller, *Eight Renais-*

status had an established niche in Neoplatonism, which maintained a category of spirit to explain the action of ideas on matter. Augustine's use of *rationes seminales* in this capacity persisted in medieval philosophy because they provided a buffer between God and nature that allowed for the immanence of divinity in nature while avoiding outright pantheism, a role that appealed to Severinus and later Paracelsians and Helmontians as well. As *semina*, *rationes seminales* formed the basis for a philosophy that was compatible with Christian thought and yet provided for the operation of regular processes in nature. In short, Severinus fused *rationes seminales*, as *semina*, with chemical philosophy in a way that was clearer and more explicit than had been expounded in Paracelsus' writings.

One of the most striking features of Severinus' *semina* doctrine was its application to pathology, where the generation and spread of disease was explained by (1) the importation into the body of disease-seeds (*semina morborum*), (2) the activation of such seeds that were already bound to the human fabric, or (3) the alteration of normal (non-morbific) seeds to become pathogenic by a process termed transplantation (*transplantatio*). The first case is attractive to modern historians of a positivist perspective, since *semina morborum*, along with Fracastoro's *fomites*, suggest that these sixteenth-century physicians were groping toward a kind of germ theory of disease, in which the aetiological agents, the pathogens, have an autonomous existence. This was also an idea that struck medical contemporaries, who in many cases adopted Severinus' theory of seminal pathogens with little emendation. However, the immediate response to Severinus' *semina morborum* was not medical, but theological. Thomas Erastus published the first parts of his attack on Paracelsianism in 1572, the year after Severinus' book was published, and in part 2 he criticized Severinus' *semina* theory for supposing that God had used *magic* to implant *semina* in their elemental wombs.[15] This was the beginning of a protracted discussion of the religious ramifications of *semina* theory, in which Severinus' critics maintained that the concept of *created* seminal pathogens, *semina morborum*, supposed God's initial creation of evil potencies, which they viewed as a Manichaean heresy.[16]

---

sance Philosophers of the Italian Renaisance (Stanford: Stanford University Press, 1964), 133.

[15]See Jole Shackelford, "Early Reception of Paracelsian Theory: Severinus and Erastus," *Sixteenth Century Journal* 26 (1995): 123–135.

[16]See Peter Niebyl, "Sennert, Van Helmont, and Medical Ontology," *Bulletin of the History of Medicine* 45 (1971): 115–137. Ambrosius Rhodius, *Disputationes supra Ideam medicinæ philosophicæ Petri Severini Dani Philosophi & Friderici II Daniæ & Septentrionalis Regis Archiatri olim felicissimi, Quibus loca illius Libri obscura & difficilia illustrantur, adversarij refutantur, & multi discursus ex inti*

In my view, the fact that semina functioned in both theological and natural contexts, and indeed provided a bridge between the two, made Severinus' theory attractive to many proponents of a unified religion and natural philosophy. Semina put divine purposefulness into the very material fabric of the cosmos. We find Severinus' ideas taken up by early-seventeenth-century authors interested in what can be called "Mosaic physics," where the principles of chemical philosophy are used to explain the account of creation in Genesis, thus providing a cosmic unity of primeval, divine physics and human physics.[17] A Christian natural philosophy of this sort, which supported biblical theology, held out promise for consensus in an age that was increasingly marked by sectarian strife over ever-narrowing definitions of orthodoxies. Such a philosophical and religious irenicism was surely appealing to mid- and late-seventeenth-century writers, too, for whom the presence of divinity in natural philosophy remained paramount.

According to Severinus, *semina* (both normal and pathogenic) operated according to the knowledge (*scientia*) that they possessed. He presented the generation of a body as a kind of Cusanian "unfolding" (*explicatio*) of the seed from potency into actuality, from generality into particularity. When the body had run its course of actual existence, which was predestined in its *scientia*, it "enfolded" back into potency, a metaphysical process that Nicholas of Cusa had called *implicatio*. Severinus did not quote Cusa, whose theory was a well-established part of the intellectual background to Paracelsian theory, nor did he use Cusa's exact terminology, but the philosophical similarity is manifest. Instead of Cusa's geometrical language, Severinus chose to refer to the "flowing forth" or "progression" of the *semina* and their "reflowing" and return to their potential dwellings; an idea that he traced to ancient philosophy: *semina* move out of what Hippocrates had called *Orcus*, the chaotic abyss, into light, and back into *Orcus*, which Orpheus had called Night.[18]

---

mis Naturæ adytis deprompti moventur (Copenhagen: Salomon Sartorius, 1643), xiii, remembered Erastus' criticism more than seventy years later: "The author [Severinus] was received and treated here and there by envious and malevolent persons, and especially badly by Erastus. [Passim a malevolis & invidis, potissimum vero ab Erasto male acceptus, & tractatus sit Author].

[17] Kort Aslakssøn drew on Severinus' ideas about spirit in his version of "Mosaic Physics," which is evident in several of his works, including one called *Physica et Ethica Mosaica* (1613), but more especially in his earlier *De natura cæli triplicis libelli tres* (Siegen, 1597); see Jole Shackelford, "Rosicrucianism, Lutheran Orthodoxy, and the Rejection of Paracelsianism in Early Seventeenth-Century Denmark," *Bulletin of the History of Medicine* 70 (1996): 181–204.

[18] On Severinus' use of Hippocratic texts and his place within the revival of Hippocratism in the sixteenth century, see Shackelford, "The Chemical Hippocrates: Paracelsian and Hippocratic Theory in Petrus Severinus' Medical Philosophy" (forthcoming).

Severinus' insistence that predestined seminal knowledge governs the development of bodies allowed a place for normal processes in nature. In this sense, his *semina* theory is compatible with the concept of natural law, inasmuch as the divine presence is an immanent predestination rather than a free agent. These processes were therefore as determined as were the activities of Boyle's late-seventeenth-century corpuscles, which form bodies by processes of aggregation that display physical laws and are regarded as "mechanical." Although very different causal models, *semina* doctrine and the corpuscular hypothesis shared this sense of ordinary development in nature. In fact, Severinus referred to the seminal process as a mechanical process (*mechanicus processus*) that was guided by mechanical knowledge (*scientia mechanica*).[19]

Mechanical Processes of Organic Development

What did Severinus mean when he used the term "mechanical process" for the unfolding of matterless, seminal potencies that were planted in material, elemental wombs? Surely he had something far different in mind than the collisions and adhesions of atoms or corpuscles that for the modern historian characterize seventeenth-century mechanical philosophy, which is commonly regarded as based on Epicurean atomism and Cartesian concepts of mechanism. Severinus also used the term *lithurgia* to describe these processes, which he then called *mechanica lithurgia*. The way he used this word *lithurgia*, and its spelling *liturgia* by later natural philosophers who commented on or adopted Severinus' ideas, has persuaded me that *lithurgia* is an ecclesiastical metaphor—liturgy—rather than the craft of stonecutting or stonemasonry, which would be suggested by the roots "lith-urgia." However, both interpretations

[19]For example, Severinus, *Idea medicinæ*, 292, refers to a "mechanical process of generations" (*in mechanico generationum processu*) in the title of chap. 13; for *scientia mechanica*, see 159: "Sane, si constantes ac perpetui sunt numeri partium numerorumque proportiones & Mixtionesordinatæ in Generationum lithurgia, casu utique non contingent, neque a posteriori: sed in Scientia Mechanica, de qua toties iam diximus, continebuntur, ubi magnitudines, figuræ, colores, sapores, & reliquæ quoque signaturæ fundantur" (Indeed, if the numbers of the parts, the proportions of the numbers, and the mixtures appointed in the process of generation, are constant and perpetual, then certainly they will not occur by accident, and not *a posteriori*, but they will be contained in the mechanical knowledge—about which we have now spoken so many times—where sizes, shapes, colors, flavors, and also the remaining characteristics, are founded); also 257: "Galenistæ ægreferentes…, causarumque evidentium & antecedentium, a quibus Inflamationes suscitantur, authoritate freti, obstinate contendent, non ex seminibus, spiritus, Tincturis, Scientia mechanica & vitali potestate præditis, sed ex sanguine solo putrescente, Inflammationes omnes produci" (The Galenist *ægreferentes* [bearers of illness]…, relying on the authority of the evident and antecedent causes, by which inflammations are aroused, will obstinately maintain that all inflammations are produced not from seeds, spirits, and tinctures endowed with mechanical knowledge and vital power, but from putrefying blood alone; my translation).

connote a kind of mechanical activity, which is what is important for the present argument.[20]

We can gain some insight into contemporary readings of these terms by examining how they were translated. In an English translation of Severinus' *Idea medicinæ* that is thought to date from the seventeenth century, *mechanica lithurgia* is rendered as a "mechanick or vitall proceedinge" of the seeds, and *mechanica* is translated as "ordenary."[21] When Severinus wrote that species carry out the liturgy of the world comedy by means of generations, transplantations, and mixtures, the English translator wrote that they "doe by meanes of generations, transplantations, & mixtions *play their parts* in this worldely commedy," rendering *lithurgia* as "parts," as in the "parts" or "roles" that actors play on stage.[22] For Severinus the metaphors of liturgy and theater intermingle; he often referred to *semina* as having vestments, and to nature as

[20]Pagel, *William Harvey's Biological Ideas*, 244, thought *lithurgia* must be a Latinization of a Greek word for stonemasonry. But the Norwegian Mauritus Petri Køning, whose work reflects the continuing interest in Severinus' ideas at the University of Copenhagen, spelled it *liturgia* in his *Dissertatio de rerum principiis et mechanica seminum liturgia* (Copenhagen: Godicchenius, 1663)—and he became a theologian. William Davidson, who wrote two commentaries on the *Idea medicinæ*, spelled it both ways; in idem, *Commentariorum in sublimis philosophi & incomparabilis viri Petri Severini Dani Ideam Medicinæ Philosophicæ ... Prodromus* (Hague: Vlacq, 1660), 207, he interprets the term *liturgia* as the continuous and orderly administration of a natural thing: "Per *liturgias* intelligit diuturnas & consuetas administraturas rerum naturalium." Note that this spelling and definition of *liturgia* differ from those given in the 1663 commentary, idem, *Commentaria in Idæam medicinæ philosophicæ Petri Severini Dani, medici incomparabilis & philosophi sublimis* (Hague: Vlacq, 1663), 150, Davidson notes that Severinus employed the term "mechanical" to draw an analogy between the seminal inner agent (*Archeus*) and the expert craftsman and that he also used the term *lithurgia* as "a metaphor taken from the mechanical arts" (Metaphora ab artificibus Mechanicis desumpta), which may have led Walter Pagel to trace the term to lith-urgy or stonecutting. However, there is an important distinction between the craftsman and the *Archeus*, namely that the latter shapes matter from within according to the seminal archetype, rather than from without.

[21]Severinus, "A Mappe of Medicyne or Philosophicall Path containinge the groundes of all the doctrines of Paracelsus, Hippocrates & Galen compiled by Peter Severine a Dane, philosopher & physician to Fredericke the II King of Denmarke & the Northerne partes." London, British Library, Sloane MS 11: fol. 30r, emphasis added; *Idea medicinæ*, 78. On one page Severinus (*Idea medicinæ*, 96) used the terms *mechanicos processus* and *spiritus mechanicos*, which were simply rendered "ordenary processes" and "workeing spirits" by the anonymous English translator; see "Mappe," fol. 35r, although the presence of "mechanicke" above the line in each case suggests that the meaning did not come easily. Quite likely Severinus took the concept of mechanical operation as a way to describe natural processes from Paracelsus, who equated "internal anatomy" (*interior anatomia*) with astral, mechanical work (*mechanica astralia opera*) and astral operation (*astralis operatio*), in *De caduco matricis*. Such mechanical skill ("Kunst *Mechanica*") was responsible for cows' conversion of grass into milk, for example; see Paracelsus, *Medici Libelli ... vorhin niemals in Truck ausgangen* (Cologne: Arnold Birkman, 1567), 78, 81, 111–115.

[22]Severinus, "Mappe," fol. 31r, emphasis added; Severinis, *Idea medicinæ*, 81: "Formæ, species ... Generationum, Transplantationum & Mixtionum ministerio mundanæ comoedia lithurgiam peragunt."

a worldly stage (*mundana scena*). This terminology reinforces the metaphor of the world as a theater, which was not uncommon in this period, as is evident from Shakespeare's observation that "all the world's a stage," in *As You Like It*, act 2, scene 7. Also implicit in this terminology is the idea that nature has a foreordained administrative process,[23] which is mechanical or routine in the same way that ecclesiastical liturgy was. The compounded impression that one gets from the manuscript translation is that the English reader understood *mechanica*, "mechanicke," to be something routine—mechanical in the sense of predictable.

The overall metaphor that runs through the *Idea medicinæ* is a Paracelsian one, where chemical activity on a subvisual, seminal level is likened to the work of the laborant or workman carrying out an alchemical process. Severinus also describes the Paracelsian *archeus* as an inner agent who is responsible for carrying out the mechanical processes, to specifically distinguish his view of generation from those philosophies that consider generation as the imposition of form onto matter by an external agent, by stellar aspects, or by chance meetings of atoms.[24] "Mechanical," then, refers to the activity of a *mechanicus* or workman, the Paracelsian chemist. But we are still left to ponder how this relates to the late-seventeenth-century concept of mechanical, which for many historians has been dominated by Cartesian conceptions of mechanism. The latter conform better to our modern sense of "mechanical" as the operation of a machine than to the "mechanical" operation of the craftsman.

One interpretation of the Paracelsian *archeus* is to focus on agency. The craftsman shapes the raw material before him into a finished product, and, since he is a human being, the worker is assigned intelligence and free will, perhaps subconsciously, by the modern historian. However, it may be that the educated virtuosi of Boyle's England, the learned gentlemen described recently by Steven Shapin and Simon Schaffer, or even the erudite middle-class Danish medical student, Severinus, viewed the craftsman in a much more mechanical sense. It seems to me that the essence of the craftsman requires efficiency, skill, and knowledge (*scientia*) of what is to be crafted and not creativity per se. The artisan unfolds in matter the plan that is in his head, and any

---

[23]The Greek root of the term "liturgy" referred to public service or ministry.

[24]As Severinus, *Idea medicine*, 81, pointed out, the advantage of the *semina* doctrine is that the form of a body is immanent, so that it "does not come from without, is not infused by a giver of forms after there is an agreeable mixture of the elements, is not dispersed from a momentary arrangement of the stars onto the lower region, is not renewed by the chance meeting of atoms, but is lying hidden in the seeds themselves: and that in various ways. These theories are Paracelsian; they are not inconsistent with Christian religion and they are close to the decrees of the Platonists."

creativity must reside there, prefigured in his knowledge. Applied to *semina*, this knowledge is not free, but is predestined, ordained, even if its actualization is contingent on other factors. The *archeus*, then, is not a gentleman dabbler, but a mechanical agent, a skilled player in the world economy—or world theater, as Severinus preferred to call it. His knowledge is therefore mechanical knowledge, and he carries out an ordered process, a liturgy, on the stage of creation.

PATHOLOGICAL PROCESS

According to Severinus, deviation from the normal, mechanical development depends on the alteration of seminal knowledge that guides it by what Severinus called a "supervening" form or impression. Such an impression was responsible for the initial appearance of diseases, when some of the seminal reasons in the world were affected by divine intention, after the Fall of Adam, and became *semina morborum*.[25] A similar mechanism accounts for diseases in the body and explains how cures are possible.

Whether *semina morborum* enter the body, exist in it from birth, or are produced in the body by the effects of supervening impressions on normal seminal processes, the end result is a hindered function or deviation from normal physiological process. Severinus was not always as clear as we would wish when describing his seminal theory of pathology, and sometimes he also referred to "seminal tinctures" as part of this process.[26] A tincture, generally speaking, is a dye, something that tints or colors something else. As such, it transfers its form—its color—to a body. Alchemists latched onto this terminology to express the multiplication of species that is evident when a small amount of tincture or elixir is used to color or transmute a base material to the nature of the tincture. In Severinus' use, a seminal tincture, sometimes called

[25]So, we see that Severinus did not maintain that the *semina morborum* were created in the beginning, but were normal (good) *semina* that were cursed by God.

[26]Severinus uses the terms semina, tincture, balsam, astra, etc., in a loose way, much as Paracelsus had used terminology, and he defends this imprecision on the grounds that the many worlds reveal many aspects of a unitary thing that defies characterization by mere human words. In his "letter to Paracelsus," *Epistola scripta Theophrasto Paracelso, in qua ratio ordinis et nominum, adeoque totius Philosophiæ Adeptæ methodus compendiose et erudite ostenditur a Petro Severino Dano Philosophiæ et Medicinæ Doctore* (Basel: Henric Petri, [1570?]), A7r, Severinus writes "Besides, it is sinful to upset the peaceful flowing of the mind with a burdensome and confused haggling over names" [Præterea, nefas est, quietum mentis fluxum, gravi et turbida vocabulorum ακριβολογια confundere]. "Vocabulorum ακριβολογια," literally "precision of terms," might be interpreted "preciseness of terminology," but the sense clearly refers to trite sophistic argumentation about terminology, when it is really the things themselves that are important to the natural philosopher.

a "mechanical tincture,"[27] imposes its mechanical knowledge onto a host. If the tincture is sufficiently powerful, or if the host is sufficiently weak and lacking the innate vital balsam needed to withstand the invading supervening form or knowledge, then a "transplantation" occurs, the host *semina* are altered, and disease sprouts in the body. Preventative therapy consists of keeping the morbific seminal tinctures (or the *semina morborum*) from reaching the host in sufficient strength to overpower the normal seminal functions and in maintaining or fortifying the host's ability to resist the supervening forms. Curative treatment entails applying drugs with the appropriate signatures (i.e. characteristics) either to hinder the mechanical tinctures of the disease, by transplanting the knowledge of the proper medicine, or to purge the *semina morborum* (or else destroy them chemically), thus ripping the sprouting disease out by its roots.[28]

All of this may seem remote from late-seventeenth-century matter theory, but the point is that readers of the *Idea medicinæ* were confronted with a well-articulated biological philosophy, which explained the pathogenic process and the curative process in terms familiar to chemical philosophers and chemical physicians, yet it was also grounded in a form of discourse with an ancient pedigree—it was Hippocratic, it was Neoplatonic, and in Severinus' eyes it was Christian. It explained biology in terms of processes that were invisible, and therefore occult, and that were tied to a metaphysics that prioritized forms over matter and viewed bodies as imperfect, inasmuch as they were already limited as concrete individuals. Yet for all that, these were mechanical processes, which explained predictable deviations from normal functions and suggested how the physician could intervene using traditional therapies and the new drugs that were prepared "mechanically" in the chemical workshop. *Semina* theory was a fairly well unified explanation and therefore a powerful explanation of the generation and corruption of animals, vegetables, and minerals alike. Consequently, it impinged on all aspects of biology, including balneology and mineralogy. It is therefore not very surprising that it was

[27]Severinus, *Idea medicinæ,* chap. 12, p. 257, does not normally use the adjective "mechanical" to describe tinctures, but the association is plain when, for example, he refers to "tinctures endowed with mechanical knowledge and vital power." Usually he refers to tinctures as seminal, spiritual, vital, radical, vaporous, or having a particular quality (subtle, strong) or chemical or medical characteristic (arsenical, epidemic, epileptic), and reserves "mechanical" for spirits. However, the two concepts are often juxtaposed and are clearly related, if not just different ways of describing the same seminal process: "Therefore, the seed is the vital principle, containing in itself the mechanical spirits and tinctures of the whole anatomy of a particular [propriæ] species"; ibid., chap. 8, p. 96.

[28]Translating *signaturæ* as signatures rather than characteristics or properties gives Severinus' writings an unnecessarily mysterious flavor, but I retain it out of convention.

considered and discussed by physicians and natural philosophers in the generations following Severinus and that it might persist in the depths of even Boyle's corpuscular hypothesis, where the light of Cartesian mechanism could not penetrate. We now turn to consider the historical fortunes of Severinus' theory in order to document its presence in seventeenth-century English discussions of medicine and matter theory.

THE DISSEMINATION OF SEVERINUS' IDEAS

The presence of "seminal principles" and vital agency as an explanation for the apparent ability of certain bodies to self-organize in Boyle's matter theory has been aptly viewed as a vestige of his youthful studies of the medical writings of Helmont and midcentury authors who were especially influenced by Helmont. Among these, perhaps Walter Charleton is most obvious. The effect of Helmont's works on English chemical medicine from the 1650s through the end of the century has been amply demonstrated by Rattansi, Debus, Gelbart, Kaplan, Clericuzio, and others.[29] In particular, Helmont's use of seminal principles, inner craftsmen (*archei*), and ferments to explain physiological processes was widely known. These include pathological processes, such as the formation of stones *in vivo* and in the macrocosm, which so captivated Walter Charleton that he wrote a book about the subject.[30] It is further evident that Helmont took these ideas from Paracelsus and his followers, but until relatively recently it was not appreciated that he took some of them directly from Severinus' *Idea medicinæ*.

In my doctoral dissertation (1989) I pointed out the striking similarity between Helmont's theories of generation and pathology and those espoused by Severinus, and since then Antonio Clericuzio has noted that Helmont's earliest treatment of these matters, a treatise that lay unpublished until the nineteenth century, was heavily inspired by his close reading of the *Idea*

[29]In addition to the works cited in n. 2 above; see Walter Pagel, *Joan Baptista Van Helmont: Reformer of Science and Medicine* (New York: Cambridge University Press, 1982); Piyo Rattansi, "The Helmontian-Galenist Controversy in Restoration England," *Ambix* 12 (1964): 1–23; Allen G. Debus, "The Chemical Debates of the Seventeenth Century: The Reaction to Robert Fludd and Jean Baptiste van Helmont," in *Reason, Experiment, and Mysticism in the Scientific Revolution*, ed. M. L. Righini Bonelli and William R. Shea (New York: Science History Publications, 1975), 18–47; Barbara Beigun Kaplan, *"Divulging of Useful Truths in Physick": The Medical Agenda of Robert Boyle* (Baltimore: Johns Hopkins, 1993); Nina Rattner Gelbart, "The Intellectual Development of Walter Charleton," *Ambix* 18 (1971): 149–168.

[30]Walter Charleton, *Spiritus Gorgonicus* (Leiden: Elsevir, 1650).

medicinæ.[31] Although the exact nature and extent of Helmont's use of Severinus' ideas remains to be determined, I will presume here that the Dane's formulation of Paracelsian metaphysics was a central influence on Helmont as he strove to understand and assimilate Paracelsian theory. What is not established is whether Helmont was the principal intermediary by which Severinus' Paracelsian ideas—and in particular Severinus' emphasis on seminal principles or organic processes—reached Charleton, Boyle, and other English chemical writers whom modern historians have associated with the rejection of occult philosophy in favor of Baconian standards and mechanical philosophy.[32] An extensive analysis of the textual construction of key Paracelsian ideas in the works of Charleton, Boyle, and their contemporaries and a comparison of these with Helmont's ideas and their formulation will be needed before a clear understanding of the sources can be had. However, I will demonstrate here that Severinus' book was well known in England before Helmont's work and continued to be read in midcentury England, when the Dane's ideas were still providing working hypotheses to the English Helmontians. The implication is that Helmont's *Ortus medicinæ* (1648) and diverse earlier publications were being read by an audience that was *already acquainted* with seminal principles and their place in the chemical operation of man and nature.

SEVERINUS' SEMINA COME TO ENGLAND

Knowledge in England of Severinus' work can be traced to a little over a decade after the *Idea medicinæ* was published and not very long after Paracelsus' name began to appear in English medical literature.[33] With the translation of Penotus' *Centum quindecim curationes experimentaque* (1582) by John Hester in 1584, English readers were introduced to the Paracelsian debates in France and also learned that Penotus regarded Severinus as chief among the Paracel-

---

[31]See Shackelford, "Paracelsianism in Denmark and Norway," 169–177, and Clericuzio, "From Van Helmont to Boyle," 307, including n. 18. Helmont's "Eisagoge in Artem Medicam a Paracelso Restitutam," which Clericuzio has identified as a commentary on Severinus' *Idea medicinæ*, was published in C. Broeckx, "Le Premier Ouvrage de J. B. van Helmont, Seigneur de Mérode, Royenborch, Oirschot, Pellines, et al., Publié pour La Première Fois," *Annales de l'Académie d' Archéologie de Belgique* 10 (1853): 327–392; 11 (1854): 119–191.

[32]I leave aside consideration of the Paracelsian heritage evident in Bacon's natural philosophy; see Graham Rees, *Francis Bacon's Natural Philosophy: A New Source* (Chalfont St. Giles: British Society for the History of Science, 1975), and idem, "Francis Bacon's Semi-Paracelsian Cosmology," *Ambix* 22 (1975): 81–101.

[33]On the early interest in Paracelsus in England, see Paul H. Kocher, "Paracelsian Medicine in England: The First Thirty Years (ca. 1570–1600)," *Journal of the History of Medicine* 2 (1947): 451–480, and Allen Debus, *The English Paracelsians* (London: Oldbourne, 1965).

sians.[34] That same year, the famous English iatrochemist and entymologist, Thomas Moffet, published *De iure et præstantia chemicorum medicamentorum* (1584), which he dedicated and sent to Severinus.[35] The two had met in Denmark in 1582, but it seems likely that Moffet already knew something of Severinus' work from his years as a student of Paracelsian medicine in Basel, where the *Idea medicinæ* was published.[36] Although Moffet's treatise was published in Frankfurt in Latin, and therefore might not have been widely read in England, it is apparent that his friends and colleagues learned of Severinus, and plausibly from him. Indeed, the acquaintance with the *Idea medicinæ* that is evident among members of England's literary elite seems to have stemmed from the circle around Moffet's patroness at Wilton House, Mary Herbert.[37]

In the meantime, Robert Bostock, the presumed author of *The Difference Betweene the Aunceient Phisicke...and the Latter Phisicke* (1585), had identified Severinus to the English-reading world as one of the leading chemical philos-

[34]John Hestus, *A hundred and fourteen experiments and cures of the famous Phisition Philippus Aureolus Theophrastus Paracelsus...collected by I. H.* (n.p., n.d. [London, 1584?]). John Ferguson, *Bibliotheca Chemica: A Catalogue of the Alchemical, Chemical and Pharmaceutical Books in the Collection of the Late James Young* (Glasgow: Maclehose, 1906), 2:180, wrote that *A hundred and fourteen experiments* was first published in 1584, subsequently in 1596 and 1652.

[35]Letter from Moffet to Severinus, May 5, 1584, Holger F. Rørdam,ed., *Kjøbenhavns Universitets Historie fra 1537 til 1621* (Copenhagen, 1868–77), vol. 4, no. 229, pp. 320–322: "Librum de Jure et præstantia chymicorum remediorum ad te dedicatum Francofurtum a Wecheli hæredibus imprimendum misi."

[36]Moffet became interested in Paracelsianism while studying on the continent from 1576 to 1580. At Basel he wrote his doctoral thesis on painkilling medicines (*Theses de anodinis medicamentis*, 1578) in which he openly criticized Erastus. As a result the medical faculty delayed his doctorate until the thesis was amended, and with the support of Professors Felix Platter and Theodor Zwinger, he was finally promoted; see Charles Webster, "Alchemical and Paracelsian medicine," chap. 9 in Charles Webster, ed., *Health, Medicine and Mortality in the Sixteenth Century* (New York: Cambridge University Press, 1979), 328, and Trevor-Roper, "The Paracelsian Movement," 163. Moffet actually met Petrus Severinus and made friends with members of the informal circle around Tycho Brahe when he accompanied an English embassy to Copenhagen in 1582.

[37]John Donne, *Ignatius his Conclave* (London, 1611), 29, included mention of Paracelsus: "Neither doth *Paracelsus* truly deserue the name of an *Innouator*, whose doctrine, *Seuerinus* and his other followers do referre to the most ancient times." Edward Herbert, *The Life of Edward, First Lord Herbert of Cherbury, Written by Himself*, ed. J. M. Shuttleworth (London: Oxford University Press, 1976), 20, not known for his love of traditional philosophy, himself recommended Severinus as a unique source of Paracelsian doctrine: "It will not bee amisse to reade The *Idea Medecinæ Philosophicæ* written by Severinus Danus there being many things considerable concerning the Paracelsian principles written in that booke which are not found in former writers." It would be reasonable to suppose that Edward Herbert was passing on his personal judgment of the *Idea medicinæ*, a copy of which he bequeathed to Jesus College Library, Oxford; see C. J. Fordyce and T. M. Knox, "The Library of Jesus College, Oxford; With an Appendix on the Books Bequeathed Thereto by Lord Herbert of Cherbury," vol. 5, *Oxford Bibliographical Society; Proceedings and Papers* (Oxford: Oxford University Press, 1940), 86.

ophers of the time.[38] *The Copie of a Letter* (1586), written by the unknown I. W., came out the following year, with its echoes of Severinian ideas about diseases as transplantations.[39] Therefore, clearly Severinus' theories were known in England among the learned and were being reflected in English medical tracts, where they were available to all literate physicians, surgeons, and natural philosophers by the beginning of the seventeenth century.

Helmont composed his "Eisagoge," which Clericuzio claims to be heavily dependent on the *Idea medicinæ*, in 1607, soon after he returned to Belgium from England.[40] This raises the possibility that Helmont learned of Severinus while in England, and immediately began to incorporate the ideas into his understanding of chemical philosophy.[41] A close study of Helmont's early works may shed more light on the genesis of his medical theory. However, one observation worth noting here is that many of the attributes that Helmont assigned to "ferments" equally well describe Severinus' *semina* and seminal tinctures, suggesting that Helmont may have adapted Severinus' ideas to the alchemical concept of fermentation, a process that figures very little into the *Idea medicinæ*.

Several of Helmont's treatises were published during his lifetime, including his *Supplementum de spadanis fontibus* (1624), in which he espoused a theory of *semina* as active principles, but most of his work lay unpublished for many years, until his son had it printed in 1648 as the *Ortus medicinæ* and *Opuscula medica inaudita*.[42] The rapidity with which these texts caught Walter

[38]R. B., *The Difference Betweene the Auncient Phisicke … and the Latter Phisicke* (London, 1585), chap. 19, sig. 12ʳ: "There bee a great number of learned Philosophers and Phisitions … which at this daie doe embrace, follow, and practice, the doctrine, methods, and wayes of curyng of this Chimicall Phisicke. As *D. Petrus Seuerinus* in Denmarcke Philosopher, and Phisition to the Kyng of Denmork now raigning."

[39]I. W., *The copie of a letter sent by a learned Physician to his friend, wherein are detected the manifold errors used hitherto of the Apothecaries* (London, 1586), unpaginated: "Neither Apoplexia, Epilepsia, …, or any other disease whatsoever, are the proper death or sicknesses of Microcosmi, but are the sicknesses and death of the fruit of Microcosmi, & that by transplantation they growe in Microcosmus." "Pluritis [is] the death of Antimonie. Prunella the death of Brimstone. [etc]." "They are the death of the fruites of the great world, & not of man, & that they grow not naturally in man but come in by transplantation, & therefore may be separated." "This is the cause that man dieth such sundry deaths, because hee eateth in his bread the death of all other things, which when perfect separation is not made, bringeth foorth fruit according to his kinde."

[40]Clericuzio, "From van Helmont to Boyle," 307, n. 18.

[41]This is just speculation, because Helmont could easily have known of Severinus from a number of continental writers, since Severinus was a leading exponent of Paracelsian theory, known to several of the major Paracelsian writers of the late sixteenth and early seventeenth centuries.

[42]Clericuzio, "From van Helmont to Boyle," 307–309, notes several treatises published in Helmont's lifetime.

Charleton's interest has been documented by Nina Rattner Gelbart, who showed that Charleton published translations of Helmont's works already in 1650, when he also published his *Spiritus Gorgonicus*.[43] In the meantime, though, Severinus' work continued to be read in England. The anonymous author of *Philiatros* (1615) took up Severinus' ideas explicitly, viewing new diseases as transplantations of old ones, "by putting upon them new Tinctures," and suggesting that new medicines might be made from old ones by transplantation.[44] Francis Bacon also knew Severinus' work, but did not particularly approve of its Paracelsian obscurity.[45] However, his own writings indicate that he accepted seminal spirits but did not give them the same scope of action as Severinus had given his *semina*.[46] Bacon realized that some kind of vital spirits—"agents and workmen that produce all the effects in the body"—were useful for explaining organic processes, but he argued that these originated from inanimate spirits, which cause "mechanical"

[43]Gelbart, "Intellectual Development of Walter Charleton," 151.

[44]*Philiatros, or The Copie of an Epistle, wherein sundry fitting Considerations are propounded to a young Student of Physicke* (London, 1615), 6r–6v.

[45]Francis Bacon, *The Masculine Birth of Time*, trans. Benjamin Farrington, in *The Philosophy of Francis Bacon* (Liverpool: Liverpool University Press, 1964), 66–67: "Only one of your followers do I grudge you, namely Peter Severinus, a man too good to die in the toils of such folly. You, Paracelsus, adopted son of the family of asses, owe him a heavy debt. He took over your brayings and by the tuneful modulations and pleasant inflexions of his voice made sweet harmony of them, transforming your detestable falsehoods into delectable fables. So I find it in my heart to forgive you, Peter Severinus, if wearying of the teaching of the Sophists, ... you gallantly sought a fresh foundation for our crumbling fortunes. When you came across these doctrines of Parcelsus recommending themselves by their noisy trumpeting, the cunning of their obscurity, their religious affiliations, and other specious allures, with one impulsive leap you surrendered yourself to what turned out to be not sources of true knowledge but empty delusions. You would have been well and truly advised if your revolt from ingenious paradoxes had taken you instead to nature's laws, which would have offered you a shorter path to knowledge and a longer lease on life."
Bacon, *Novum Organum*, book 1, aphorism 116, in Francis Bacon, *The Works of Francis Bacon*, ed. James Spedding, Robert Leslie Ellis, Douglas Denon Heath, 7 vols. (London: Longmans, 1857–74; rpt. New York: Garrett, 1969), 4:103: "First, then, I must request men not to suppose that after the fashion of ancient Greeks, and of certain moderns, as Telesius, Patricius, Severinus, I wish to found a new sect in philosophy. For this is not what I am about."

[46]Francis Bacon, *Novum Organum*, book 1, aphorism 23; in Spedding, ed., *Works of Francis Bacon*, 4:51: Bacon referred to *ideas* in the divine mind as corresponding to "the true signatures and marks set upon the works of creation as they are found in nature."
Bacon stopped short of equating spirit with seminal forms or reasons, referring rather to spirit as a "pneumatic matter" that is *weightless*, highly active, and possessed of dimension and location. If we put these characteristics into a Severinian frame, we can see that Bacon's "pneumatic matter" (spirit) is like immaterial body (weightless, but extended). Furthermore, in *De augmentiis scientiarum*, Bacon said that this spirit springs from the wombs of the elements (*e matricibus elementorum*), a decidedly Paracelsian and Severinian formulation; see Rees, *Francis Bacon's Natural Philosophy*, 42.

changes in the inorganic world.[47] Bacon's reduction of the operation of *vital* workmen to the *mechanical* operations of inorganic spirits indicates an overlap of various concepts of agency and underscores the fluidity of the terminology.

Severinus' *semina* theory was also applied to the field of balneology, and therefore geology, with Edward Jorden's treatise on mineral waters. Jorden explained both the heat and the curative virtues of mineral waters on the basis of *semina* theory. He explicitly used the *Idea medicinæ* in the first edition of his *Discovrse of Natvrall Bathes, and Minerall Waters* (1631), but removed several references to the Dane when he revised the work the following year, for reasons that are not clear.[48] Jorden's work seems to have helped spread *semina* theory, inasmuch as William Simpson's *Zymologia Physica* (1675) echoed Severinus' formulations of "mechanical and efficient principles," which explain the fermentation of mineral juices in spa waters. This work was strongly influenced by Jorden's *Discovrse*, as was Simpson's earlier *Hydrologia Chymica* (1669).[49] John Webster, who cited Severinus in his *Metallographia* (1671), also quoted Severinus, using textual citations taken from Jorden's treatise.[50]

Roughly contemporary with Jorden's *Discovrse*, a Scotsman named William Davidson was teaching chemistry at the Jardin des Plantes in Paris, a course that was attended by at least one well-known English student.[51] Davidson had studied chemistry in France and likely developed an interest in Severinus through his acquaintance with Guy de la Brosse, the intendant at the Jardin, who was very enthusiastic about Severinus' ideas.[52] Davidson included

[47]Bacon, *Historia vitæ et mortis*, trans. Spedding, ed., *Works of Francis Bacon*, 5:268.

[48]Edward Jorden, *Discovrse of Natvrall Bathes, and Minerall Waters* (1631; reprint, Amsterdam: Theatrum Orbis Terrarum, 1971); idem, *A Discourse of Naturall Bathes, and Minerall Waters* (London: Thomas Harper, 1632). Debus, *Chemical Philosophy*, 2:344–359, places Jorden's balneology in the context of Helmontian philosophy. However, as I have shown here by examination of the first edition of Jorden's book, Jorden clearly received many of his ideas about *semina* directly from the *Idea medicinæ*, rather than through Helmont's interpretation.

[49]William Simpson and W. S., *Zymologia Physica* (London, 1675), 19, 35–36, 66–67, 101–102; William Simpson, *Hydrologia Chymica* (London, 1669), esp. sigs. A4r, A7vff., 267–269. Of course, these ideas could have come from Helmont, too.

[50]John Webster, *Metallographia: Or, An History of Metals* (London: A. C., 1671), 61–68. Webster, *The Displaying of Supposed Witchcraft* (London: J. M., 1677), 9, notes that Severinus was one of the "most strong and invincible Champions," to have defended Paracelsus against "the malevolent Pen of *Erastus*" and others who have laid "horrid and abominable false scandals" on Paracelsus.

[51]At least we know from John Aubrey's copy of the 1641 edition of *Philosophia pyrotechnica* that Thomas Hobbes "went through a course of chymistrie" with Davidson at Paris; see John Read, "William Davidson of Aberdeen," *Ambix* 9 (1961): 77–78.

[52]In 1628 Guy wrote that he had been testing the assertions of Severinus and Paracelsus for twenty-five years, so he must be reckoned as active while Quercetanus and Mayerne were still in Paris; see Henry Guerlac, "Guy de La Brosse and the French Paracelsians," in Allen Debus, ed., *Science, Medicine, and Society in the Renaissance* (New York: Science History Publications, 1972), 185–

Severinus in his published chemical curriculum, which was largely concerned with laboratory preparations and methods rather than theory. It was very popular and both reprinted in Latin and translated into French.[53] But Davidson's interest ran deeper than this and eventually compelled him to publish *two* lengthy commentaries on the *Idea medicinæ*, the third edition of which accompanied Davidson's first commentary in 1660.[54]

Chemical medicine in Paris was discouraged at the university, which was staunchly anti-Paracelsian, but enjoyed great popularity at the Jardin, which was patronized by the crown and by the Paracelsian physicians in royal service. It is therefore not surprising that Severinus' ideas were also known generally in France in this period. Chemical philosophers would already have been familiar with the Dane's ideas either directly or from their adaptation by Joseph Duchesne (Quercetanus),[55] so it is not surprising that C. de Sarcilly commended Severinus in his preface to his translation of several of Paracelsus' treatises in 1631, in which he noted that Galenist opposition to the new medicine really began in Paris after the publication of Severinus' *Idea medicinæ*.[56] But other French philosophers, ones that we do not normally associate with

---

186. La Brosse felt that the Paracelsians, except Severinus, accepted Paracelsus' ideas without putting them to the test. For a more recent study of Guy de la Brosse, see Rio Howard, *Guy de La Brosse: The Founder of the Jardin des Plantes in Paris* (Ann Arbor: UMI, 1981).

[53]William Davidson, *Philosophia pyrotechnica seu curriculus chymiatricus* (Paris: Bessin, 1633–35), was published in parts in Paris from 1635 to 1640, and a second edition came out in 1642. A French translation by Jean Hellot, a Parisian surgeon, *Les elemens de la philosophie de l'art du feu ou chemie*, appeared in Paris in 1651 and again in 1657. Even Isaac Newton owned a copy, though it does not appear on the list of books he annotated; see John Harrison, *The Library of Isaac Newton* (New York: Cambridge University Press, 1978), 130, 271–272.

[54]William Davidson, *Commentariorum in sublimis philosophia incomparabilis viri Petri Severini Dani Ideam Medicinæ Philosophicæ...prodromus* (The Hague: Vlacq, 1660), and *Commentaria in Idæam Medicinæ Philosophicæ Petri Dani, Medici incomparabilis & Philosophi sublimis* (The Hague: Vlacq, 1663).

[55]Andreas Libavius, *Alchymia* (2d ed. of *Alchemia*) (Frankfurt, 1606), sig. Aa5r, noted Quercetanus' use of Severinus: "In Quercetanus' books I indeed find more from Severinus' *Idea* than from the teaching of Riolan, and indeed [it is] largely excellent; largely Hippocratic. And he is perhaps not so peculiar in deeds as in words and comparatively more an iatrochemist or Hermetist than an addict to the school of Paracelsus."

[56]Paracelsus, *Les XIV Livres des Paragraphes de Ph. Theoph. Paracelse Bombast, Allemand ... Prince des Hermetiques & Spagyriques*, ed. C. de Sarcilly (Paris: Jean Guillemot, 1631), 20: "Quiconque vondra voir la verite de ces choses à face descouuerte, peut lire les liures du tres-docte Petrus Seuerinus Danus, en son idée Medicinale, pour la deffence de la doctrine de nostre Paracelse, apres lequel ie n'attends pas grande gloire de me rendre icy son Aduocat." I am grateful to Susan Alons for providing me a photocopy of the relevant pages of this rare book; see also Allen G. Debus, *The French Paracelsians: The Chemical Challenge to Medical and Scientific Tradition in Early Modern France* (New York: Cambridge University Press, 1991), 74.

Paracelsian ideas and chemical medicine, also had heard of Severinus. Gassendi, for example, knew of Severinus' *semina*, and one can wonder if something of their "mechanical" knowledge and predestination was not transferred to the atoms that Gassendi was "baptizing" to allow them divine inspiration.[57]

Given the strong presence of Severinus' ideas and reputation in the works of La Brosse and Davidson, English natural philosophers and physicians could readily have learned of the Dane from French sources if they had not read about him in the English literature. But they could also have become acquainted with Severinus' ideas from reading Libavius' lengthy criticism of the chemical philosophy of Johannes Hartmann, which Libavius thought had been taken directly from Severinus, or from the works of a number of other continental philosophers who commented on Severinus' ideas.[58] Of the possible German sources, two stand out: Gregor Horst and Daniel Sennert. Both were influential teachers and both recognized the importance of *semina* theory in their extensive writings.[59] Sennert, in particular, was read by the English,

[57]Among Guy de La Brosse's friends in Paris, Severinus' doctrine was known to at least Etienne de Clave and Pierre Gassendi (Oliver Rene Bloch, *La Philosophie de Gassendi: Nominalisme, Materialisme et Metaphysique.* (The Hague: Martinus Nijhoff, 1971), 445–446: "Nous avons dit que la notion de *semina rerum*, principes des choses organisées, empruntée vers 1636 par Gassendi aux chymistes, en particulier à de Clave, et sans doute, par son intermédiaire, à Pierre Séverin le Danois." Bloch, ibid., 259, also calls Severinus "disciple de Paracelse et lui-même un des inspirateurs de Clave." De Clave mentioned Severinus in the preface to book 2 of his *Paradoxes, ou Traittez Philosophiques des Pierres et Pierreries, contre l'opinion vulgaire* (Paris: Pierre Chevalier, 1635), 199. However, according to Debus, *French Paracelsians*, 71, De Clave rejected both the Aristotelian elements and Paracelsus' *tria prima* as fundamental principles.

It is difficult to tell whether the inner principles of motion that Gassendi permitted his atoms to possess were inspired by Severinus' *semina*, but Webster, *From Paracelsus to Newton*, 69, argued that Gassendi used the idea of *semina* to reconcile vitalist and materialist philosophy. Following up on Webster's lead, Clericuzio, "Redefinition of Boyle's Chemistry," 587, notes that Gassendi attributed the fecundity of seeds to a plastic principle that he called an *animula* or *flammula*. Osler, " Intellectual Sources," 180, refers to Gassendi's alterations to atomism as a "baptized version."

[58]Libavius saw Hartmann as a Severinian, as is clear from the title of his treatise: *De philosophia vivente seu vitali Paracelsi iuxta P. Severinum danum ex repetitione I. Hartmanni Chymiatri Marburgensis* ("On the living or vital philosophy of Paracelsus, according to P. Severinus Danus, from the repetition of I. Hartmann, Iatrochemist at Marburg"), 88, in Andreas Libavius, *Prodromus vitalis philosophiæ Paracelsistarum Examen philosophiæ novæ, quæ veteri abrogandæ opponitur: in quo agitur de modo discendi novo: De veterum autoritate; De magia Paracelsi ex Crollio; De philosophia vivente ex Seuerino per Johannem Hartmannum; De philosophia harmonica magica Fraternitatis de Rosea Cruce* (Frankfurt, 1615), which was bound with other tracts and issued under the title *Syntagmatis selectorum undiquaque et perspicue traditorum alchymiæ arcanorum, tomus primus* (Frankfurt, 1615).

[59]Gregor Horst (1578–1636) drew heavily on the *Idea medicinæ* in his treatment of generation and transplantation and mentions Severinus frequently in *De morborum differentiis et causis, exercitatio I* (Geissen: Caspar Chemlinus, 1612), and *De natura humana libri duo…Cum præfatione de Anatomia vitali & mortua pro conciliatione Spagyricorum & Galenicorum plurimum inseruiente*

and his critical evaluation of Severinus' Paracelsian philosophy may have contributed to the acceptability of seminal principles as a part of the corpuscular hypothesis. Sennert's matter theory is regarded as largely shaped by the Aristotelian ideas of *minima naturalia*, but he was an eclectic and drew on diverse schools of thought for his ideas.[60]

By the 1650s, English natural philosophers could have known of Severinus' work from a variety of continental and domestic sources, including the works of Helmont. And they were also familiar with the *Idea medicinæ* itself. Walter Charleton, who translated Helmont's *Magnetic Cure of Wounds* in his *Ternary of Paradoxes* (1650), included Severinus among those to whom he referred the reader.[61] Charleton also cited Severinus in *Spiritus Gorgonicus*, a Latin book about the formation of stones in the human body. Despite his criticism of Severinus on page 45, he found worth repeating his idea that stones generated in the human body arise from foreign seeds or rudiments of diseases that are lodged in the human anatomy. This serves as at least one example that the Dane's ideas were being read and taken seriously in England in the transition from vitalism to mechanism as the dominant philosophical framework for understanding nature.[62] About that same time, Thomas Vaughan

---

(Frankfurt am Main: Erasmus Kempfer, 1612).

Sennert gave Serverinus' doctrines special attention in his *De chymicorum cum Aristotelicis et Galenicis consensu ac dissensu Liber* (Wittenberg, 1919), 57, where he singled out Severinus as an important Paracelsian exponent: "In the yeqr 1493, in Switzerland, Philippus Theophrastus Paracelsus was born… whom Alexander of Suchten, Dorn, Phaedrus, Thurneisser, and P. Severinus Danus have followed. Yet even these do not quite agree, either with Paracelsus or among themselves. Nevertheless, most of those who today would be called iatrochemists follow Petrus Severinus, who has undertaken to bring the doctrines thrown out here and there by Paracelsus into a learned form, better than Paracelsus himself. For this reason I recognize today that a school, as it were, has been born, which can be called Severinian."

Although Sennert recognized Severinus' efforts to correct some of the doctrines of Paracelsus, in the end he regarded many of the Paracelsian terms that Severinus had used as merely new words for old concepts and thought that much of Severinus' metaphysics was but a recent version of "a common doctrine about forms, especially of living things, which are called souls; ibid., 181.

[60]William R. Newman, "Boyle's Debt to Corpuscular Alchemy," in *Robert Boyle Reconsidered*, ed. Michael Hunter (New York: Cambridge University Press, 1994), 107–118, treats Boyle's use of the concept of the *minima naturalia*, a concept developed in the Pseudo-Gerberian *Summa perfectionis*. Clericuzio, "Reconsideration of Boyle's Chemistry," 586 points to Sennert's implication of seminal forms in atomic matter, an idea also associated with Gassendi's "baptism" of Epicurus' atomism in order to make it amenable to Christian thought. I suspect that a fuller analysis of Sennert's large corpus will eventually result in him receiving a larger place in the development of seventeenth-century matter theory than he currently holds.

[61]Gelbart, "Intellectual Development of Walter Charleton," 152.

[62]Charleton, *Spiritus Gorgonicus* (Leiden: Elsevir, 1650) 78, cites chap. 12 of the *Idea medicine*. Charleton first referred to Severinus on p. 33, in connection with explanations for the formation of stones from solutions, noting that this can be accounted for by heat and cold or by some stone-

also cited Severinus in his *Anthroposophia Theomagica* (1650).[63] We know that John Webster owned a copy of the *Idea medicinæ*, as did Robert Child, who sent it to John Winthrop, Jr., in New England.[64] Elias Ashmole had also read the *Idea medicinæ*, which he cited in a gloss on Thomas Norton's *Ordinall of Alchemy*.[65] Even Boyle knew of Severinus, as is evident from his reference to Severinus as one of the "innovators" of natural philosophy in his *The Excellency of Theology Compared with Natural Philosophy* (1674), where Boyle contrasted the fame of theologians with the relative obscurity of natural philosophers:

> And accordingly we see, that the writings of *Socinus Calvin, Bellarmine, Padre Paulo, Arminius,* & cet. are more famous, and more studied, than those of *Telesius, Campanella, Severinus Danus, Magnenus,* and diverse other innovators in natural philosophy.[66]

Therefore, even if Boyle took his knowledge of seminal principles mainly from his reading of Helmont, it is evident that he at least knew of Severinus and his reputation as an important innovator. Whether directly or via the works of Helmont or some other writer, Boyle and his contemporaries were in possession of a salient doctrine of the *Idea medicinæ*, the doctrine of *semina mechanica*.

---

forming seminal power, as Helmont would have it. He said that some such explanation must exist for the concretion of minerals from liquids, but thought that it was madness to hope to determine whether such a concretion is caused by the qualities or, as Severinus said, by the action of a seminal form constructing a corporeal shelter for itself.

[63]Thomas Vaughan, *Anthroposophia Theomagica* (London, 1650), 26. I thank Lawrence Principe for drawing my attention to this treatise.

[64]William Jerome Wilson, "Robert Child's Chemical Book List of 1641," *Journal of Chemical Education* 20 (1943): 123–129. "Severini *Idea*" is entry 63 on p. 127; Ronald Stearne Wilkinson, "The Alchemical Library of John Winthrop, Jr. (1606–1676) and His Descendants in Colonial America," *Ambix* 11 (1963): 33–51; 13 (1965): 139–186, entry no. 251 for Severinus on p. 182.

[65]Among the tracts that Ashmole reprinted is that English favorite, Thomas Norton's *Ordinall of Alchemy*. In the gloss to Norton's phrase "And for the *Red Stone* is preservative, Most precious thinge to length my Life," Ashmole referred to chap. 12 of Severinus' *Idea medicinæ*: "It is apparent that our *Diseases proceed chiefly from Transplantation*…for, by what we *Eate* or *Drinke* as *Nourishment*; the corrupt and harmfull, nay deathfull qualities…is removed from them into our *Bodyes*, and there grow up and multiply till (having heightened the *Sal, Sulphur,* and *Mercury,* into an irreconcileable *Contestation,* through the impurities wherewith they are loaded and burthened) they introduce a miserable *decay,* which consequently become a *Death*"; see Elias Ashmole, *Theatrum Chemicum Britannicum* (1652; New York: Johnson Reprint, 1967), 88, 448. The reference to the *Idea medicinæ* is in the margin adjacent to the text here quoted.

[66]Robert Boyle, *The Excellency of Theology Compared with Natural Philosophy,* in *The Works of the Honourable Robert Boyle: In Six Volumes,* ed. Thomas Birch (London, 1772), 4:63. I thank Rose-Mary Sargent for bringing this passage to my attention.

BOYLE, SEMINAL FORMS, AND MECHANICAL PHILOSOPHY

Robert Boyle commands the center field in attempts to understand the development of mechanical philosophy and the establishment of experiment and ocular demonstration as the proper methods of determining scientific facts upon which to base and evaluate hypotheses. Certainly his numerous writings set a standard for public discourse in English natural philosophy in the second half of the seventeenth century, and his influence on Restoration chemistry was acknowledged by his contemporaries, warranting modern attention to his place in the mechanization of chemistry.[67] Boyle's singular status as a prolific writer on the cusp of the transition from Renaissance to modern science has accordingly made him the focus of differing views about the nature of English mechanical philosophy and changing attitudes within the chemical community towards alchemy and occult philosophy. William Newman's recent assessment of Boyle's dependence on medieval alchemical theory, combined with Lawrence Principe's revelations about Boyle's alchemical practice, have placed the skeptical chemist squarely in the tradition of English alchemy, which influenced Newton's speculations.[68] Investigating a slightly different chemical heritage, John Henry and Antonio Clericuzio have aired their differing conclusions about the nature of the vestiges of chemical philosophy in Boyle's matter theory—whether corpuscles were associated with active principles or were themselves active corpuscles.[69] The difference, a slight one in my view, hinges less on corpuscularism or mechanical philosophy than it does on the role of divinity within mechanical philosophy, but in any case, Boyle's incorporation of vitality into his matter theory is established.

Part of Boyle's success in forging links between mechanical philosophy and chemical philosophy rests on the nature of his corpuscles, which owe their attributes to the *minima naturalia* of Aristotelian alchemy as well as to Gassendi's renovation of Epicurean atomism.[70] Boyle's corpuscles are also

[67]Clericuzio, "From Van Helmont to Boyle," 327–328, makes a case for the importance of Boyle for unifying mechanical philosophy and chemistry.

[68]Newman, "Boyle's Debt to Corpuscular Alchemy," and Lawrence M. Principe, "Boyle's Alchemical Pursuits," in *Robert Boyle Reconsidered*, 91–105. William Newman, *Gehennical Fire: The Lives of George Starkey, an American Alchemist in the Scientific Revolution* (Cambridge, Mass.: Harvard University Press, 1994), has placed Boyle's researches firmly in studies of alchemical processes that occupied English adepts in the middle of the century.

[69]Clericuzio, "Redefinition of Boyle's Chemistry," 572, 583 n. 107, rejects Henry's claim that Boyle viewed matter as "imbued with activity" (572). However, Henry, on the page cited by Clericuzio (368), did not claim that Boyle thought that matter was inherently active, "imbued with activity," but rather "imbued with occult active principles."

[70]On *minima naturalia*, see Newman, *Gehennical Fire*; on Gassendi's atomism, see Clericuzio, "Redefinition of Boyle's Chemistry," 579.

indebted to the theory of seminal principles, the legacy of Paracelsian chemical philosophy. These three streams of thought flowed together in Boyle's theory to accommodate divinely predestined, secondary causation with a hypothesis that on the experimental level conformed to the requirements of materialism.[71] This is to say that Boyle's seminal forms, like Severinus' *semina*, permitted divine, predestined purpose a place in the everyday workings of matter.[72] I turn now to investigate Boyle's use of seminal principles in the Severinian-Helmontian tradition and how these fit into his conception of "mechanical."

Boyle's interest in Helmontian chemistry has been traced back to 1648, the year that Helmont's *Ortus medicinæ* was published.[73] In the next dozen years, Boyle mulled over Helmontian and alchemical ideas and joined them to a corpuscular scheme that is explained in Walter Charleton's *Physiologia Epicuro-Gassendo-Charletoniana* (1654), which in turn had been taken from Gassendi's *Syntagma Philosophiæ Epicuri* (1649).[74] The result was a four-level hierarchy of material organization, in which (1) *minima naturalia*, which were endowed with chemical properties in Boyle's early works, but strictly mechanical properties in his later writings, came together to form (2) primary clusters or concretions, which were the smallest particles to possess distinguishable chemical characteristics. These primary clusters, or corpuscles, could in turn be joined together to form (3) sensible compound bodies, which could then form a higher class of mixtures called (4) decompounded bodies.[75] During the early development of this corpuscular hypothesis, Boyle was willing to allow the primary clusters of primitive atomic matter to possess "the formative power of the seeds of things." These seminal principles or seminal faculties were responsible for organic growth, and appear in an early draft of Boyle's famous *Sceptical Chymist*.[76] An echo of this idea survived in the published version, *Sceptical Chymist* (1661), where Boyle refers to "the pecular fabrics of the bodies of plants and animals (and perhaps also of some metals and minerals)

---

[71]Kaplan, *Medical Agenda of Robert Boyle*, 72, characterizes Boyle's mechanical philosophy as "chemical dynamics" to distinguish it from Cartesian "positional dynamics," which requires that the mechanical motions of particles be inertial translations and rotations instead of chemical "motions" or changes (motions in the general sense).

[72]Such predestinations do not infringe on God's will, since presumably God wills things to be the way they are (i.e. normal development), unless he chooses to will them otherwise (intervention).

[73]Clericuzio, "From Van Helmont to Boyle," 304–305.

[74]Clericuzio, "Redefinition of Boyle's Chemistry," 579, 583; see also Kaplan, *Medical Agenda of Robert Boyle*, 57.

[75]Kaplan, *Medical Agenda of Robert Boyle*, 59.

[76]Marie Boas, "An Early Version of Boyle's *Sceptical Chymist*," *Isis* 45 (1954): 153–168, 167; see also Clericuzio, "Redefinition of Boyle's Chemistry," 584.

which I take to be effects of seminal principles."[77] There is no convincing evidence that Boyle got these ideas directly from Severinus' *Idea medicinæ*, but it is likely that they are Severinian in origin, perhaps derived from Helmont's works or some other intermediary. Moreover, in another unpublished manuscript, Boyle considered that mineral generation was possibly caused by "seminal principles...lodg'd in Individualls themselves or which is in most cases more probable, in pregnant and prolifick wombs," which sounds as if could have come directly from the *Idea medicinæ*.[78]

Boyle's mature mechanical philosophy spoke less about seminal principles, but instead materialized them in the form of "effluvia." If one examines the role that Boyle assigned to "effluvia" in his philosophy, one can understand why he might find Severinus' *semina* acceptable. Boyle held that effluvia, with chemically defined characteristics and sometimes possessing electric and magnetic properties, too, are thrown off by animals, plants, minerals, and even celestial bodies, accounting for the influence of one thing upon another.[79] These effluvia are invisible and leave either friendly or hostile impressions on the bodies onto which they impinge. If they are hostile, they can produce disease in the recipient, depending on the number of incident effluvial particles.[80] Boyle thought that this explanation could account for the toxic effects of subterranean effluvia on miners, the sudden appearance of epidemic diseases, and the action of specific drugs in the body.[81] All of this sounds like a corpuscular version of Severinus' pathology, where *semina* and the impressions of their supervening, mechanical tinctures have been replaced by particulate effluvia and their impressions. The operation of both Severinus' *semina morborum* and Boyle's effluvia is "mechanical," and both *semina*—as they exist in nature—and effluvia are material units. The main difference is that for Severinus, *semina* were intrinsically immaterial, "mechanical" agents that were inseparably bound to elemental matter, whereas Boyle's effluvia were intrinsically material, although endowed with divinely ordained motion.[82] The inescapable conclusion is that Paracelsian *semina* theory, by

[77]Robert Boyle, *Sceptical Chymist* (*Works*, 1:571). Boyle cites these instances as exceptions to his by then general rejection of Helmontian seminal causation.

[78]Quoted by Clericuzio, "Redefinition of Boyle's Chemistry," 585.

[79]Kaplan, *Medical Agenda of Robert Boyle*, 105–107.

[80]Ibid., 107–108, 110–111.

[81]Kaplan, *Medical Agenda of Robert Boyle*, 57. Clearly the model could be used to explain the traditional astrological aspects of disease and medicine, too, as well as the sympathetic action of amulets.

[82]Boyle says that seminal particles possess an ordained generative texture, which is programmed by God to reproduce; see Kaplan, *Medical Agenda of Robert Boyle*, 62, 67.

whatever intermediary, found a material place in Boyle's corpuscular hypothesis, which has been taken as a model for the development of English mechanical philosophy.[83] We might well return, then, to reconsider how Boyle might have interpreted Severinus' references to "mechanical" principles and tinctures endowed with the "mechanical" knowledge to carry out "mechanical" processes, and draw some tentative conclusions about the nature of the concept of "mechanical" in the genesis of the mechanical philosophy.

Recent studies by Malcolm Oster and J. A. Bennett have again drawn attention to the possibility that Boyle's concept of mechanical philosophy developed from a "mechanical" tradition that was espoused by instrument makers and mathematicians beginning in England in the sixteenth century.[84] Edgar Zilsel and those persuaded by a Marxist approach to history put forth this idea earlier this century, but Oster has taken it out of the context of Marxist economic determinism and made it an intellectual-historical proposition. Oster sustains the opinion that Boyle grafted what Francis Bacon had called the "maker's knowledge" onto corpuscular philosophy, and he documents Boyle's references to learning techniques from artisans and tradesmen, whose opinions about processes are less likely to be influenced by theory than are those of the virtuosi.[85] But what is the maker's knowledge? According to Antonio Pérez-Ramos, the maker's knowledge is "an internalization of operational skills" that the maker of a thing draws on in the process of fabrication; it is the "knowledge which *determines* its object in the way in which a cobbler's knowledge of a shoe determines his activity in producing one."[86] He attributes this conception of knowledge to Francis Bacon, in contrast to

---

[83]For example, Malcolm Oster, "The Scholar and the Craftsman Revisited: Robert Boyle as Aristocrat and Artisan," *Annals of Science* 49 (1992): 225: idem, "Robert Boyle, a leading advocate of Mechanical Philosophy at the Restoration," and Gary B. Deason, "Reformation Theology and the Mechanistic Conception of Nature," 167–191 in David C. Lindberg and Ronald L. Numbers, eds., *God and Nature: Historical Essays on the Encounter between Christianity and Science* (Berkeley: University of California Press, 1986), 180: Boyle as "one of the strongest advocates of the Mechanical Philosophy." Clericuzio, "Redefinition of Boyle's Chemistry," 573, 577, however, considers Boyle to have developed a moderate version of mechanical philosophy, which attributed chemical properties to corpuscles without attempting to reduce them to mechanical principles.

[84]Oster, "Scholar and the Craftsman Revisited," and J. A. Bennett, "The Mechanics' Philosophy and the Mechanical Philosophy," *History of Science* 24 (1986): 1–28.

[85]Oster, "Scholar and Craftsman Revisited," 268, 274. Boyle's reliance on artisans' opinions to be more faithful than those that have been filtered through the virtuoso's philosophical lens raises some interesting questions about the validity of Shapin and Shaffer's claim that truth was socially constructed by witnesses of high social rank.

[86]Antonio Pérez-Ramos, *Francis Bacon's Idea of Science and the Maker's Knowledge Tradition* (New York: Oxford University Press, 1988), 50, 150.

knowledge in the Cartesian sense, which aims to understand the artifact or machine from the point of view of the "beholder" rather than the maker.[87]

Boyle distinguished between the mechanical knowledge of the artisan, "hand knowledge," and the rational, philosophical knowledge possessed by the virtuosi landowners, like himself.[88] Artisan was socially synonymous with "mechanic," as is explained by Stephen Pumfrey, who has recently examined the social stratification between tradesmen or mechanics and gentlemen virtuosi in Boyle's time and the barriers it erected for people like Robert Hooke, who sought to cross the border.[89] According to Boyle, the mechanics often cannot give a good explanation of what they do; they just do it.[90] It seems to me that the working advantage that the artisan has over the virtuoso who wishes to learn the artisan's process, is that he has a knowledge of the process that is implanted in him by years of craftsmanship, which enables him to carry out that process with predictable results.[91] This is exactly what Boyle (and Severinus) demand from seminal principles, namely that they produce generation with "uniform regularity."[92] Now, I do not deny that Boyle, and especially Newton and later mechanical philosophers, usually spoke of "mechanical" in the Cartesian sense, as characterizing the mechanisms of inert mechanical contrivances (the clockwork model), yet I submit that in the formative phases of mechanical philosophy, "mechanical" had a broader meaning, one that was in part conditioned by social hierarchy. Thus, when Boyle

[87]Ibid., 152: "The Cartesian knower is a 'maker' only in that remote analogical sense, for the ultimate goal of his science is to 'understand' the machine of the world in the sense of grasping or comprehending it. What he really seeks is beholder's knowledge (conceptual grasp) and not, like the alchemical magus, to reproduce the world's processes at will."

[88]Ibid., 270.

[89]Stephen Pumfrey, "Ideas above His Station: A Social Study of Hooke's Curatorship of Experiments," *History of Science* 29 (1991): 1–44, esp. 10–11, 16. That the term *mechanicus* was applied to artisans in this period is further borne out by William Petty's 1648 plan for a *gymnasium mechanicum*, a "college" of artisans for the progress of all the mechanical arts and of the manufactures"; quoted by Paolo Rossi, *Philosophy, Technology, and the Arts in the Early Modern Era*, trans. Salvator Athanasio (New York: Harper Torchbooks, 1970), 123.

[90]Ibid., 260–261, at 266.

[91]Thomas Sprat, *The History of the Royal-Society of London* (1667), contrasted the "Tradesmen" or "*Mechanick Laborers*" from gentlemen virtuosi ("men of freer lives"): the former carry out their trades as "dull, and unavoidable, and perpetual *employments*," while the latter are only interested in them as diversions; after Pumfrey, "Ideas above His Station," 17.

[92]Clericuzio, "Redefinition of Boyle's Chemistry," 584; see Boyle, *Works*, 2:44. Pérez-Ramos, *Francis Bacon's Idea of Science*, 159, has also captured the overlap in conceptions of natural process and artificial process when he writes, "On the one hand, Nature seems to operate like a craftsman, but, on the other, the real craftsman, whenever any *theoretical* discussion of his products is at stake, has 'internalized' his craft in such a way that he himself 'works' with the automatism attributed to natural processes."

wrote that the "mechanical possibility of any corporeal agent" can be considered in natural philosophy,[93] we must admit that the concepts of machine and agent are interleaved, and that the mechanical part in some way is analogous to the human cog in the social machinery, the "mechanic" who carries out the routine business of the economy. For the term agent was in medieval and early modern philosophy inextricably connected with the idea of actor and not given the modern "mechanical" reading that we associate with "chemical agents" and "active ingredients" in household cleansers.[94] The Maker's knowledge was thus "science" in the sense that Severinus and Paracelsus used the term *scientia*—a knowledge of a process that enabled the artisan or archeus to carry out a chemical (or mechanical) activity, whether in the workshop or at the atomic level. In this context it is interesting to note that William Davidson described this process in his second commentary on Severinus' *Idea medicinæ*, published just two years after Boyle's *Sceptical Chymist*, as an orderly mechanical process, much as Severinus had, but now Davidson calls it "scientific" as well, no doubt reflecting Severinus' use of the term *scientia* to refer to the seminal plan that is used by the *archeus* to carry out the seminal predestination. This combination of "mechanical" and "scientific" reinforces the argument of this paper.[95] This was not the "new science" of the Royal Society until the virtuosi appropriated it and made it part of their program.

CONCLUSION

Given the subtleties and shades of meaning evident in the various uses of such concepts as "mechanical," "workmen," and "inner artisan," and the persistence of organic metaphors of seed and ferment in corpuscular philosophy, it is understandable that there should be some interpenetration of the "occult" philosophy of the Paracelsians and the "mechanical" philosophy of Gassendi, Charleton, Boyle, and their contemporaries. Whether this represents a persistence of occult qualities in late-seventeenth-century mechanism, or a mechanical reading of Paracelsian "mechanics" (workers), it is clear that no abrupt, decisive shift occurred at the metaphysical basis of matter theory between the Renaissance Paracelsus and the Scientific Revolution's Robert Boyle. This is

[93]Boyle, *Works,* 4:72, "The excellency and grounds of the corpuscular or mechanical philosophy" (1574); after Henry, 346.

[94]The point I am making here is that it is no harder to imagine the seventeenth-century writer attributing mechanical activities to active principles than it is to understand that we attribute activity (agency) to what we conceive to be mechanical, i.e. purely lifeless, chemicals. In both cases the meanings of the words must be sought in the philosophical contexts.

[95]See Davidson, *Commentaria in Idæam medicinæ philosophicæ,* 151: "*Ordinata corporum explicatione Mechanico & scientifico processu.*"

not to say that there were no important changes in this period, merely that any claim for a revolution in science is going to have to accommodate the historical record, interpreted in ways appropriate to the sources, and this demands attention to how the sources were read.

We seem to be in such a situation now, where attempts to rebuild an explanatory "grand narrative" or paradigm are coexisting with studies that continue to break down the old model. A grand narrative is arguably necessary to the identity of the history of early modern science, and I do not oppose its creation, so long as it does not run roughshod over the historical evidence, ignoring matters of importance to seventeenth-century writers for the sake of demonstrating a break between the old and the new.

Recent contributions to a reassessment of Robert Boyle's place in the history of science collectively impress upon us that many diverse fields of inquiry—medicine, mathematics, chemistry, physics, moral philosophy, politics, and theology—come together in seventeenth-century speculations about the nature of matter and the causes of change in nature, and that all of these disciplines must be considered in explaining the rise of modern science. The survival of Paracelsian *semina*, with their predestined, purposeful knowledge and impressions, into the natural philosophy of members of the Royal Society, should signal to us that there were powerful concerns associated with matter theory that occupied the inventors of the new science, concerns that could preserve and subsume elements of a rejected paradigm even as a new one was in the ascendant. These are the phenomena that a new grand narrative will of necessity address, if it is to achieve any acceptable degree of consensus.[96]

---

[96]A recent presentation by Peter Dear at a colloquium at the University of Wisconsin alerted me to new attempts to establish a canonical Scientific Revolution by again focusing on the role of mathematics in early modern science. This reinforces the message of Bennett's "The Mechanics' Philosophy and the Mechanical Philosophy," which defines a commonality between sixteenth-century engineers and instrument makers and seventeenth-century mechanical philosophers in mathematics, and gives the mathematization of natural philosophy a prominent place in the Scientific Revolution.

Charles D. Gunnoe, Jr.

ERASTUS AND PARACELSIANISM

THEOLOGICAL MOTIFS IN THOMAS ERASTUS' REJECTION OF PARACELSIAN NATURAL PHILOSOPHY

Ich schreib christenlich und bin kein heide,
ein Teuscher nicht ein Welscher,
ein interpres und nit ein sophist
— Paracelsus, *Astronomia Magna* [1]

Impurissimae sunt blasphemiae, quas
in hoc libro eructavit impius Sannio
— Thomas Erastus on the *Astronomia Magna* [2]

IN THE SIXTEENTH CENTURY, two "reformations" of natural philosophy took place in central Europe. The first occurred when Martin Luther's close associate Philip Melanchthon at the University of Wittenberg began the project of setting forth a distinctly Protestant natural philosophy based largely on Aristotle, Plato, and Galen.[3] This tradition did not represent a radical break with the scholastic past but a reorientation brought on by changes in theological assumptions and humanist method. Universities like Wittenberg, Tübingen, and later Heidelberg fostered this Protestant natural philosophy, and it soon became the new establishment in much of central Europe. While the new Protestant natural philosophy was yet emerging, Theophrastus Bombastus von Hohenheim, commonly known as Paracelsus, proposed a more radical

---

[1] Karl Sudhoff, ed., *Theophrast von Hohenheim genannt Paracelsus: Sämtliche Werke,* 1 Abt., 14 vols. (Berlin and Munich: Oldenbourg 1923–33) (hereafter cited as PI), 12:10.

[2] Thomas Erastus, *Disputationum de medicina nova de Philippi Paracelsi Pars Prima* (Basel: Perna, [1571]), 255.

[3] Sachiko Kusukawa, *The Transformation of Natural Philosophy: The Case of Philip Melanchthon* (Cambridge: Cambridge University Press, 1995).

reformation of natural philosophy. Paracelsus advocated the abandonment of ancient authorities of natural philosophy and the development of a new experimental learning which integrated themes from alchemy, natural magic, and a spiritualistic brand of Christianity.[4] Paracelsus's new philosophy made its public debut in his meteoric rise and fall at the University of Basel in 1527–28, which was signaled by his unprecedented medical lectures in the vernacular and the perhaps legendary account of his burning of Avicenna's *Canon*.[5] After his fall from prominence in Basel, Paracelsus led an itinerant life until his death in 1541, at which time most of his works remained unprinted. Although a full-scale Paracelsian revival was afoot by the 1570s, Paracelsians did not represent the establishment, but rather the vibrant counterculture in sixteenth-century natural philosophy. Though Paracelsus had clearly thrown down the gauntlet with his explicit rejection of Galen and Aristotle, the two paradigms of natural philosophy were not always in conflict, and figures such as Theodor Zwinger sought to mediate between the competing traditions.[6] Alternatively, there were times when the divisions between the two schools of natural philosophy seemed absolute, as in Thomas Erastus' comprehensive rejection of the Paracelsian system. In this paper, I will examine Erastus' refutation of Paracelsian conceptions of creation and mortal flesh as presented in the first volume of *Disputations on the New Medicine of Paracelsus* (see title page, fig. 1) before attempting some preliminary observations regarding the nature of Erastus' rejection of the Paracelsian worldview. I add the qualification that while I have tried to measure Erastus' portrayal of Paracelsus's ideas with reference to Paracelsus' own writings as well as modern scholarship, my goal has been to fathom Erastus' interpretation of Paracelsus as opposed to a strictly internal reading of Paracelsus or the heroic Paracelsus-image of his late-sixteenth-century followers. It is my hope to contribute to our understanding of the conflict between established Protestant natural philosophy and Paracelsianism by

---

[4]Paracelsus' religiosity defies simple categorization. He is now generally considered something of a radical spiritualist reformer, though he never formally broke with the Catholic church; see Ute Gause, *Paracelsus: Genese und Entfaltung seiner frühen Theologie* (Stuttgart: Mohr, 1993).

[5]Walter Pagel, *Paracelsus: An Introduction to the Philosophical Medicine in the Era of the Renaissance*, 2d ed. (Basel: Karger, 1982), 19–22.

[6]Johannes Winther von Andernach also tried to mediate between Paracelsian medical theory and Galenism; see Allen G. Debus, "Guintherius, Libavius and Sennert: The Chemical Compromise in Early Modern Medicine," in *Science, Medicine and Society in the Renaissance: Essays to Honor Walter Pagel*, ed. Allen G. Debus (New York: Science History Publications, 1972); Carlos Gilly, "Zwischen Erfahrung und Spekulation: Theodor Zwinger und die religiöse und kulturelle Krise seiner Zeit," *Basler Zeitschrift für Geschichte und Altertumskunde* 77 (1977): 57–137; 79 (1979): 125–233.

DISPVTATIONVM
DE MEDICINA
NOVA PHILIPPI
PARACELSI
Pars Prima:
IN QVA, QVAE DE REMEDIIS SVPERSTI-
tiofis & Magicis curationibus ille prodi-
dit, præcipuè examinantur.
A
THOMA ERASTO, MEDICINAE
in Schola Heydelbergenfi profeffore.

AD ILLVSTRIS. *Principem, D. Auguftum Saxo-*
niæ Ducem & Electorem,&c.

Liber omnibus,quarumcunq; artium & fcientiarum ftu-
diofis apprimè cum neceffarius tum vtilis.

Cum Indice locupletißimo.

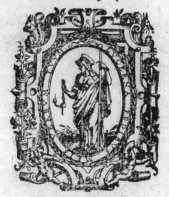

BASILEÆ,
APVD PETRVM PERNAM.

Fig. 1. Title page of the first volume of Thomas Erastus' *Disputationum de medicina nova de Philippi Paracelsi Pars Prima[-Quarta]* (Basel: Peter Perna, [1571]–1573). Note that no date of publication appears on the title page. (Bernard Becker Medical Library, Washington University School of Medicine.)

examining why Erastus found that the heretical implications of Paracelsus' natural philosophy made a rapprochement impossible.

Recent scholarship has significantly enhanced our knowledge of the religious dimension of Paracelsianism. Not only is Paracelsus' theological corpus receiving fresh attention,[7] but scholars such as Carlos Gilly and Charles Webster have displayed the importance of the accusation of heresy in the early reaction to Paracelsian ideas among intelligentsia of the Holy Roman Empire.[8] In the early phase, men such as Johann Oporinus and Konrad Gesner, who had been contemporaries of Paracelsus, spread vague accusations of irreligiosity and heresy concerning Paracelsus and his followers. After their deaths, Johannes Crato von Krafftheim, an imperial physician and protégé of Melanchthon, became the principal agitator against the Paracelsian sect.[9] Until the Paracelsian revival had reached an advanced stage, however, there had been little sustained reflection on the religious implications of his natural philosophy. The publication in 1570 of Bartolomäus Reußner's *A Short Explanation and Christian Refutation of the Unheard Blasphemies and Lies, which Paracelsus has poured out Against God, His Word and the Praiseworthy Art of Medicine in the Three Books of Philosophy to the Atheniens* inaugurated a new era in the reaction to Paracelsus with the study of theological implications of Paracelsian texts.[10] Ironically, Paracelsus' specifically theological

[7]For an orientation regarding the state of the research, see Hartmut Rudolph, "Paracelsus' Laientheologie in traditionsgeschichtlicher Sicht und ihrer Zuordnung zu Reformation und katholischer Reform," in *Resultate und Desiderate der Paracelsus-Forschung*, ed. Hartmut Rudolph and Peter Dilg (Stuttgart: Steiner, 1993); see also Katrin Biegger, *De invocatione beatae Mariae virginis: Paracelsus und die Marienverehrung*, Kosmosophie, vol. 6 (Stuttgart: Steiner, 1990); Bruce T. Moran, "Paracelsus, Religion, and Dissent: The Case of Philipp Homagius and Georg Zimmermann," *Ambix* 43 (1996): 65–79.

[8]Carlos Gilly, "Theophrastia Sancta: Der Paracelsismus als Religion im Streit mit den offiziellen Kirchen," in *Analecta Paracelsica: Studien zum Nachleben Theophrast von Hohenheims im deutschen Kulturgebiet der frühen Neuzeit*, Heidelberger Studien zur Naturkunde der frühen Neuzeit, vol 4, ed. Joachim Telle (Stuttgart: Steiner, 1994), 425–488; Charles Webster, "Conrad Gessner and the Infidelity of Paracelsus," in *New Perspectives on Renaissance Thought*, ed. J. Henry and S. Hutton (London: Duckworth, 1990), 13–23; see also Charles D. Gunnoe, Jr., "Thomas Erastus and His Circle of Anti-Paracelsians," in *Analecta Paracelsica*, ed. Joachim Telle (Stuttgart: Franz Steiner, 1994), 127–148; idem, "Letters of Erastus," in *Documenta Paracelsica*, ed. Joachim Telle (Stuttgart: Franz Steiner, forthcoming).

[9]See Charles D. Gunnoe, Jr., and Jole Shackelford, "Johannes Crato von Krafftheim," in *Documenta Paracelsica*, ed. Joachim Telle (Stuttgart: Franz Steiner, forthcoming).

[10]Bartholomäus Reußner, *Ein kurtze Erklerung und Christliche Widerlegung/Der unerhörten Gotteslesterungen und Lügen/welche Paracelsus in den dreyen Büchern Philosophiae ad Athenienses hat wider Gott/sein Wort und die löbliche Kunst der Artzney außgeschüttet* (Gorlitz: Ambrosius Fritsch, 1570). Reußner, a city physician of Zittau (Lausitz), concentrated his attack on the Paracelsian conception of creation. Reußner was born March 11, 1532, in Lemberg where his father was a member

corpus was not known to his early religious opponents.[11] Thus, the late-six-teenth-century theological reaction to Paracelsus was not a rejection of his religious writings per se, but an attack upon the religious implications of this natural philosophy.

Close on Reußner's heels, Thomas Erastus (1524–1583) entered the arena as the new champion of the anti-Paracelsian crusade. With his Swiss-German background and close connections to Basel, one might imagine that Erastus would have possessed a native appreciation for Switzerland's great medical innovator. However, though they shared a common national heritage, the two occupied diametrically opposed intellectual universes. Erastus was born in Baden (Canton Aargau) and attended the University of Basel before moving to the University of Bologna where he obtained his doctorate in medicine in 1552. From Basel he imbibed the spirit of the Zwinglian Reformation; from Bologna a passion for a philosophically oriented Galenism of the medical Renaissance. After a brief tenure as personal physician to the counts of Henneberg in central Germany (1555–1558), he landed a position on the medical faculty of the University of Heidelberg in 1558. Erastus's participation in the revision of the medical faculty's statutes in 1558 and his election as rector of the university in 1559 marked his rapid rise to academic and political prominence in Heidelberg. He soon found himself more deeply imbedded in church politics than in academic work. He helped to orchestrate the expulsion of the Gnesio-Lutheran church superintendent Tilemann Heshuss and was instrumental in the conversion of Elector Frederick III, the Pious (1559–1576), to a Reformed interpretation of the Lord's Supper through his personal impact on the Heidelberg disputation (1560). As a member of the church council, Erastus helped reorganize the Palatine church and in all probability took part in composition of the Heidelberg Catechism (1563), which bears motifs similar to his contemporaneous theological tracts.[12] Erastus lost much of his prestige

---

of the city council. He practiced medicine in Breslau before moving on to become city physician (*Stadtartz*) in Zittau. He died on October 23, 1572. Given Reußner's interests and locus of activity, it is difficult to imagine that he was not an acquaintance of Johannes Crato von Krafftheim, through whom he could have easily come into contact with Erastus. I have yet to find a clear reference to Reußner in Erastus' work or correspondence. *Allgemeines Gelehrte-Lexicon,* ed. C. G. Joecher (Leipzig, 1751; reprint, Hildesheim: Georg Olms, 1961), vol. 3, cols. 2031–2032; Gunnoe, "Letters of Erastus."

[11]Gilly, "Theophrastia Sancta," 434. Erastus likewise quotes from all of Paracelsus' major medical and natural philosophical works but did not know Paracelsus' theological works, the bulk of which existed only in manuscript in 1570.

[12]See, especially, Thomas Erastus, *Gründtlicher bericht/ wie die wort Christi/ Das ist mein leib/ etc. zuverstehen seien* (Heidelberg, 1562).

in the controversy regarding church discipline which divided the Heidelberg Reformed into two camps in 1568. In this debate, Erastus opposed the effort of his Calvinist rivals to establish church discipline independent from state control and thus gave his name to the concept of "Erastianism," a term which implies that the state should exercise sovereignty over the church though Erastus' chief motivation at the time had been to avoid the reimposition of what he regarded as arbitrary clerical tyranny.[13] The elector opted for the Calvinist system, and Erastus' anti-disciplinist party was completely discredited when it was discovered that two of his close associates were Antitrinitarians seeking to emigrate to Transylvania.[14] Erastus would also be accused of Antitrinitarianism and, rather predictably, excommunicated by his rivals. Now virtually excluded from church affairs, Erastus sought solace in academic life. In the decade of the 1570s, Erastus engaged in a number of academic controversies. Beyond his refutation of Paracelsus, his rebuttal of Johann Weyer's appeal for clemency for those accused of witchcraft was perhaps his most important work though he published a number of medical treatises including a piece on the occult powers of medicines.[15] After the Lutheran elector Ludwig VI forced the university faculty to sign the Lutheran Formula of Concord in 1580, Erastus moved to University of Basel where he spent the three remaining years of his life.[16]

It was at the time of his deep humiliation after defeat in the controversy over church discipline and his subsequent withdrawal from church affairs that Erastus undertook the refutation of the work of Paracelsus. To this point Erastus' published corpus consisted mostly of theological treatises, though he was never an ordained minister or member of the theology faculty, and a couple of works against astrology. Erastus recounted that Johannes Crato von Krafft-

[13]See Ruth Wesel-Roth, *Thomas Erastus: Ein Beitrag zur Geschichte der reformierten Kirche und zur Lehre von der Staatssouveränität* (Lahr/Baden: Moritz Schauenberg, 1954).

[14]Christopher J. Burchill, *The Heidelberg Antitrinitarians.* Bibliotheca Dissidentium XI, ed. André Séguenny (Baden-Baden: Editions Valentin Körner, 1989).

[15]Thomas Erastus, *Repititio disputationis de lamiis seu strigibus* (Basel: Peter Perna, 1578); idem, *De occultis pharmacorum potestatibus* (Basel: Peter Perna, 1574).

[16]Gunnoe, "Erastus and His Circle"; J. Karcher, "Thomas Erastus (1524–1583), der unversöhnliche Gegner des Theophrastus Paracelsus," *Gesnerus* 14 (1957): 1–13; Wilhelm Kühlmann, and Joachim Telle, "Humanimus und Medizin an der Universität Heidelberg im 16.Jahrhundert," in *Semper Apertus: Sechshundert Jahre Ruprecht-Karls-Universität Heidelberg 1386-1986,* vol. 1, ed. Wilhelm Doerr et al. (Berlin: Springer, 1985), 1:255–289; Walter Pagel, "Thomas Erastus," in *Dictionary of Scientific Biography;* idem., *Paracelsus: An Introduction to Philosophical Medicine in the Era of the Renaissance,* 2d ed., (Basel: Karger, 1982); Eberhard Stübler, *Geschichte der medizinische Facultät der Universität Heidelberg 1386–1925* (Heidelberg, 1926); Lynn Thorndike, *A History of Magic and Experimental Science,* 8 vols. (New York: Columbia, 1923–1958).

heim and the ducal Saxon physician Johann Hermann persuaded him to take on the task. Though Erastus was well placed in terms of physical location and acquaintances to have been well informed regarding Paracelsus, it seems that he had been such a serious-minded Aristotelian-Galenist physician that he had almost completely ignored Paracelsus before 1570.[17] The fruit of Crato's encouragement was Erastus' four-volume *Disputations on the New Medicine of Paracelsus,* which offered an exhaustive rejection of Paracelsus' views based on nearly the entire published corpus of Paracelsus.[18]

CREATION

Perhaps taking his clue from Reußner, Erastus opened his attack in the first volume of *Disputations on the New Medicine of Paracelsus* on the Paracelsian notion of creation. Before addressing Erastus' specific objections, it is fitting to outline the nature and difficulties of Paracelsus' theory of creation. Paracelsus taught that creation largely consisted in a divine or angelic separation of preexisting matter. The central question regarding the Paracelsian theory of creation, which has intrigued commentators since the sixteenth century, is whether this primeval material—which he alternatively called "*materia prima*," "*materia ultima*," and "*mysterium magnum*"—was itself created by God or whether it was uncreated.

Since Walter Pagel was able to show that many of Paracelsus' ideas appeared to have been influenced by Gnostic conceptions, we might imagine that Paracelsus would have advocated the existence of uncreated matter before "creation" in line with Gnosticism.[19] There are passages in the Paracelsian corpus that appear to bear out this Gnostic interpretation. For example, in *Das Buch de Mineralibus,* Paracelsus taught that *materia ultima* was "bei Gott" in

[17]I follow these connections more fully in "Erastus and His Circle"
[18]Thomas Erastus, *Disputationum de medicina nova de Philippi Paracelsi Pars Prima: In qua, quae de remediis superstitiosis & Magicis curationibus ille prodidit, praecipuè examinantur* (Basel: Peter Perna, [1571] (hereafter cited as *De Medicina nova*); idem, *Disputationum de nova Philippi Paracelsi medicina Pars Altera: In qua Philosophiæ Paracelsicæ Principia & Elementa explorantur* (Basel, Peter Perna, 1572); idem, *Disputationum de nova Philippi Paracelsi Medicina Pars Tertia* (Basel: Peter Perna, 1572); idem, *Disputationum de nova medicina Philippi Paracelsi Pars Quarta et Ultima* (Basel: Peter Perna, 1573). As the titles suggest, the first two volumes of the work were largely occupied with the religious and philosophical topics. A word of caution: Paracelsus was not always the target of Erastus' critiques in the first volume. For example, Erastus used this opportunity to publish a brief disputation on witchcraft which was a response to Johann Weyer rather than Paracelsus. On other occasions Erastus engages the ideas of figures such as Pomponazzi and Avicenna.
[19]Walter Pagel, "Paracelsus in the Neoplatonic and Gnostic Tradition,"*Ambix* 8 (1960): 125–166; idem, "The Prime Matter of Paracelsus,"*Ambix* 9 (1961): 117–135; Walter Pagel and Marianne Winder, "The Higher Elements and Prime Matter in Renaissance Naturalism and in Paracelsus," *Ambix* 21 (1974): 94–127.

the beginning. From it, *materia prima* was made. Pagel argued that this passage clearly assumed that there was some type of primeval matter that existed alongside God at creation.[20] While this passage was the most positive affirmation of the existence of uncreated matter among the genuine works of Paracelsus, other passages could be adduced to argue that he definitely taught that all matter was first created by God. For example in *De Meteoris*—in a passage that did not directly address the question of primeval matter—he did say that each of the four elements had bodies which were made "from nothing."[21] Thus, the works in which Paracelsus' authorship is not questioned offer a split decision on the question of the createdness of prime matter.

The spurious works in the Paracelsian corpus speak with no more unanimity on the issue of created or uncreated prime matter than the authentic works. On the one hand, the *Secretum magicum* suggested that God created the *materia prima*.[22] On the other hand, the *Philosophia ad Athenienses,* a text labeled Pseudo-Paracelsian by Karl Sudhoff but widely accepted as authentic in the sixteenth century (see title page, fig. 2), offered a definitive affirmation of the preexistence of uncreated matter.[23] Here our unknown author spoke of

[20]*Das Buch de Mineralibus*, PI, 3:34: "Nun ist das erst gewesen bei got, der anfang, das ist ultima materia, die selbige ultimam materiam hat er gemacht in primam materiam." One should note that judging this reference is further complicated by the fact that Paracelsus here spoke of "materia ultima" rather than "materia prima"; Walter Pagel, "Paracelsus in the Neoplatonic and Gnostic Tradition," 142.

[21]*Liber Meteororum,* PI, 13,:134: "nun sollent ir aber wissen, das alle vier corpora der vier elementen gemacht seind aus nichts, das ist alein gemacht durch das wort gottes, das fiat geheißen hat." Pagel did not find this reference a definitive rejection of the preexistence of matter since Paracelsus was speaking here of a later stage of creation; Pagel, "Paracelsus in the Neoplatonic and Gnostic Tradition," 144–145.

[22]Pagel, "Paracelsus in the Neoplatonic and Gnostic Tradition," 146.

[23]Karl Sudhoff treats the question of the authenticity of the *Philosophia ad Athenienses* in the introduction to PI, 13:xi–xiii. Sudhoff's first complaint against this text was the lack of manuscript attestation for it by its sixteenth-century editors. Neither its original publisher, Theodor Birckman, nor Johann Huser, who included it in his authoritative collection, made any reference to a manuscript source. Sudhoff lamented, "Auch haben wir ausschließlich diesen Kölner Druck [of Birckman] unserem Texte…augrunde legen müssen, da uns keine einzige handschriftliche Überlieferung dieser Schrift bekannt geworden ist." The second major complaint against the work stems from its fragmentary nature. It is obviously incomplete (e.g., it starts with the second "*paras*") and shows signs of having been worked over by an editor. The most obvious indication of the latter is the fact that the introductions refer to "the Prince Theophrastus" in the third person. Thus, Sudhoff considered it a work of questioned authenticity but did not rule out the possibility that the work might contain "einen echten Kern" which stemmed from Paracelsus. Later scholars have been more sanguine regarding its potential authenticity, and Josef Strebel regarded the text as a preliminary draft of the *Astronomia Magna*. Kurt Goldammer also raised objections to Sudhoff's earlier critique and referred to it as "die den echten Paracelsus gedankenreich paraphrasierende und interpretierende 'Philosophia ad Athenienses'" though he still labeled the work "deu-

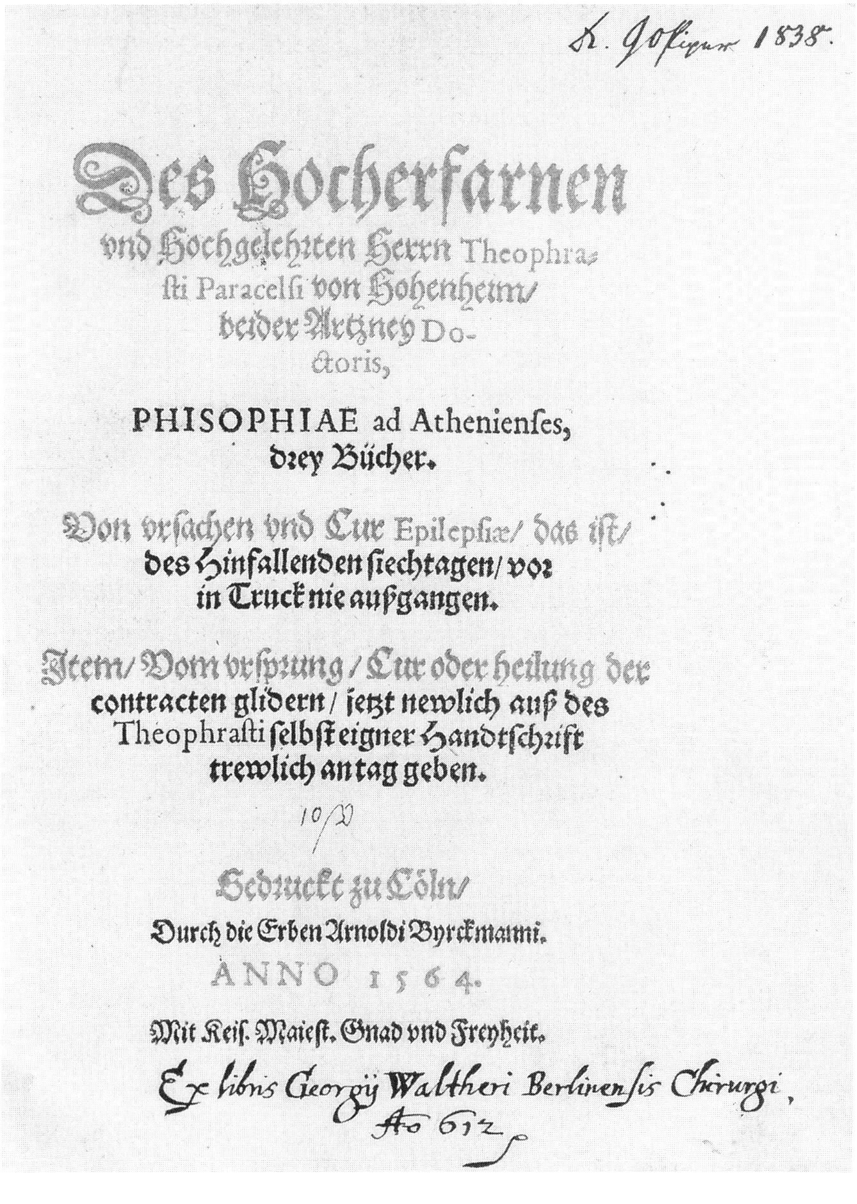

d. Jofinur 1838.

Des Hocherfarnen

vnd Hochgelehrten Herrn Theophrasti Paracelsi von Hohenheim/
beider Artzney Do-
ctoris,

PHISOPHIAE ad Athenienses,
drey Bücher.

Von vrsachen vnd Cur Epilepsiæ/ das ist/
des Hinfallenden siechtagen/vor
in Truck nie aufgangen.

Item/ Vom vrsprung / Cur oder heilung der
contracten glidern/ jetzt newlich auß des
Theophrasti selbst eigner Handtschrift
trewlich antag geben.

10/X

Gedruckt zu Cöln/
Durch die Erben Arnoldi Byrckmanni.
ANNO 1 5 6 4.

Mit Keis. Maiest. Gnad vnd Freyheit.

Ex libris Georgij Walthei Berlinensis Chirurgi,
Ao 672

Fig. 2. Title page of the [Pseudo?-]Paracelsian *Philosophia ad Athenienses* (Cologne:
Arnold Birckmann's Erben, 1564). Note that the title is misspelled "Phisophiae" in this
edition. (Bernard Becker Medical Library, Washington University School of
Medicine.)

a *mysterium magnum* from which all things were separated. Along with Paracelsus' sixteenth-century critics, Pagel asserted that it was clear that the *Philosophia ad Athenienses* taught that *mysterium magnum* was uncreated.[24]

It was precisely on the concept of uncreated prime matter that Erastus focused his attack. Like his patristic and scholastic predecessors, Erastus asserted that the proposition that God created the world *ex nihilo* was a non-negotiable item for Christians. He claimed that Paracelsus had expressly taught in *Philosophia ad Athenienses* that the *mysterium magnum* was uncreated and that Paracelsus did not believe in "creation" per se but only in the "separation" of previously existing material. Erastus interpreted Paracelsus's theory of creation to be nothing other than the chaos which existed in the beginning of the world as described by Presocratic philosopher Anaxagoras.[25] Erastus went on to claim that Paracelsus's teaching was actually much worse than Anaxagoras' since at least the Presocratic philosopher had taught in that this

---

tero-Paracelsian." Pagel often mined the *Philosophia ad Athenienses* as a source for "Paracelsian" ideas. With his extensive use of the work, Pagel appears to have been a de facto advocate of the authenticity of the *Philosophia ad Athenienses* even if he was forthcoming about the questions of its genuineness. Following Pagel, many Anglo-American writers have traced the impact of "Paracelsian" ideas in a broad sense, rather than limit their studies to works which can be concretely proven to have come from Paracelsus' pen. While we can agree with Pagel and his followers that the work was universally regarded as "Paracelsian," nevertheless, the fundamental reservations regarding the work's authenticity raised by Sudhoff have not been overturned. Given the fact that a later redactor edited the text and that it contains an apparent accretion of materials that are not in close harmony with the rest of Paracelsus' works, the *Philosophia ad Athenienses* cannot in the final analysis be regarded as a faithful representation of Paracelsus' own thought however much it became an integral part of the "Paracelsian" heritage; see Sudhoff, PI, 13:xii; Pagel, *Paracelsus*, 89–91; Kurt Goldammer, "Zur philosophischen und religiösen Sinngebung von Heilung und Heilmittel bei Paracelsus," in *Paracelsus in Neuen Horizonten: Gesammelte Aufsätze*, Salzburger Beiträge zur Paracelsusforschung, vol. 24 (Vienna: Verband der Wiss. Ges. Österreichs, 1986), 343–357, esp. 353.

[24]*Philosophia ad Athenienses*, PI,13:404ff. However, Pagel cannot prove that Pseudo-Paracelsus was definitely thinking in Gnostic terms in this passage. Pagel also noted the disagreement among Paracelsians regarding whether *materia prima* was uncreated. For example, Robert Fludd assumed that Paracelsus taught the materia prima was uncreated, though Fludd himself preferred to think of it as created by God. Alternatively both Heinrich Khunrath and Joseph Duchesne appear to have regarded the chaos as created; Pagel, "Paracelsus in the Neoplatonic and Gnostic Tradition," 143, 147–148.

[25]Anaxagoras of Clazomenae (ca. 500–428 B.C.) had rejected the notion of generation and passing-away; cf. G. S. Kirk, et al., *The Presocratic Philosophers* (Cambridge: Cambridge University Press, 1983), 352ff. It reveals much about Erastus' intellectual background that he connects this notion with Anaxagoras rather than the hermetic tradition. Erastus no doubt knew Anaxagoras as mediated through Aristotle. He likely had passages in mind like this one from the *Physics* where Aristotle characterizes Anaxagoras' position with: "The upshot of all this is that everything must once have been mixed together and must have started changing at some point in time"; see Aristotle, *Physics*, trans. Robin Waterfield (Oxford: Oxford University Press, 1996), p. 64 [203b].

separation was accomplished by God whereas Paracelsus suggested that "mortal gods" had completed this process of separation.[26] Thus Paracelsus had denied the fundamental principle of creation *ex nihilo* and, worse yet, had suggested that God employed demonic powers to complete creation.

Erastus rejected the theory of the *Philosophia ad Athenienses* and embarked on a discourse on his own theory of creation, which interpreted the Genesis narrative within Aristotelian categories. According to Erastus there were two clearly distinguishable types of creation, both of which only God had the power to perform. The first kind was absolute creation—the creation of the world *ex nihilo*.[27] In Erastus' conception, in the first moment of creation all the *materia* on earth received its particular *forma* by God's command: "For in the same moment that he commanded that they should exist by his omnipotent word, he mixed and arranged the parts of the *materia* and also differentiated and adorned them with many potentials and dispositions so that the different and manifold *forma* appeared in the same moment."[28] This first moment of creation was described in the first sentence of Genesis: "In the beginning, God created heaven and earth." Being a good Aristotelian, Erastus had to clarify that here Moses must have included all the terrestrial elements— including water, air, and fire, in the word "earth." After the initial creation, "the earth (i.e., the mass of the elements) existed empty and void."[29] This "prime matter" of Erastus lacked the *forma* of later composite *materia* and was equally suitable to be molded into any one type of *materia* as another.[30]

Following the vocabulary of Genesis, Erastus was able to distinguish a second type of creation as well. The second type was a nonabsolute creation, in which God made new compounds and creatures from the prime matter of his first act of creation. The most obvious example of this second type of

[26]Erastus, *De Medicina Nova*, 1:4.

[27]Of course Aristotle himself had not taught creation *ex nihilo* but maintained the eternity of the world. For Aristotle's conception, the thought of the early church fathers, and the scholastic tradition, see respectively, G. E. R. Lloyd, *Aristotle: The Growth and Structure of His Thought* (Cambridge: Cambridge University Press, 1968); Jaroslav Pelikan, "Creation and Causality in Christian Thought," *Journal of Religion* 40 (1960): 246–255; David C. Lindberg, *The Beginnings of Western Science* (Chicago: University of Chicago, 1992).

[28]Erastus, *De Medicina Nova* 1:11: "Etenim momento eodem quo, ut haec existerent, iussit, tam variè omnipotente suo Verbo materiae partes miscuit at temperavit, tamque multiplicibus potentiis & dispositionibus distinxit & exornavit, quam variae multiplicesque formae in eadem subitò apparverunt."

[29] Erastus, *De Medicina Nova* 1:7: "Disertè namque dicitur, terram, id est, elementorum massam, inanem & vacuam extitisse, hoc est, formis istis compositarum rerum caruisse, quae simul atque Deus esse iussit, eodem illo momento perfectae extiterint."

[30]Ibid., 1:15: "Quoniam potentia, quam tunc habuit solam, generalissima fuit, per quam ad rerum omnium creationem æquè idonea erat, ad nullam magis apta, quam ad aliam quamlibet."

creation was the creation of Adam, who, Erastus noted, was called a "creature" only when he received the spirit of life. Eve likewise was created when God formed her from Adam's rib.[31] In this line of thought, something must be called "creation" if it required divine agency for its existence.[32] Erastus criticized what he described as the scholastic view of creation which only viewed the first "type" of creation as creation per se; the second action of creating the various compounds of the world (i.e., the other five active days of creation) was only considered "adornment and definition" by God.[33] Erastus placed two qualifications on this notion of creation. First, to have been rightly considered a creation, the new creature or compound could not have originated out of its own innate power. Thus, when a seed grows into a tree, it is no "creation" but rather, the seed has simply developed out of its inborn potential. The second qualification was that it must have been made immediately and without movement or change.[34] In this second phase of creation, God transformed the *materia prima* of the first creation into composites: "Out of these elements before any alteration then," claimed Erastus, "God created diverse kinds of things through his omnipotent word."[35]

Seen in the light of Erastus' interpretation of Genesis, Paracelsus denied both the initial creation *ex nihilo* as well as God's role in the secondary acts of creation in giving composite materials their set forms. The Paracelsian notion that angelic or demonic forces were at work in this separation troubled Erastus, and he surmised that Paracelsus had really believed that Christ was one of these minor deities but Paracelsus did not have the courage to say it. In this connection, he accused Paracelsus of Arianism in placing the son in a subordinate position to the father.[36]

This condemnation of Paracelsus' theory of creation expressed as it was in an Aristotelian vocabulary was ironic considering the fact that contemporary Paracelsians such as Gerhard Dorn and Richard Bostocke were hailing Paracelsus precisely for avoiding the pernicious influence of Aristotle and Galen. To them, Paracelsus had freed natural philosophy from the pagan ancient philosophers and had set forth a restored, Christian natural philosophy.[37] Alternatively, Erastus continued in the tradition of the scholastics in

---

[31]Ibid., 1:8.

[32]Erastus, *De Medicina Nova*, 1:6. [33]Ibid., 1:7. [34]Ibid., 1:6. [35]Ibid., 1:7. [36]Ibid., 24.

[37]Gerhard Dorn, *De natura luce physica ex genesi desumpta....*, in *Theatrum Chemicum*, ed. Lazarus Zetzner (Strasbourg, 1659–61); R. B. [Richard Bostocke], *The difference betwene the auncient Phisicke, first taught by the godly forfathers, consisting in unitie peace and concord: and the later Phisicke proceding from Idolaters, Ethnikes, and Heathen: as Gallen, and such other consiting in dualitie, discord and contrarietie. And wherein the naturall Philosophie of Aristotle doth differ from the trueth of Gods worde, and is iniurous to Christianitie and sounde doctrine* (London: for Robert Walley, 1585).

explaining the doctrine of creation with an Aristotelian vocabulary and building a bastion around the concept of creation *ex nihilo*, though not restricting "creation" to solely *creatio ex nihilo*. Whereas Dorn and Bostocke regarded Paracelsus as the restorer of Godly natural philosophy, Erastus condemned him as "blinder than the heathens."[38]

ADAM'S FLESH AND THE RESURRECTION OF THE BODY

At the 1571 Lenten Frankfurt Fair, Erastus came upon a text which caused him to put the publication of the first volume of his anti-Paracelsian disputations on hold. This book was Michael Toxites' *editio princeps* of Paracelsus' *Astronomia Magna oder die gantze Philosophia sagax der grossen und kleinen Welt*[39] (see title page, fig. 3). Erastus not only recoiled from the "horrible heresies" of the work; he also marveled that Toxites had been so audacious as to dedicate it to the pious Lutheran elector August of Saxony. Erastus wrote a special refutation of the *Astronomia Magna* which he appended to the end of the first volume of his *Disputations on the New Medicine of Paracelsus*.[40] He also dedicated the work to elector August and wrote him a personal letter gently instructing him of the manifold blasphemies contained in the *Astronomia Magna* and warning him of ill-reputed patronage seekers who would sully his glorious reputation.[41]

Whereas Erastus' critique of the *Philosophia ad Athenienses* had focused on Paracelsus' conception of creation, here Erastus objected to Paracelsus' anthropology and its broader theological implications. First, Erastus rejected the three-part division of humans which Paracelsus had outlined in the *Astronomia Magna*. According to Paracelsus, a human consisted of three components: elemental, sidereal, and divine. This notion related the composition of humans—the microcosm—to the composition of the universe—the macrocosm. Conceptualizing humans in this manner had clear utility for medical therapy. For example, the part of humans which was made of elements would

---

[38]Erastus, *De Medicina Nova*, 1:25: "quo videas ipsis Ethnicis coeciorem fuisse."

[39]A loose translation would be: *Great Astronomy or the Complete Adept Philosophy of the Macrocosm and the Microcosm*. Paracelsus, *Astronomia Magna: Oder die gantze Philosophia sagax der grossen und kleinen Welt* (Frankfurt: Sigmund Feyrabend: 1571). Karl Sudhoff, *Versuch einer Kritik der Echtheit der Paracelsischen Schriften*. I. Theil: *Bibliographia Paracelsica: Besprechung der unter Hohenheims Namen 1527–1893 erscheinenen Druckschriften* (reprint, Berlin, 1894; Graz, 1958), no. 131. For Toxites, see C. Schmidt, *Michael Schütz genannt Toxites* (Strasbourg, 1888); Rudolf Zaunick, "Michael Toxites (Schütz) und Kurfürst August von Sachsen," *Sudhoffs Archiv* 36 (1943): 90–99.

[40]Erastus, *De Medicina Nova*, 1:243–267.

[41]Erastus to Kurfürst August von Sachsen, Heidelberg, Sept. 9, 1571. Sächsisches Hauptstaatsarchiv (Dresden), Geheim. Rat (Geheim. Archiv), Loc. 8523, Sechs unterschiedliche Bücher, Bd. 1; 1570–1574, fols. 1867r–1877v.

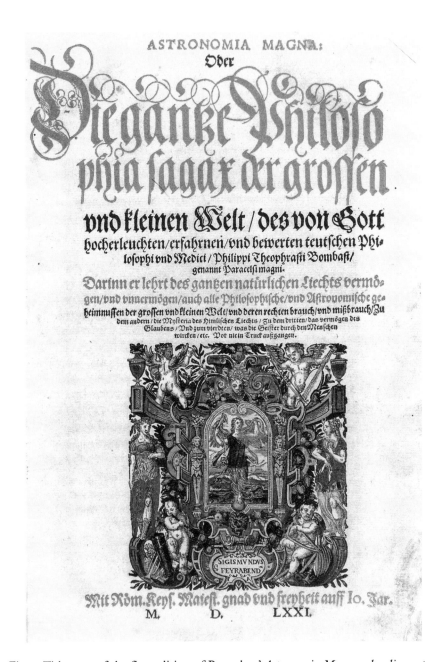

Fig. 3. Title page of the first edition of Paracelsus' *Astronomia Magna oder die gantze Philosophia sagax der grossen und kleinen welt, ed. Michael Toxites* (Frankfurt: Siegmund Feyrabend, 1571). (Bernard Becker Medical Library, Washington University School of Medicine.)

58

respond to chemical medicines. Likewise, the sidereal or celestial part of humans was the part which was most under the influence of the powers of the stars. Finally, there were spiritual maladies that could only be treated by the divine physician.

As successful as this division may have been in explaining how the micro-cosm was related to the macrocosm and likewise harmonized with Paracelsian medical theory, Erastus recoiled from the heretical implications of what he considered to be a three-substance anthropology and interpreted this theory as an attack on the traditional Christian belief in the resurrection of the body.[42] Unlike Platonic thought, which had emphasized only the existence of the immortal soul in the afterlife, the New Testament writers taught that the human person, a union of soul and body, would itself be resurrected at the last judgment. While later Christian writers incorporated the notion of an immor-tal soul into their theology, nearly all held that the body would itself be mate-rially resurrected at the last judgment.[43] In Paracelsus' conception, however, only the divine part of humans could be received by God into paradise. Paracelsus termed this divine aspect alternatively "living flesh," "heavenly flesh," and flesh "from the Holy Spirit" and maintained that it was given to humans in baptism.[44] Paracelsus argued that only things which have their ori-gin in God can return to God. Alternatively, neither the elemental nor even the celestial part of humans could be resurrected.[45] At death, the elemental part of humans returned to earth, the sidereal to the stars, and the divine to God. Erastus interpreted what Paracelsus termed the elemental and sidereal dimension of humans to be nothing other than the human body.[46] Since such discussion suggested that actual human flesh could not be resurrected, Erastus concluded that Paracelsus' theory was a manifest denial of the Christian doc-trine of the resurrection of the body. This threefold composition would have

---

[42]Paracelsus did not speak of substances but of "parts" (*Theilen*) or "beings" (*Wesen*); *Astro-nomia Magna*, PI, 12:10.

[43]Oscar Cullmann, *Immortality of the Soul or Resurrection of the Dead?* (New York: Macmillan, 1964), Caroline Walker Bynum, *The Resurrection of the Body in Western Christianity, 200–1336* (New York: Columbia, 1995), 5–14. While Paul's discussion of the resurrection in 1 Corinthians 15 does emphasize the spiritual nature of the resurrected body (v. 12: "It is sown a physical body, it is raised a spiritual body"), it is also clear that he taught a continuity between the earthly body and the heav-enly body (v. 53: "For this perishable nature must put on the imperishable, and this mortal nature must put on immortality."); quotations from the Revised Standard Version.

[44]*Astronomia Magna*, PI,12:308–309.

[45]Ibid., PI, 12:288: "doch so kompt nichts gen himel, weder der elementisch noch der side-risch leib, alein der mensch der ein geist ist und nemlich der geist der von got ist." Erastus, *De Medicina Nova*, 1:245.

[46]Erastus, *De Medicina Nova*, 1:251.

been more readily harmonized with Christian theology if one understood Paracelsus to mean properties or qualities of the human body that corresponded to earthly, celestial, and divine existence. Since Erastus interpreted Paracelsus from the perspective of Aristotelian categories, however, Erastus insisted that Paracelsus must here be understood to refer to substances rather than qualities.[47] The fact that Paracelsus at other times taught that there were two bodies in humans (mortal and immortal) rather than three parts (elemental, sidereal, divine) did not soften Erastus' criticism, since Paracelsus still maintained that the earthly body returned to earth while only the eternal body entered the kingdom of God.[48] Erastus offered the standard critique of the inconsistent and self-contradictory nature of Paracelsus' works and at one point counted up the various ways that Paracelsus had divided the human person and exclaimed: "Thus you have a three-bodied monster of a man composed out of nine parts."[49]

Naturally Paracelsus would not have accepted this accusation of heresy but would have asserted that he too believed in the resurrection of the body. In the *Paramirum,* Paracelsus had taught that human flesh could not enter the kingdom of God until it was regenerated. Erastus conceded that Paracelsus' conception of the sanctification of human flesh necessary for it to enter heaven was fundamentally orthodox in the *Paramirum.*[50] However, Erastus argued that Paracelsus' teaching in the *Astronomia Magna* went beyond the bounds of orthodoxy. Here, rather than maintain that human flesh had simply to be sanctified to enter paradise, Paracelsus suggested that humans must receive new spiritual flesh by the agency of the Holy Spirit. Paracelsus thus distinguished between two types of flesh: the first, "Adam's flesh," which could not enter paradise, and a second, flesh incarnate through the Holy Spirit, which

[47]In this light, it is interesting to observe Erastus' translation of Paracelsus' sentence, "So doch Got zwei wesen im menschen gemacht hatt, das irdisch und das ewig und seind zusammen vermelet bis an die auferstehung?" with "Deus duas essentias in homine fecit, terremam & eternam: quæ coniunctæ manent usque ad resurrectionem." In Erastus' translation, Paracelsus' "Wesen," which could suggest a number of nuances, has been translated with "essentia" which Erastus correlates with the Aristotelian category of "substance" or "οὐσία." *Astronomia Magna,* PI, 12:10; Erastus, *De Medicina Nova,* 1:251.

[48]Erastus, *De Medicina Nova,* 1:251.

[49]Ibid., 1:261: "Sic monstrum tricorporeum hominis habebis ex partibus novem compositum." Regarding the competing anthropological conceptions in Paracelsus' work, see H. C. Erik Midelfort, "The Anthropological Roots of Paracelsus' Psychiatry," in *Kreatur und Kosmos,* ed. Rosemarie Dilg-Frank (Stuttgart: Fischer, 1981), 67–77; Gause, *Paracelsus,* 85; Kurt Goldammer, "Paracelsischer Eschatologie: Zum Verständnis der Anthropologie und Kosmologie Hohenheims," in *Paracelsus in Neuen Horizonten: Gesammelte Aufsätze,* Salzburger Beiträge zur Paracelsusforschung vol. 24 (Vienna: Verband der Wiss. Ges. Österreichs, 1986), 87–152 , here 108.

[50]Erastus, *De Medicina Nova,* 1:248.

since it had its origin in God, could return to God.[51] Here Paracelsus appeared to have attempted to reconcile a Neoplatonic notion of the migration of the incorporeal soul to the divine with the Christian notion of the resurrection of the body. Kurt Goldammer has suggested that Paracelsus was torn between a spiritualist-dualistic pneumatology and an authentic faith in the resurrection. This led Paracelsus to adopt what Goldammer has termed a "paradoxical compromise-formula."[52] Although Paracelsus offered a plausible, if paradoxical, reinterpretation of the doctrine of the resurrection of the body, Erastus asserted that such a spiritualistic interpretation of the resurrection of the body with "heavenly flesh" substituted for "Adam's flesh" was tantamount to an outright rejection of corporeal resurrection. Likewise, Paracelsus' application of this distinction between heavenly flesh and Adam's flesh to his understanding of Christ opened the door to extensive criticism of Paracelsus' christology and soteriology.

Erastus' attack on Paracelsus' christology began with Paracelsus' depiction of the Virgin Mary's role in the incarnation. What follows is the passage from the *Astronomia Magna* which Erastus found most unsettling:

> From the Virgin comes the new birth and not from woman. From this it follows, that the Virgin, from whom the new birth has proceeded and been born, has been a daughter of Abraham according to the promise and not from Adam; that is, she has been born from Abraham without male seed, in the power of the promise without all mortal nature. From the Virgin, who thus is not from Adam, not from his seed, only out of his flesh, Christ was born, who was conceived by the Holy Spirit and was made incarnate from holy flesh, not according to the order of the mortal flesh, but according to the new birth which thus proceeds from the Holy Spirit. From this you should consider the fact that [he is] *out of* Adam's flesh in much the same way that you might consider wine which was stored in a vat; it is *out of* the vat, but it

---

[51]*Astronomia Magna*, PI, 12:306ff. Hartmut Rudolf, "Kosmosspekulatin und Trinitätslehre: Ein Beitrag zur Beziehung zwischen Weltbild und Theologie bei Paracelsus, in *Paracelsus in der Tradition*, Salzbürger Beiträge aus Paracelsusforschung, no. 21, ed. Sepp Domandl (Vienna, 1980), , 32–47, here 42, suggests that this teaching was also present in Paracelsus's earlier theological work *De geneologia Christi*, a work which Rudolf maintains bears many resemblances to the later *Astronomia Magna*.

[52]In contrast to Goldammer, Harmut Rudolf has asked whether Paracelsus actually held a negative view of the "earthly-material body." Rudolf suggests that it was the mortality of the body which Paracelsus held in low regard, rather than flesh and blood itself. I am inclined to agree with Goldammer that Paracelsus' notion is at least implicitly dualistic, since it would seem to preclude any real continuity between the "mortal flesh," which humans received as descendants of Adam, and the "heavenly flesh" that they are given by Christ. The Paracelsian notion does not represent a simple material/immaterial dualism. For example, the sidereal part of humans is itself invisible, but, like the elemental body, it cannot be resurrected. Goldammer, "Paracelsischer Eschatologie," 111; Rudolf, "Kosmosspekulation und Trinitätslehre," 43.

is not *of* the vat. From this it follows that that which is incarnate from the Holy Spirit is from heaven and will return again to heaven; that, however, which is not incarnate from the Holy Spirit, that will not return to heaven.[53]

To save Mary from the blemish of original sin, Paracelsus argued that Mary was not descended from Adam but rather from Abraham and was thus not born of Adam's seed though he does not explicitly deny that she still possessed Adam's flesh.[54] Erastus did not follow the full subtlety of this point and asserted that Paracelsus taught that Mary's flesh was not derived from Adam and that therefore she did not possess normal human flesh.[55] Here was a rare occasion where Erastus as a Reformed Protestant could criticize a Catholic motif in Paracelsus' thought. Erastus, however, chose not to dwell on the exalted view of Mary which undergirded Paracelsus' theory and focused instead on the fundamental christological issue. Like Mary, Christ was not born of Adam's seed but was made incarnate by the Holy Spirit in Mary's womb. To illustrate this theory, Paracelsus claimed that Christ had only dwelt in Mary's womb as wine filled a barrel.[56] She had only been a channel for Christ's holy flesh; he became incarnate in her, but did not assume her flesh.[57]

---

[53]*Astronomia Magna*, PI, 12:308–309: "aus der jungfrauen gehet die neue geburt und nicht aus der frauen. aus dem folgt nun, das die jungfrau, aus der ausgangen und geboren ist die neu geburt, ein tochter ist gewesen von Abraham nach der verheischung und nicht aus Adam, das ist sie ist gewesen von Abraham on menlichen samen geborn, in kraft der verheischung on alle tötliche natur. aus der jungfrauen, die also von Adam nit ist, nit von seinem samen, nur aus seinem fleisch, ist geboren Christus, der empfangen ist vom heiligen geist und vom heiligen fleisch incarnirt/ nicht nach der ordnung des tödlichen fleischs, sonder nach der neuen geburt, die da gehet aus dem heiligen geist. darin verstanden aus Adams fleisch nich anderst, dann sovil als ihr verstehen möget von einem wein, der in ein faß gelegt wird, der ist auß dem faß, aber nicht vom faß. iezt folgt auf das, was von dem geist incarniert wird, das ist vom himel und kompt wider gen himel; das aber von dem geist nicht incarnirt wird, das kompt nit gen himel."

[54]*Astronomia Magna*, PI, 12:307–309. At first sight it might appear difficult to understand why Paracelsus had argued that Mary was not born of Adam's seed, since he also maintained that Christ received no flesh from Mary but was made incarnate by the Holy Spirit in Mary's womb. The answer to this puzzle is that Paracelsus had taught that both Christ *and* Mary bore human nature only as a covering. In this sense, Mary shares more in common with Christ than normal mortals. Gause, *Paracelsus,* 45.

[55]Erastus, *De Medicina Nova*, 1:255.

[56]Paracelsus had used this same analogy to illustrate how the Virgin Mary grew in the womb of her mother Saint Ann without receiving the stain of her fallen nature; Gause, *Paracelsus,* 44–45.

[57]*Astronomia Magna*, PI, 12:309: "aus der jungfrauen, die also von Adam nit ist, nit von seinem samen, nur aus seinem fleisch, ist geboren Christus, der empfangen ist vom heiligen geist und vom heiligen fleisch incarnirt nicht nach der ordnung des tödlichen fleischs, sonder nach der neuen geburt, die da gehet aus dem heiligen geist. darin verstanden aus Adams fleisch nich anderst, dann sovil als ihr verstehen möget von einem wein, der in ein faß gelegt wird, der ist auß dem faß, aber nicht vom faß."

Since Mary had not been born of Adam's seed and Christ did not assume flesh from Mary, it would seem that Paracelsus had double-insulated Christ from the taint of original sin. While Paracelsus denied that Christ received flesh from Mary, he taught that Christ possessed "holy flesh" made incarnate by the Holy Spirit. In Erastus' view, to assert that Christ did not assume Adam's flesh was to say that he possessed some other type of flesh than that of normal humans; in short, that Christ was not truly human.[58] Erastus argued that not only did this clash with the Apostles' Creed, but it also called into question whether Christ could have actually died for humans on the cross if he did not possess mortal flesh.[59] Thus, Paracelsus' attempt to apply his "spiritualist" natural philosophy to the doctrine of Christ necessarily called into question the means of salvation.

The idea that it was possible that all humans did not inherit their flesh from Adam led to many novel conceptions in Paracelsus' thought which Erastus considered to be strange heresies. Paracelsus taught that the blessed actually possessed two bodies: a mortal one, born of Adam's flesh, and an immortal one, made incarnate by the Holy Spirit. Following this distinction, he speculated that the apostles in New Testament times performed miracles by their "new bodies" rather than by their "old bodies." Erastus thought that Paracelsus attributed immaterial bodies to nymphs, wild men, and giants.[60] Paracelsus had also suggested that the inhabitants of the New World were not necessarily descended from the Adam of Genesis but had perhaps descended from "another Adam."[61] Later Spanish writers vehemently condemned this notion of Paracelsus when grappling with the question of whether American Indians were fully human. Like Erastus, they also asserted that Paracelsus'

---

[58]Erastus, *De Medicina Nova*, 1:247, 252. Interestingly it was precisely this "heretical" notion of Christ's flesh that Valentin Weigel found attractive; see Moran, "Paracelsus, Religion and Dissent," 69.

[59]Erastus, *De Medicina Nova*, 1:255.

[60]Erastus, *De Medicina Nova*, 1:254; *Astronomia Magna*, PI, 12:113–114, 244–249, 362–363; see also *Liber de nymphis, sylphis, pygmaeis et salamandris et de caeteris spiritibus*, in PI, 14: 115–151. For an English translation, see Paracelsus, *Four Treatises*, ed. Henry E. Sigerist (Baltimore: Johns Hopkins, 1996).

[61]*Astronomia Magna*, PI, 12:35: "und so mag ich nit underlassen, von denen ein kleine meldung zu tun, die in verborgenen insulen gefunden seind worden, und noch verborgen sind, das sie von Adam zusein geglaubt mögen werden, mag sichs nit befinden, das Adams kinder seind kommen in die verborgenen insulen, sonder wol zu bedenken, das dieselbigen leut von einem andern Adam seind; dan dahin wirt es schwerlich komen, das sie fleish und bluts halben uns gefreundt sein. und das ist auch wol zu gedenken, were Adam im paradeis bliben, es were villeicht ein anderer Adam worden, doch villeicht nit mit der bildtnus gottes, als dan die neuen insulen seind."

suggestion, if followed to its natural conclusion, might well call into question the salvation of Western Christians as well.[62]

The final error that Erastus cited in reference to "Adam's flesh" was that Paracelsus' theories were an attack on divine omnipotence. Erastus distilled this charge from Paracelsus' description of how immortal bodies were created. According to Paracelsus, God the Father had only been responsible for the creation of mortal flesh, like the flesh of Adam. However, the immortal flesh of those who enter heaven was created and given by Christ. Erastus considered the mere notion that God the Father was unable to transform mortal flesh into immortal flesh an affront to divine omnipotence.[63]

CONCLUSION

In both the case of Erastus and Reußner, orthodox Protestant physicians were at least as exercised at the religious heresy of Paracelsianism as they were at the novelty of Paracelsian medical theory. Erastus, like Reußner before him, directed much of his animus against the likely Pseudo-Paracelsian *Philosophia ad Athenienses*. This fact allows the tentative conclusion that the reception of Paracelsian ideas by mainstream Protestant natural philosophers was further complicated by the more hermetic orientation of the Pseudo-Paracelsian corpus.[64] In the case of the *Astronomia Magna*, Paracelsus had offered a radical reinterpretation of human anthropology, the nature of Christ's flesh and the resurrection of the body. Although animated by a unique largely biblical spiritualistic vision, by most any sixteenth-century standard, Paracelsus was a heretic many times over. Like Paracelsus' more sympathetic interpreter Bostocke, Erastus had been able to conceptualize ways in which the Paracelsian natural philosophy could be reconciled with an orthodox Christian position. Unlike Bostock, however, Erastus chose to emphasize the cacophony and heterodoxy of Paracelsus's teachings rather than their unity and orthodoxy. Although Erastus was generally an honest critic of Paracelsus, his tendency to examine Paracelsus's teaching through Aristotelian lenses compounded the difficulty of reconciling Paracelsus's natural philosophy with orthodox Protestantism.

[62]See Anthony Pagden, *The Fall of Natural Man* (Cambridge: Cambridge University Press, 1982), 22–23.

[63]Erastus, *De Medicina Nova*, 1:254–255.

[64]Here I follow the suggestion of Charles Webster that "a more hermetic view of the magus ideal of Paracelsus derives from the corpus of doubtful or spurious writings attributed to Paracelsus, and to the works of early Paracelsians, sources which have deeply influenced historical accounts of Paracelsus himself and which prove that the Paracelsian movement was swept up in the hermetic tide which engulfed Europe in the late sixteenth century"; Charles Webster, *From Paracelsus to Newton: Magic and the Making of Modern Science* (Cambridge: Cambridge University Press, 1982), 57.

Though this paper has focused on specific theological objections, Erastus's attack was as much directed at Paracelsus's natural magic as it was his theology. While Erastus's work only offered a blunt "No!" to Paracelsus's entire system of natural philosophy, the end-result of his exchange with the Paracelsian corpus was likely more productive. In delivering an acid critique of Paracelsus's religious and magical concepts, he paved the way for the future separation of Paracelsus's progressive medical ideas from their original heretical milieu in later writers like Andreas Libavius and Daniel Sennert.[65]

[65]Cf. Debus, "Guitherius, Libavius and Sennert"

ACKNOWLEDGMENTS

I would like to thank Conrad Bult and Kathleen Struck of the Hekman Library for their help in procuring materials for this article and Bruce Moran for his timely bibliographical suggestions.

388

suos naenos habeant, tamen eorum authoritatem, miniſtri
tueri, non ex illis publica ſpectacula facere debent. Ro-
go autem Excell. tuam, vt aliquando priuatim de tota hac
cauſa cum D. Eraſto, viro pietate & eruditione ſingulari
prædito, conferat, neque eos audiat, qui optimè meritum
oderunt & perſequuntur, adeóque ex ijs locis electum vo-
lunt, in quibus ipſi fortaſsis vix nidum inuenturi fuiſſent,
niſi alij primam glaciem fregiſſent, inter quos iſtius viri
eruditio & ſtudium præcipuè eluxit. Scripſit hic ſub initi-
um iſtius Tragœdiae Theſes aliquot, quibus totum hoc
negotium complexus eſt. Probauit has D. Bullingerus
cum toto noſtro collegio. At confutationem earundem
D. Beza inſtituit: ſed quod tanti viri pace dixerim, parùm
profecit. Nolim tamen apud vos nouas turbas excitari. Hoc
potius opto, vt quae per nouatores aliquos inuecta eſt con-
fuſio, paulatim aboleatur. Quod facilè fiet, ſi qui rectius
& moderatius ſentiunt, tutò per illos agere, & quod ani-
mo ſentiunt, modeſtè proponere alijſque dijudicanda
proponere poſſunt: Theologi verò à Reipub. guberna-
tione & bellorum conſilijs atque aulicis negotijs ad ſugge-
ſtum & ſcholas remittantur: quæ propria eorum arena &
palaeſtra eſt, in qua ſeſe exerceant. &c.

Rodolphus Gualtherus.

Clariſſ. viro D. Thomæ Eraſto Doctori
medico, D. meo honorando, & fratri
charisimo. Heidelbergam.
S. D.

HOrreo ſanè ad commemorationem eorum quæ nar-
ras de excommunicatoribus, verùm vt-ut res ceci-
derit, ſemper deteriora metui. Vnde & illuſtriſſ. Principi
ſcripſi, ne ſe huic aeſtuoſo credat pelago. Ac mirum eſt ho-
mines iſtos Principi inſtillaſſe, non tam meo conſilio, quàm
Gual-

Bruce T. Moran

LIBAVIUS ᵀᴴᴱ PARACELSIAN?

MONSTROUS NOVELTIES, INSTITUTIONS,
AND THE NORMS OF SOCIAL VIRTUE

ON JANUARY 29, 1609, there arrived in the German city of Coburg a book published a few months before by a doctor at Paris named Pierre Le Paulmier (Petrus Palmarius, 1568–1610). The book was called *Lapis Philosophicus Dogmaticorum* (The Philosophical Stone of the Dogmatists)[1] and the fact that it should have found its way to Coburg was no accident since much of the book's contents centered upon the alchemical and pharmaceutical practices of one of the town's more recent residents, the physician, chemist, and director of the Coburg *Gymnasium Casimirianum Academicum,* Andreas Libavius (ca. 1540–1616).[2] Outside Coburg Libavius' reputation rested more upon the

---

[1]Petrus Palmarius, *Lapis Philosophicus Dogmaticorum: Quo paracelsista Libavius restituitur, Scholae Medicae Parisiensis iudicium de Chymicis declaratur, Censura in adulteria et fraudes Parachymicorum deffenditur, asserto verae Alchemiae honore. Per P. Palmarium Doctorem Parisiensem Galenochymicum* (Parisiis: Apud Davidem Dovlcevr, 1608). On Palmarius and Libavius' problems with other French physicians see Allen G. Debus, *The French Paracelsians: The Chemical Challenge to Chemical and Scientific Tradition in Early Modern France* (Cambridge: Cambridge University Press, 1991), 59 ff.

[2]Concerning the life and work of Andreas Libavius see Gottfried Ludwig, *Ehre des Hoch-Fürstlichen Casimiriani Academici in Coburg* (Coburg: Paul Günther Pfotenhauer und Sohn, 1725). J. Ottmann, "Erinnerung an Libavius in Rothenburg ob der Tauber," *Verhandlung der Gesellschaft Deutscher Naturforscher und Ärzte* 65 (1894): 79–85. R.P. Multhauf, "Libavius and Beguin," in *Great Chemists,* ed. Eduard Farber (New York/London: Interscience Publishers, 1961), 65–79. J.R. Partington, *A History of Chemistry,* vol. 2 (London: Macmillan, 1961), 244–270. Pietsch, Kotowski, Rex, eds., *Die Alchemie des Andreas Libavius, ein Lehrbuch der Chemie aus dem Jahre 1597* (Weinheim: Verlag Chemie, 1964). Lynn Thorndike, "Libavius and Chemical Controversy," in *History of Magic and Experimental Science* (New York: Columbia University Press, 1964), vol. 6, 238–253. Allen G. Debus, "Guintherius-Libavius-Sennert: The Chemical Compromise in Early Modern Medicine," in *Science, Medicine and Society in the Renaissance,* ed. Allen Debus (New York: Science History Pub-

books he had written than upon his skills in teaching or in the practice of medicine. His best-known work, the *Alchymia,* had been published in 1597 and was thereafter enlarged by the addition of commentaries, partially inspired by disputes at Paris. Other polemical treatises, three volumes of letters, and another major alchemical work, his *Alchymia Triumphans,* had, by 1609, placed the Coburg chemist near the center of a cultural maelstrom that swirled together issues relating to religious orthodoxy, Renaissance magic, pharmacy, and Paracelsian medical philosophy. Underneath it all, however, there was a different sort of confusion and another kind of struggle in which Libavius also played a leading role. This was a struggle over language as well as a contest over which institutional authorities would legitimize its use.

When he saw Palmarius' book Libavius recounts that he laughed at the author's madness and pitied him. Libavius also cursed the enormity of Palmarius' vices, his trickery, and his lies. Among other things, Palmarius had accused the Coburg gymnasiarch of having defined alchemy in a way that threatened the public good and then had labeled Libavius a Paracelsian. The book did not seem worthy of a response and, indeed, Libavius' allies were divided about what to do. Since their friend had already for several years been involved in debates with the Paris faculty of medicine over the use of chemical preparations, some warned against responding in a way that might further offend the Paris school. Even Joseph Duchesne (Quercetanus) (ca. 1544–1609), whose books had helped initiate the Parisian debate, wrote (shortly before his death) to advise Libavius to moderate his reply so as not to provoke further controversy. Others called for a rough response, advising that one could hardly be silent in the face of such atrocious vices and that the course of such depravity had to be hammered back. By May Libavius had heard from the younger Martin Ruland (1569–1611), chief physician at the imperial court, and learned that Ruland too was considering a refutation. By October Ruland was writing that those things which he had written against Palmarius for the sake of truth and

lications, 1972), 151–165. Wolf-Dieter Müller-Jahncke, "Andreas Libavius im Lichte der Geschichte der Chemie…," *Jahrbuch der Coburger Landesstiftung* 17 (1972): 205–230; also, "Libavius, Libau, Andreas," *Literaturlexikon: Autoren und Werke deutscher Sprache,* ed. Walther Killy (Gutersloh: Bertelsmann Lexikon, 1990), 262ff. Owen Hannaway, *The Chemists and the Word: The Didactic Origins of Chemistry* (Baltimore: Johns Hopkins University Press, 1975). Wlodzimierz Hubicki, "Libavius," in *Dictionary of Scientific Biography* (1975). Bettina Meitzner, *Die Gerätschaft der Chymischen Kunst: Der Traktat "Se Sceuastica Artis" des Andreas Libavius von 1606: Übersetzung, Kommentierung und Wiederabdruck* (Stuttgart: Franz Steiner, 1995).

in Libavius' defense would be seen on future market days.[3] In the end, Libavius decided upon a personal counterassault and published, finally, his own tract, *De Igne Naturae* (Concerning the Fire of Nature), printed as part of his much larger book, the *Syntagmatis Arcanorum Chymicorum* (1613).

Palmarius' book had displeased the medical school at Paris as much as it had annoyed the gymnasium director at Coburg, but not for the same reasons. In fact, the Paris faculty had condemned the text, declaring it to be full of errors, frauds, impostures, and lies, shortly before the book made its appearance in Libavius' new hometown. Palmarius was ordered to acknowledge his errors in writing within six months and to profess that he would conform thereafter to the doctrines of Hippocrates and Galen and follow the teachings of the Parisian school. Until then he would be deprived of all emoluments from the school which would, instead, be dispersed to the poor of the local hospital. If the conditions were not met, it would be worse for him. He would lose all privileges of the Academy and be expunged from the register of regent doctors as well. The dean of the school ordered the decree to be read aloud in the presence of all in attendance and to be printed "so that all people … and posterity may understand that the school of physicians of Paris considers nothing to be of greater antiquity than its retention of the old and true method of healing, and its conservation in unimpaired form of the doctrine and ancient teachings of Hippocrates and Galen."[4]

One need not look far to find this decree. Libavius republished it at the beginning of his own Palmarian rebuttal. Moreover, so that his fellow Germans might become better acquainted with it, he had additional copies printed at Coburg and sent them by means of friends into Bohemia, Austria, and other regions.[5] The opinion of the Paris faculty clearly mattered to Libavius. But we should also remember that this was the same school that had recently condemned Quercetanus for introducing what Quercetanus called the spagiric art into medicine. One of the school's most distinguished members, Jean Riolan (the elder) (1539–1606), had just three years before written a

[3]Andreas Libavius, *D.O.M.A. Syntagmatis Arcanorum Chymicorum, Tomi Secundi, Tractatus Primus, De Igni Naturae* [i.e. De Igne Naturae] *In Qvo Accvrate Investigantvr, Et Ad Trvtinam Veritatis Expendvntvr Solertissimorum Chymicorum de eo sententiae, et cum P. Palmarii D. Medici Parisiensis quondam, placitis conferuntur, iudicanturque*… (Frankfurt: Nicolaus Hoffmannus, impensis Petri Kopffii, 1613), *Prooemivm*, 5–7.

[4]Libavius, *De Igne Naturae,* "Censura in Librum M. Petri Palmarii de Lapide Philosophico Dogmaticorum, exscripta ex Commentariis facultatis medicinae," 8. Hoc decretum in commentarios facultatis referatur, et typis excudatur, ut omnes atque adea posteri intelligant Medicorum Parisiensium scholam nihil antiquius habere, quam ut antiqua, et vera medendi ratio retineatur, Hippocratis, Galenique doctrina, et vetus disciplina conseruetur illibata.

[5]Ibid.

stinging attack against Libavian alchemy, and had accused Libavius, who had earlier fought for the principles of Hippocrates against those of Paracelsus, of having now altered his course and of raising to the heavens the defenders of such (Paracelsian) principles. Thus, Riolan had claimed, "you used to give bread to the students of medicine, now you give stone."[6]

Why, then, should Libavius now have been so eager to make public use of any decree of the Paris medical school? To understand that we need to bear in mind that medical categories and terminology were anything but pure in the early seventeenth century. No one understood better than Libavius the linguistic complications brought about by so many shadings of medical and pharmaceutical practice in which chemical preparations might be joined with Galenic and Hippocratic traditions on the one hand and, on the other, combine with popular practices and Paracelsian notions outside the purview of institutionalized learning. Nowhere did the Paris decree even mention alchemy, but since Palmarius had written against "Libaviana" and Palmarius had been condemned, Libavius seems to have interpreted the decree as institutional support, in the most Catholic and Galenic of medical faculties, for his own variety of medical chemistry. Although at odds with the strict Galenism endorsed at Paris, Libavius never questioned the authoritative power of the institution itself. His difficulties had been with individuals, not with the school. The school was important because the school, among other things, functioned as the best social force for distancing his own practices from those of the so-called "moderns" (*recentiores*) — those who depended upon their own inventions, who relied upon secrets as a means of establishing their medical authority, and who may or may not have been outright frauds. In the turbulence Libavius not only argued for an epistemology of openness and didactic utility in chemistry (a claim articulated so well by Owen Hannaway years ago)[7] but elevated the moral and political power of didactic institutions in defining the social norms of a particular way of gaining knowledge and in determining what was legitimate to medicine and what was not.

CONFUSING TERMS: ALCHEMY AND PARACELSUS

"I saw that this Libavius," Palmarius wrote, "the deserter of true medicine, a most base traitor, fled to the factions of the Paracelsians."[8] On the surface, one

---

[6]Jean Riolan, *Ad Libavi Maniam, Ioan Riolani Responsio pro Censura Scholae Parisiensis contra Alchymiam lata* (Paris: In officina Plantiniana, apud Adrianum Perier, 1606), 10–11.

[7]Hannaway, *The Chemists and the Word*, 1975.

[8]Palmarius, *Lapis Philosophicus Dogmaticorum, Lectori Palmarius*. Vidi Libauium desertorem veritatis medicae, transfugam turpissimum, ad factionem Paracelsistarum deuolasse.

might be led to believe that Libavius had decided to put his critical reservations aside and adopt the speculative medical philosophy of Paracelsus. After all, the Coburg physician was not opposed to everything that might be called Paracelsian and seems to have accepted some form of a relationship between the macro- and the microcosm.[9] But this would not be the Libavius portrayed in most discussions. Certainly not the Libavius of the long-winded assault on Paracelsian medical practice known as the *Neoparacelsica* (1594).[10] Simply commending efficacious essences separated from useless chemical dregs did not, after all, make one a Paracelsian. If it did, Libavius explained, one would have to include Avicenna, Bulcasis, and even the Parisian school itself in that company.[11] Thus it was Palmarius's own ignorance of traditions and of what was appropriate to medicine, chemistry, physics, and Paracelsianism that had resulted in confusing terms relating to natural philosophy (medicine) and alchemy. The result was an inability to discern between what was real and what was illusory. Referring to Horace, one of his favorite authors, Libavius notes that Palmarius had failed to distinguish between bronze and lupines, that is, between real coins (bronze) and lupine seeds which were used sometimes instead of money in playing games.[12]

Not only had Palmarius blindly created, in this way, something hideous by inappropriately defining Paracelsianism and by painting the chemist at Coburg with the same definitional colors; he had also given birth to something quite monstrous by creating a new term linking alchemy and medicine. This was, according to Libavius, a certain freakish offspring that could proclaim from one mouth, "Whatever physicians seek is in the humors," and "Whatever the wise seek is in Mercury." The name of the monster was *Galenochymia*. Thank heaven it had died soon after being born.[13] The Paris medical faculty had seen to that and had also made sure that its creator did not survive the birth struggle unscathed. Its reprimand had been both an intellectual and a moral censure. Palmarius himself died soon thereafter, suffocated, Libavius

---

[9]Libavius, *De Igne Naturae*, 9. Paracelsi et Paracelsistarum foeditates detestamur. Parabolicos vero autores, si caetera sint sani, tolerandos putamus. Non enim negari potest harmonia maioris, et minoris mundi.

[10]Libavius, *Andreae Libavi Halensis Sax. Med. D. Po. Laur. Physici Rotenburgici ad Tubarim, Neoparacelsica...* (Frankfurt: Ioannes Saur, impensis Petri Kopfij, 1597).

[11]Libavius, *De Igne Naturae*, 33.

[12]Ibid., 33; cf. Horace, *Epistles* I.vii.23. *Horace: Satires, Epistles and Ars Poetica*, trans. H. Rushton Fairclough (1926; reprint, Cambridge, Mass.: Harvard University Press, 1991), 296–297.

[13]Libavius, *De Igne Naturae*, 8–9.

exclaims, by apoplexy,[14] stripped of the honors and privileges of the school. "Would that his soul may be saved."[15]

Palmarius had lost his honor and maybe his eternal life, but the school's decision to reject Galenochemistry amounted also, in Libavius' opinion, to nothing less than a personal moral victory. The school, in his view, had chosen to hold onto "its study and profession of genuine alchemy" while condemning Palmarius' definition. At the same time it had recognized that God had provided the material for curing illnesses and that such material might be chemically prepared.[16]

If Palmarius had not understood Paracelsianism, he had also gone about linking alchemy to Galenic and Hippocratic medicine in an altogether misguided and fraudulent manner. Galenochemistry meant producing a universal panacea by means of possessing what Palmarius called the "Fire of Nature." This was the elixir of the philosophers, the metaphysical stone, the practically pure fire of heaven. It was this fire that instantly perfected metals, made the stars shine, and gave things below their vigor. It was the quintessence confined in everything. Thanks to it chemistry reigned over pharmacology and by its means all things in nature were converted into desirable medicines.[17] Galenochemistry meant finding the philosophers' stone. Ironically, in this Libavius noticed a position that itself could be considered Paracelsian. Did not Palmarius, like Paracelsus, claim to possess a single universal medicine, a fire of nature which was a unique instrument of chemistry and an elixir to be used against all diseases? On the basis of his own reasoning then he must himself be a Paracelsian.[18]

In alchemical matters Libavius seems to have accepted the possibility of transmutation in some sense and notes in his Palmarian response several figures, including Hermes, Geber, Edward Kelly, Michael Sendivogius, and Alexander Conthonius, who had made the philosophers' stone.[19] He also admitted the metaphorical opaqueness of some alchemical texts. But Palmarian Galenochemistry was not just practically opaque. It was a fraud. Chemistry did in fact make use of what Libavius called sophistries or adulterations (*sophismata*) and these might serve to benefit the whole community, but only when understood for what they were and not veiled in deceit. Palmarian Galenochemistry, however, was a sophistry lacking any possibility of virtue or usefulness since it appeared to be what it was not. "Ingenious adulterations,"

---

[14]Ibid., *Prooemivm*, 2.
[15]Libavius, *De Igne Naturae*, 9.   [16]Libavius, *De Igne Naturae*, 9.
[17]Palmarius, *Lapis Philosophicus Dogmaticorum*, 24–27. Cf. Libavius, *De Igne Naturae*, 12.
[18]Libavius, *De Igne Naturae*, 33.   [19]Ibid., 34.

Libavius writes, "which are made without any effort to defraud, and are sold for what they are, are far from being prohibited. They are a matter of public right and were celebrated in antiquity.... In this way temples, houses, and the family were adorned, and by the sparing use of gold and silver the household economy makes great savings.... [However] if anyone sinks to such a level that he willingly puts out these sophistries/adulterations with an intent to deceive the naive, he is at once found out by means of many [chemical] tests, and, if he is caught, is compelled to pay legal penalties."[20]

In accordance with the nature of alchemical sophistry Galenochemistry treated solely of the universal sort of *magisteria* in which one dreamt of a universal elixir. To Palmarius, any other pursuit, like extracting oils, essences, waters, and salts, was simply dross work and empty ostentation. The problem was that just these other sorts of extracts were Libavius' bread and butter, and these were what the Paris condemnation had, in his view, preserved as medically acceptable. Such preparations required careful attention to method, but Palmarius, Libavius complained, described no procedure nor did he provide any example of true elaboration in his workshop. "If you ask about his labors, Palmarius replies that there is no need to describe everything one by one.... We are commanded to distill or sublimate, but how many times are we to sublimate or distill? He responds, learn that among the artisans."[21]

Alchemical procedures and pharmaceutical practice are often closely related in Libavian texts, and that relationship is especially intimate in the tract following *De Igne Naturae* in the *Syntagmatis,* a tract written still with Palmarius very much in mind, *De Alchymia Pharmaceutica* (1613). There Libavius notes that alchemy is composed of two factions: one medical, the other, what he calls metallurgic. Of the metallurgic sort it was not necessary to say much since this kind of alchemy stood open only to the knowledgeable and to sons of the doctrine who possessed the art either by a sensible idea readily at hand (*informatione praesente, sensibilique*) or through divine revelation. In either case, instruction was not altogether clear, and, Libavius notes, from such a sea of enigma it would be impossible to extricate oneself even if furnished with

---

[20]Ibid., 35. Ingeniosa metallorum sophismata, quae fiunt sine studio fallendi, et pro eo, quod sunt, venduntur, adeo non sunt in hac arte prohibita, vt etiam publici sint iuris, et a vetustate eximie celebrata.... Ita ornantur templa, et domus, et familia, parciturque auro et argento magno rei familiaris compendio.... Quod si quis eo malitiae deuenerit, vt sophismata illa studio fallendi velit proponere, simplicesque decipere; is statim redarguitur examinibus pluribus, cogiturque dare poenas legibus si deprehendatur.

[21]Libavius, *De Igne Naturae,* 119. Si queras de laboribus respondet Palmarius, no[n] opus esse singulari descriptione... vt cu[m] iubemur destillare, sublimare, etc. At quid est, et quotuplex sublimare, destillare, etc. R. Disce apud artifices.

Delian industry.[22] The type of alchemy called *pharmaceutica,* on the other hand, was more lucid and could be described more plainly in words. As opposed to mysteries and *arcana* that could not be shared with anyone else, pharmaceutic alchemy claimed a long didactic tradition, and Libavius refers to ancient teachers who had joined alchemy to pharmacy and who had cultivated alchemy for the sake of preparing medicaments. These had found, through all manner of extractions, the hidden forms within things.[23]

PROFESSIONAL BOUNDARIES AND INSTITUTIONAL VIRTUES

Clarity about alchemy in general and pharmaceutic alchemy in particular might be hindered as a result of linguistic relativism and deceitful rhetoric, but Libavius also perceived problems emerging from indistinct disciplinary boundaries and a lack of institutional control over the laws and precepts that defined professions. "Are philosophy and wisdom *amethodos*? Are they," he asks, "so fickle and hindered by threats that they can be kept in no enclosures without any laws being written for them? Is their license so loose that however one represents oneself, whether without art, without fortune, practiced or unpracticed, just as long as he calls himself an arcane chemist, that is enough to be a chemist? The ancients knew better. The person who was truly wise surrounded himself with his peculiar barrier, and not only separated himself from other arts or sciences, but also separated its parts so that he might distinguish its divisions as in the members of the human body."[24] Here was one of the central problems with Paracelsus and the Paracelsians. After claiming for himself the monarchy of chemistry, Paracelsus had decreed that he should found a new alchemy as well as a new medicine. In doing so, however, he opened doors to fashioning by whatever method you will (*quidvis quovismodo*) and of proclaiming all manner of chemical and medical *arcana*. Hence it comes about that hardly anyone agrees with anyone else, and each person wants to seem to have brought forth *something new* (*aliquid novi*), the knowledge and art of which they lay claim to only for themselves. "Thus finally one ends up with a hodgepodge of things composed and elaborated as one pleases

[22]Libavius, *D.O.M.A. Syntagmatis Arcanorum Chymicorum, Tomi II: Tractatus Secundus De Alchymia Pharmaceutica, Praefatio,* 122.

[23]Libavius, *D.O.M.A. Syntagmatis Arcanorum Chymicorum,* 122.

[24]Ibid., 127: Num philosophia, et sapientia sit amethodos, tamque vaga et interminata vt nullis claustris coherceatur, nec vllas sibi praescripserit leges, data licentia tam laxa, vt *quod quisque fingit, sive arte, sive fortuna, perite, imperite, si dicat chymicum esse arcanum, statim sit chymicum?* Antiquissimam eam faciunt. Tantis mundi spaciis nemo fuerit sapiens, qui septis eum circumdederit propriis, et non tantum ab aliis siue artibus, siue scientiis separauerit; verum etiam eius partes sic digesserit vt suis articulis, tanquam in humano corpore membra, distingueretur?

and not according to [any] prescription of the art. These are thrown together in *schedulas* [and] marked with the monstrous names of their more-monstrous authors," and, thanks to the typographic art, are sent forth to the public in a far larger number than the health of anyone requires.[25]

If chemical medicine of the Paracelsian type was *amethodos* and amounted to a hodgepodge of recipes and claims, how was one to study it? Since 1609, however, the study of what was called *chymiatria* had gained a foothold within the medical curriculum of at least one institution of traditional learning, the German university at Marburg.[26] The man appointed as public professor of the new discipline was Johannes Hartmann (1568–1631), and it is probably while thinking of both the man and the institution that Libavius complained that chemiatric studies had progressed to the point where a youth sent into the academy need no longer worry about having to learn and labor over the decrees of philosophy and medicine. Instead he could inquire into the novelties of those who otherwise hid their art from view. What a student actually received was something from an impostor. When that same student returned home he could then display *indices* and ponderous *Sympegmata,* but no one dare see those things called *arcana.* If this should happen the arrogance of such foreign wisdom would immediately perish because all would see that the only things really mysterious were names and titles.[27]

New things are so attractive to the youth, and yet young people have generally no knowledge of the *chymia* of Avicenna, Mesua (Mesue), Rhasis, Serapton (Serapion), and Bucasis (Albucasis). Instead they admire illegitimate novelties born scarcely yesterday from furnace smoke.[28] But nothing good, says Libavius, is really unique. In fact the claim to uniqueness is the ultimate fraud since it allows a person to agree with no one, while, at the same time, granting him license to contradict everyone else and to condemn all the writings, sayings, and deeds of others.[29]

It was here that the Coburg gymnasium director made his stand, as much against Palmarius as against institutions that broke with traditional didactic practices. At Marburg the study of *chymiatria* was a private matter with

---

[25]Ibid.: Componuntur farragines rerum: elaborantur ad libitum, et non ad praescriptum artis. Coniiciuntur artificia illa arbitraria in schedulas. Praesiguntur nomina monstrosa monstrosiorum autorum....

[26]See Wilhelm Ganzenmüller, "Das Chemische Laboratorium der Universität Marburg im Jahre 1615," *Angewandte Chemie* 54 (1941): 215–217; also Bruce T. Moran, *Chemical Pharmacy Enters the University: Johannes Hartmann and the Didactic Care of Chymiatria in the Early Seventeenth Century* (Madison: AIHP, 1991).

[27]Libavius, *De Alchymia Pharmaceutica,* 127–128

[28]Ibid., 128.   [29]Ibid., 122.

chemical preparations contractually kept secret between teacher and students. *Chymiatria* meant something institutionally unique. From Libavius' point of view that amounted to a contradiction of terms. Paris, for all its troubles, had at least never wavered in its insistence upon traditional studies based upon common scholastic virtues. In contrast to those offering private *arcana*, Libavius defined himself and his task within a public domain. "It is publicly clear," he says, "what has fallen to us and still falls to us." We labor at the general understanding of the ancients and at tearing [that understanding] out of the darkness.... We collect the practices (*artificia*) of antiquity and the commentaries of those who came later, and so that we may have some form in the art [of chemistry] we adorn these techniques by providing them with a methodical arrangement (*dispositione methodica*).[30]

Bringing back what he called "form" to the art of chemistry is what had disturbed the entire *lerna* (the marshy abode of the hydra) of the Paracelsians. And what had been their reaction? The adherents to novelties had wrinkled their noses and ridiculed the whole undertaking. "Are we recalled to order and bound to laws by precepts which are eternal and consistent? What? If this should happen, then *arcana* shall perish. There would be no admirer of unique inventions, and no purveyor of the same."[31]

It is one of the curious features of Libavius' writings that from time to time he takes on the voice of his opponents. The rhetorical aim, of course, is to cast even more into relief the truths of his own perceptions and the supposed errors of his enemies. This man Libavius they say has nothing of his own; he knows no secret (*arcanum*). He collects everything and these are long since despised and obsolete. He is not an astrologer. He neither knows nor cares for the constellations (*constellata*) of Paracelsus. He does not understand the *arcana* of Suctenius (Seton) concerning antimony. He relates his own dreams about the philosophers' stone. He ignores the Palmarian fire of nature. Therefore, he is a nobody in alchemy. "These things and others they growl at our labors," Libavius remarks, "and thus they repudiate the art discovered and proven through much experience and reason. In its place they offer only their own accidental experiments...[and] bring forth monsters of words."[32]

[30]Ibid., 122.

[31]Ibid., 128: Nosne in ordinem redigi, et ad vlla praecepta, legesque constantes, et perpetuas alligari? Quid? Si hoc fieret, peristent arcana. Nullus esset singularium inuentorum admirator: nullus redemptor.

[32]Ibid., 128: Haec et similia multa ogganiunt nostris laboribus, et vt...repudiant artem longa experientia, et ratione inuenta, et comprobatam, tantumque fortuitis suis experimentis...monstra vocabulorum proferunt.

WORDS, TRADITIONS, AND SOCIAL LEGITIMACY

Libavius had much to say about the creation of new words,[33] but neologisms were not by definition bad. In chemistry, if an artisan of proven ability met with something new he might assign a convenient term to the discovery, whether a new word or an old one. In fact, Libavius recognized that the use of older terms could also be misleading and he notes that the ancients, in order to hide their *arcana,* did not all speak about their procedures in one manner.[34] Indeed, those who pursued the Hermetic art followed a practice similar to that of the Egyptians who hid their esoteric teachings in hieroglyphics and the diverse coverings of nature. The Paracelsians, on the other hand, invented new terms every day and subjected the chemical art to criticism. For the most part, however, there was nothing more in those new terms, whether thought up yesterday or given an application beyond the meaning of the ancients, than a plastering over of Paracelsian ignorance and impostures.[35]

Elsewhere Libavius was more precise about how new terms should be chosen. It is not uncommon for necessity to compel the construction of a word, he writes; however, this should never occur arbitrarily, but should be derived from Greek, especially in any subject matter that is devoid of Latin words.[36] One example may serve for others. The term "Echeneis," which means literally ship-detaining and which is connected to a sort of sea slug or fish that impedes the motion and direction of a ship or causes it to stop altogether, would be applicable to astringents, to things that stop the flow of humors, as in the case of hemorrhages and catarrhs.[37]

Clearly, Palmarius had not fashioned his terms in this way. With the destruction of *Enchiria,* Libavius observes, Palmarius the "corrector" contrived the "stone of the dogmatists" and Galenochymia, and gave his own names to *spagyria* and chemistry.[38] Libavius would now take back the names as part of a linguistic strategy to preserve the social norms and established discursive practices of traditional institutionalized learning. The term *Spagyrus,*

---

[33]See the discussion by William Newman, "Alchemical Symbolism and Concealment: The Chemical House of Libavius," in *The Architecture of Science,* ed. Peter Galison and Emily Thompson (MIT Press, forthcoming).

[34]Libavius, *De Igne Naturae,* 27.   [35]Ibid., 26–27.

[36]Libavius, *D.O.M.A. Vita, Vigor et Veritas Alchymiae Transmvtatoriae in Syntagmate Arcanorum non Per dubias coniecturas, sed Philosophemata solida explicatae et traditae, Illabefacta Infracta et constans* in *D.O.M.A. Appendix necessaria Syntagmatis Arcanorum Chymicorum Andreae Libavii...* (Frankfurt: Excudebat Nicolaus Hoffmannus, Impensis Petri Kopffij, 1615), 172. Also, Libavius, *Neoparacelsica,* 694. Cf. Horace, *Ars Poetica,* 52–53 [et nova fictaque nuper habebunt verba fidem, si Graeco fonte cadent parce detorta]. *Horace: Satires, Epistles and Ars Poetica,* 454–55.

[37]Libavius, *De Igne Naturae,* 27.

[38]Libavius, *De Alchymia Pharmaceutica,* 123.

for instance, had come to be associated with the dishonest practices of Paracelsians who touted wondrous medicines which contained nothing more than ordinary ingredients. The word had become tainted by common usage, but Libavius did not deny that it also possessed a healthier sense, one that comprehended the art of extraction and coagulation.[39] The same term, depending upon its cultural heritage, could thus conceal different meanings. Perhaps to underscore the point and to highlight the nature of the competition for cultural authority in the Paracelsian debate, Libavius asks his reader to consider the words *Spagirus* and *Spagyrus*. There is really no obvious difference between the two terms except that, in this case, the first word is spelled with an *i*, the second with a *y*. The former, says Libavius, derives from the Greek meaning to separate and to gather together, which is to dissolve and to coagulate—two operations important in making the *magisterium* of the Stone. The latter word, however, is a word of ill omen. It is cognate with the Greek terms for crowd and mendicity. As such it defines Paracelsian alchemy as an art without art, whose goal is to go begging.[40]

Was Libavius just playing with words? Perhaps so, and yet there is something even in that, something so trifling and yet so important that in passing by too quickly we miss the possibility of finding a valuable ancestral bone among the rocks. It is the insistence upon the value of cognates, or common original forms possessing similar natures and qualities. For Libavius words as well as ideas and practices had their own ancestral roots. The power to mediate their meanings and to legitimize their use had to be invested in cognates of a social and cultural kind, in institutions, in schools.

Conclusion

In his diatribes against Palmarius and others, Andreas Libavius pursued goals that were social as well as intellectual. If he worried about upholding a certain epistemology of openness, he also sought to preserve a means for the social accreditation of that epistemic view. Knowledge based upon a particular procedural, epistemological, and linguistic style required a prescribed set of social values and virtues. It did not, however, require conformity of intellectual opinion. After the death of Joseph Duchesne (Quercetanus), Libavius reminisced that Duchesne was of such a noble spirit that he could stand to be admonished by those who conducted studies in the same art, and was prepared to refute and to be refuted. In what amounts to a rare tender moment

[39]Libavius, *De Igne Naturae*, 33.
[40]Ibid., 33. Paracelsica alchymia est ars sine arte, cuius finis mendicatum ire.

in Libavian discourse, he added that friendship, to be sure, was not a conformity of judgment but an identity of feeling in minds that were joined in virtue.[41] The notion comes from Aristotle's *Nicomachean Ethics*,[42] but the sense of conforming to norms and virtues may have been as important in defining the true link between individuals in the struggle for chemical truths as it was in defining friendship. Establishing the reliability and legitimacy of a certain epistemology was, after all, different from the work of establishing the epistemology itself. Guarantees of reliability required social virtues—virtues that defined an entire style of life, one that was settled, dependable, predictable, and measured.[43] The salvos of thick books launched by Libavius against Palmarius and others who dwelt in different, less precise cultural spaces aimed in part at rendering explicit the social basis of linguistic authority in chemistry and medicine. Such an authority would replace personal nomination by official definition, and would be particularly helpful to those suffering the inappropriate labels of others—such as being called a "Paracelsian" when one was not.

[41]Ibid., 10. Amicitia non est opinionum conformitas, sed cum virtute coniuncta animorum consensio.

[42]Aristotle, *Nichomachean Ethics*, 1156b7. "Perfect friendship is the friendship of men who are good, and alike in virtue." From *The Basic Works of Aristotle*, ed. Richard Mckeon (New York: Random House, 1941), 1061.

[43]For a discussion of the relationship between cultural styles and "scientificity" see Pierre Bourdieu, *Homo Academicus*, trans. Peter Collier (Stanford: Stanford University Press, 1988), 28ff.

ACKNOWLEDGMENTS

I wish to express my sincere thanks to Michael McArthur and J. Mark Sugars for translation assistance. All errors regarding texts, misapprehensions, and misjudgments are, of course, entirely my own.

Samuel Clarke N.º 660

Apophthegmes

NEW AND

OLD. *LE,19*

COLLECTED BY
THE RIGHT HO-
NOVRABLE,

Francis

L O. V E R V L A M,
Viscount
S^t. A L B A N.

L O N D O N,
Printed for *Hanna Barret*, and
Richard Whittaker, and are to be
sold at the Kings Head in
Pauls Church-yard. 1625.

William R. Newman

ALCHEMICAL ᴬᴺᴰ BACONIAN VIEWS ᴼᴺ ᵀᴴᴱ ART/NATURE DIVISION

SINCE THE PUBLICATION OF PAOLO ROSSI'S *Francis Bacon: From Magic to Science* in 1957, it has been widely accepted that the famous lord chancellor owed a debt to alchemical literature, for Rossi cogently argued that Bacon's theme of human domination over nature was inspired by writings on alchemy and natural magic.[1] Despite Rossi's perception that alchemical authors supplied Bacon with some of his technological optimism, he viewed Bacon's ruminations on the *limits* of human power as forming a watershed of a different sort. Both in his *Francis Bacon* and in *Philosophy, Technology, and the Arts*, Rossi promotes the view that Francis Bacon was the prime mover in overthrowing an age-old division between art and nature.[2] Indeed, Rossi maintains that the deep impression made on Bacon by such artificial contrivances as the mariner's compass, gunpowder, and the printing press encouraged him to deny any schism between nature and art. According to Rossi, it was the early modern ascendancy of the mechanical arts, not alchemy, that led Bacon to this new position.[3]

[1]Paolo Rossi, *Francis Bacon: From Magic to Science* (London: Routledge and Kegan Paul, 1968), 16–22.

[2]Rossi reaffirmed his position more recently: Paolo Rossi, "Bacon's Idea of Science," in Markku Peltonen, ed., *The Cambridge Companion to Bacon* (Cambridge: Cambridge University Press, 1996), 25–46; esp. 31–43. For the relevant passages in Rossi's earlier works, see idem, *Francesco Bacone, dalla magia alla scienza* (Torino: Einaudi, 1974), 39–40; idem, *I filosofi e le macchine (1400–1700)* (Milan: Feltrinelli, 1962), 139–147.

[3]Rossi, *Francis Bacon*, 26: "But Bacon saw the development of the mechanical arts as a new and exciting cultural event, and his reappraisal of their social and scientific significance and of their aims enabled him to disprove some of Aristotle's theories concerning the relation of art to nature."; see also ibid., 93–97, and "Bacon's Idea of Science," 31–43.

Rossi's analysis of the Baconian attack on the art/nature distinction has been adopted and championed by a host of more recent authors, including Peter Dear, Lorraine Daston, and Antonio Pérez-Ramos. These authors share the view that the "New Science" of the seventeenth century depended on the erasure of an Aristotelian credo that art and nature were distinct and inviolable realms which could not interact, and that Bacon was a key player in bridging this dichotomy. Dear and Pérez-Ramos develop the argument to maintain that experiment was effectively prohibited by the Aristotelian position.[4] The notion that the ancients and medievals erected an insurmountable barrier between art and nature finds support in the *Physics* II.1 (192b.9–19), where Aristotle distinguishes natural products from artificial ones on the basis of the fact that the natural have an innate *principle of movement (or change)* [*echonta en heautois archnē kineseōs*], whereas the artificial have *no inherent trend towards change* [*oudemian hormēn echei metabolēs emphyton*].[5] For this reason, Aristotle says (193b.8–9), "men propagate men, but bedsteads do not propagate bedsteads." The artificial product is static, having received no intrinsic principle of development.

According to Rossi's thesis, this fundamental divide between natural and artificial products, expressed in the Aristotelian belief that man-made artifacts are mere imitations of natural exemplars, implied that it would be futile to look to the artificial for knowledge about nature. In a similar fashion, Lorraine Daston has argued that it was only in the early modern period that the chasm between art and nature was finally bridged, primarily by Bacon, who importantly assimilated works of art to those of nature, a view which is said to have contributed to the Royal Society's sponsorship of the mechanical philosophy, with its notion "that nature was actually composed of microscopic machines."[6] In Daston's view the Baconian overthrow of Aristotle's distinction between art and nature led to a new view of nature *as* art: a view underlying the formation of modern science.

---

[4]The argument is expressed very succinctly by Antonio Pérez-Ramos, "Bacon's Forms and the Maker's Knowledge Tradition," in Peltonen, *Cambridge Companion*, 112: "What is the point, gnoseologically speaking, of making or constructing something in order to gain insight into Nature's mysteries if we posit from the very start that no productions of human technology can remotely equal or even approach the essence and subtlety of natural processes?" On the other hand, Daston, "Baconian Facts, Academic Civility, and the Prehistory of Objectivity," *Annals of Scholarship* 8 (1991): 337–363, esp. 340–341, argues that Aristotle was unconcerned with experiment because of his interest in generalities rather than "particulars." Her argument is equally problematic, but must be considered elsewhere.

[5]Aristotle, *The Physics,* trans. Philip H. Wicksteed and Francis M. Cornford (London: Heinemann, 1929), 106–115.

[6]Lorraine Daston, "The Factual Sensibility," *Isis* 79 (1988): 452–470; esp. 464.

Peter Dear's *Discipline and Experience* offers much the same viewpoint though more explicitly linked to the development of experiment or "contrived experience."[7] The theme of Dear's book, that "modern experimental science [first] appears in the seventeenth century,"[8] draws support from his analysis of the Aristotelian division between art and nature. Dear argues that the seventeenth-century view of the world as a machine, embodied in the "mechanical philosophy," implied a breakdown of the art/nature division.[9] Following the lead of Rossi, Dear argues that the art/nature division had impeded the development of experimental science because it had reduced all "contrived experience" to the status of artifact.[10] Any active meddling with natural processes could therefore be written off as unable to tell us anything about the natural world.

Dear credits Bacon with playing an important part in overcoming the art/nature distinction: "Bacon argued that art was only a matter of setting up situations in which nature will produce a desired result—so that art is the human exploitation of nature rather than an activity outside of nature."[11] Yet as Dear also points out, the art/nature division was "eminently breachable" even without Bacon's vaunted collapsing of the two categories.[12] Drawing on seventeenth-century sources, Dear points out that it was a commonplace of the period that artisans could "improve on nature" by "utilizing the natural properties of natural materials."[13] In a passage of admirable concision Dear states, "Experimental contrivance was permissible when the goal was operational knowledge rather than teleological knowledge of nature."[14] By implication it was not possible in the context of the natural philosophy of Aristotle. Using seventeenth-century Jesuit sources, Dear then develops an elaborate argument that the category of mixed mathematics, which included optics and astronomy among other pursuits, allowed authors such as Christopher Clavius and

---

[7]Peter Dear, *Discipline and Experience: The Mathematical Way in the Scientific Revolution* (Chicago: University of Chicago Press, 1995).

[8]Ibid., 13.   [9]Ibid., 151.

[10]Ibid., 153: "The art/nature distinction impinged on the use of artificial contrivances in the making of natural knowledge—that is, it compromised the legitimacy of using in natural philosophy the sorts of procedures used by mathematicians"; see also 155: "The natural course of a process could [only] be subverted by man-made, artificial causes, because art replaced nature's purposes with human purposes. An aqueduct, for example, is not a natural watercourse; it reveals the intention of the human producer, which thwarts that of nature.... *The Aristotelian distinction between art and nature depended on seeing human purposes as separate from natural ones and hence irrelevant to the creation of a true natural philosophy*" (my emphasis).

[11]Ibid., 155.   [12]Ibid., 161.   [13]Ibid., 156.   [14]Ibid., 158.

Christopher Scheiner to obviate the issue of teleology altogether in favor of efficient causality.[15]

The net result of Dear's argument is to broaden the cultural context of the disintegrating division between art and nature, but hardly to expand its chronological dimension.[16] He either downplays or ignores the diachronic dimension of the claim that art can perfect nature. Let us remember, after all, Aristotle himself said in the *Physics* (II.8.199a.16) that "the arts either, on the basis of Nature, carry things further than Nature can, or they imitate Nature," thus opening up an avenue for the argument that art can improve on nature.[17] I shall expand on this point presently.

Just as Aristotle was not so hidebound as Rossi and his followers suppose, so Bacon was considerably less radical. The very passage from Bacon's *Descriptio globi intellectualis* (and *De augmentis scientiarum*) often used to support the claim that he rejected the distinction between nature and art is immediately followed in the Baconian text by these comments:

> and not only that, but another and more subtle error finds its way into men's minds; that of looking upon art merely as a kind of supplement to nature; which has power enough to finish what nature has begun or correct her when going aside, but no power to make radical changes, and shake her in the foundations; an opinion which has brought a great deal of despair into human concerns. Whereas men ought on the contrary to have a settled conviction, that things artificial differ from things natural, not in form or essence, but only in the efficient; that man has in truth no power over nature, except that

[15]Ibid., 162: "Because mathematics had to do only with quantity, not with process and teleology, the Aristotelian dichotomy of natural and artificial did not apply. The mathematician did not seek to reveal essential natures, and could therefore interfere with natural processes quite legitimately; to do so, however, required a constant policing of the disciplinary boundary between mathematics and natural philosophy." Dear seems to be following a lead supplied by John Heilbron, *Electricity in the 17th and 18th Centuries* (Berkeley: University of California Press, 1979), 104.

[16]Dear, *Discipline*, 51–53, does acknowledge early in the book that the eleventh-century optical writer Ibn al-Haytham *did* employ contrived experiences, but does not see this as a problem for his main thesis, since he argues that the Arabic philosopher did not view himself as an Aristotelian and was therefore unconcerned with the art/nature division *ab initio*: "Although Alhazen used a special technical term, apparently drawn from astronomy, to designate an active production or construction of phenomena, he did not worry about the problems of casting optics as an Aristotelian science. Methodologically, he saw himself within a properly optical tradition stemming from Euclid, who is his main source of reference on such matters. For Alhazen, contrived experiences were techniques; they did not constitute a cognitive category. Both Aguilonius and Scheiner, by contrast, wanted to establish optics as a science fulfilling Aristotelian canons ...."

[17]Aristotle, *Physics*, 173.

of motion—the power, I say, of putting natural bodies together or separating them—and that the rest is done by nature working within.[18]

What Bacon is objecting to here is an overly narrow interpretation of the view represented by Aristotle in *Physics* (II.8.199a.16), cited earlier, where the Stagirite argued that art can either imitate nature or complete its unfinished processes. In accordance with his general anti-Aristotelianism, Bacon has chosen to give an uncharitable reading to this passage, whereby Aristotle is made to say that art can only coax nature to arrive at quite limited goals, rather than induce her to undergo "radical changes." Does Bacon then go on to say that nature and art are the *same*, as our modern commentators would lead us to suspect? Emphatically not—instead Bacon says that art and nature *differ* in the *efficient causes* that they employ, although the things produced in either case can have the same "form or essence." Bacon's concluding comment, that art acting on nature consists in associating and dissociating natural bodies, is entirely traditional, indeed a commonplace among the medieval scholastics.[19] More than this, I shall argue in the following pages that virtually the entire Baconian program of reducing the distinction between nature and art to one of efficient causality is already found in alchemical writings of the high Middle Ages. In fact, these treatises formed the *locus classicus* for discussion of the art/nature division up to the time of Bacon.[20]

Discussions of art and nature are strikingly evident in medieval works of alchemy.[21] This theme acquired the status of a *locus classicus* in alchemical writings, in reaction to the *De congelatione et conglutinatione* of the Persian philosopher Avicenna (980–1037), a work that was misleadingly attached to

---

[18]Francis Bacon, *Descriptio globi intellectualis*, trans. James Spedding, et al., vol. 5 in *The Works of Francis Bacon* (London: Longmans & Co., 1870), 506. See also Bacon, *De augmentis Scientiarium*, vol. 4, in *The Works of Francis Bacon*, 294

[19]The twelfth-century writer on the arts and sciences, Hugh of Saint Victor, epitomized this view in *The "Didascalicon" of Hugh of St. Victor*, trans. Jerome Taylor (New York: Columbia University Press, 1961), 55: "the work of the artificer is to put together things disjoined or to disjoin those put together..."; see also Thomas Aquinas, *In quatuor libros sententiarum* in his *Opera omnia curante Roberto Busa S. I*, vol. 1 (Stuttgart: Frommann-Holzboog, 1980), 145, where it is said that demons act like artisans, in that both operate on nature only insofar as they "can join agents to determinate passive subjects."

[20]Mary Richard Reif, *Natural Philosophy in Some Early Seventeenth-Century Scholastic Textbooks* (Ph.D. diss., Saint Louis University, 1962), 238: "One final question briefly touched upon by several authors concerns the possibility of producing a truly natural product by means of human skill. The question is usually posed in this way: 'Can art effect certain works of nature?' The specific problem which they almost always have in mind is the transmutation of baser metals through the art of alchemy."

[21]William Newman, "Technology and Alchemical Debate in the Late Middle Ages," *Isis* 80 (1989): 423–445.

Aristotle's *Meteors* by Alfred of Sareshel at the beginning of the thirteenth century.[22] Under the involuntary pseudonym of Aristotle, Avicenna there debunked alchemy, by claiming generally that "art is inferior to nature, and cannot equal it, however much it strive."[23] It is imperative to realize that this attack on alchemy is thus embedded in a strongly worded *ne plus ultra* concerning technology as a whole. Avicenna's statement of the limits of art was far more forceful than the rather docile comments made by Aristotle in the *Physics*. Avicenna's attack, which terminates with the phrase *sciant artifices alkimie species metallorum non posse transmutari* ..., came to be known in Latin simply by the incipit *sciant artifices*. The *sciant artifices* was a challenge to alchemy that could not be ignored; as such it was taken up by the army of subsequent alchemists, and rebutted in many an alchemical *Theorica*. Let us consider one such example.

An influential *Book of Hermes* that circulated already in the thirteenth century is organized around a succession of attacks upon alchemy and their subsequent rebuttals.[24] One of these attacks takes up the cudgels of Avicenna, saying, "Metallic bodies, inasmuch as they are works of nature, are natural, but human works are artificial, and not natural."[25]

The opponent of alchemy here merely states the distinction between natural works and human works: the implication, obviously, is that these are two radically different realms which cannot lead to the same products. "Hermes" replies with the following rebuttal:

> But human works are variously the same as natural ones, as we shall show in fire, air, water, earth, minerals, trees, and animals. For the fire of natural lightning and the fire thrown forth by a stone is the same fire. The natural ambient air and the artificial air produced by boiling are both air. The natural earth beneath our feet and the artificial earth produced by letting water sit are both earth. Green salt, vitriol, tutia, and sal ammoniac are both artificial and natural. But the artificial are *even better than the natural* [my emphasis], which anyone who knows about minerals does not contradict. The natural wild tree and the artificially grafted one are both trees. Natural bees and artificial bees generated from a decomposing bull are both bees. Nor does art make all these things; rather it helps nature to make them. Therefore the assistance of this art does not alter the natures of things. Hence the works of man can be both natural *with regard to essence* and artificial *with regard to mode of production*.[26]

---

[22]William Newman, "Technology and Alchemical Debate in the Late Middle Ages," *Isis* 80 (1989): 423–445, see 427.

[23]William Newman, *The Summa Perfectionis of pseudo-Geber* (Leiden: Brill, 1991), 49: "ars est debilior quam natura et non consequitur eam quamvis multum laboret."

[24]Ibid., 6–15; for the Latin text, see 52–56.   [25]Ibid., 11.

[26]Newman, *Summa Perfectionis*, 11–12 (my emphasis).

The response of "Hermes" begins with a set of empirical examples provided by the four elements, fire, air, water, and earth. The author wants to show that man can produce "artificial elements" which are fully identical to the naturally occurring forms. In like fashion he can make artificial forms of "green salt" (perhaps verdigris—copper acetate), vitriol (copper or iron sulfate), tutia (zinc oxide or carbonate), and sal ammoniac (ammonium chloride). These artificially produced minerals will not only be equivalent to their natural counterparts—they will be better. Finally, new types of trees produced by grafting and bees "spontaneously produced" out of dead livestock are identical to their natural exemplars. "Hermes" concludes from this barrage of empirical evidence that art makes these multifarious products only by aiding nature. In a line that is astonishingly close to Bacon's *Descriptio globi intellectualis*, "Hermes" says that human works and natural works are identical as to essence (*secundum essentiam*), even if they differ according to their means of production (*secundum artificium*). This is identical to Bacon's claim that the works of art and nature diverge "not in form or essence, but only in the efficient."

The similarity between "Hermes" position and that of Bacon is not limited to their mutual conclusion that nature and art differ only in the efficient cause. Both authors extol the power of art not merely to help nature attain her proper end, as in the passage earlier quoted from Aristotle's *Physics*, but even to surpass that end. Hence, "Hermes" claims that his artificial minerals are better than the natural, and Bacon wanted to make art perform "radical changes." Similar claims that alchemy can make products more excellent than the natural are found in the works of other thirteenth-century authors. Roger Bacon, for example, argues in his *Opus minus* that alchemical gold can be made to exceed the twenty-four carats of the best natural gold, and that the ingestion of this gold can prolong human life to a length approximating that of Adam and Eve.[27]

From the examples cited it should be clear that alchemical texts from the high and late Middle Ages already were enunciating an attitude toward the art/nature division that was strikingly similar to the operative view of nature held by Francis Bacon and others in the Scientific Revolution.[28] And yet these authors were for the most part avowed admirers of Aristotle trained in the

[27]Roger Bacon, *Opera hactenus inedita* (Oxford: Clarendon, 1909–41), vol. 9, *Liber sex scientiarum,* ed. a. G. Little, 183–184.

[28]See also the *Alterum exemplar Rosarii philosophorum,* bearing the incipit "Desiderabile desiderium impretiabile pretium...," in Manget, *BCC* 2:119–133. On 120 the author says in rebutting the *sciant,* "non est differentia inter naturam & artem nisi quod ars agit exterius, natura vero interius; ars enim tanquam organum administrat motum, natura autem ipsa per se agit quoniam ad suam nititur perfectionem."

scholastic natural philosophy of the medieval university.[29] This fact should cast serious doubt on the common view that an Aristotelian orientation necessarily excluded the possibility of intervening with natural processes.

Before concluding I would like to point out that the close similarity between Bacon's viewpoint and that of traditional Latin alchemy is echoed in several places by Robert Boyle. This is not surprising, since as Rose-Mary Sargent shows in her important book on Boyle, his philosophy of experiment was in many ways a response to Bacon.[30] All the same, several passages that Sargent has extracted from Boyle suggest strongly that he augmented Bacon with a direct consultation of alchemical texts.[31] Given Boyle's deep immersion in alchemical literature, which Lawrence Principe, Michael Hunter, and Antonio Clericuzio have demonstrated, perhaps this is not surprising.[32] Let us consider an important passage from Boyle's *Usefulness of Experimental Philosophy*, where he is intent on denying the validity of the art/nature distinction:

> And I consider, in the first place, that the phaenomena afforded by trades, are (most of them), a part of the history of nature, and therefore may both challenge the naturalist's curiosity, and add to his knowledge. Nor will it suffice to justify learned men in the neglect and contempt of this part of natural history, that the men, from whom it must be learned, are illiterate mechanicks, and the things that are exhibited are works of art, and not of nature. For the first part of the apology is indeed childish, and too unworthy of a philosopher, to be worthy of a solemn answer. And as for the latter part, I desire that you would consider, what we elsewhere expressly discourse against, the unreasonable difference that the generality of learned men have seemed to fancy betwixt all natural things and factitious ones. For besides, that many of those productions that are called artificial, do differ from those that are confessedly natural, not in essence, but in efficients; there are very many things made by tradesmen, wherein nature appears manifestly to do the main parts of the work: as in malting, brewing, baking, making of raisins, currans, and other dried fruits; as also hydromel, vinegar, lime, &c. and the tradesman does but bring visible bodies together after a gross manner, and then leaves

---

[29]For example, Roger Bacon, Albertus Magnus, and Paul of Taranto, for whom see Newman, "Technology and Alchemical Debate," 423–445.

[30]Rose-Mary Sargent, *The Diffident Naturalist: Robert Boyle and the Philosophy of Experiment* (Chicago: University of Chicago Press, 1995), passim.

[31]Ibid., 160–161.

[32]Lawrence Principe, "Boyle's Alchemical Pursuits," in Michael Hunter, ed., *Robert Boyle Reconsidered* (Cambridge: Cambridge University Press, 1994), 91–105; Michael Hunter, "Alchemy, Magic and Moralism in the Thought of Robert Boyle," *British Journal for the History of Science* 26 (1990): 387–410; and Antonio Clericuzio, "A Redefinition of Boyle's Chemistry and Corpuscular Philosophy," *Annals of Science* 47 (1990): 561–589.

them to act one upon another, according to their respective natures; as in making of green and coarse glass, the artificer puts together sand and ashes, and the colliquation and union is performed by the action of the fire upon each body, and by as natural a way, as the same fire, when it resolves wood into ashes, and smoak unites volatile salt, oil, earth, and phlegm into soot; and scarce may any man think, that when a pear is grafted upon a white thorn, the fruit it bears is not a natural one, though it be produced by a coalition of two bodies of distant natures put together by the industry of man, and would not have been produced without the manual and artificial operation of the gardener.[33]

Although Boyle mentions numerous artisanal examples here, he focuses on the production of glass and the grafting of pear trees. Grafting was a traditional example often invoked by alchemical authors both to demonstrate the equivalence of natural and artificial products and to show that species can be transmuted, as we saw in the passage from the *Book of Hermes* above. Similarly, the example of glassmaking was a veritable *locus classicus* among authors of alchemy. The fourteenth-century *Rosarium philosophorum* attributed to Arnald of Villanova, for example, uses it explicitly to rebut the *sciant artifices*—

Therefore Aristotle says that alchemists cannot transmute the bodies of metals unless they be first reduced to their prime matter, for then they are indeed rendered into another form than they were before. For reason does not oppose this, since with one form destroyed, another is immediately introduced, as appears from the works of rustics, who make calx out of stone, and glass out of cinders.[34]

The example of making glass is here used to support the belief that radically different forms can be imposed by man on nature. The author intends this as an empirically based attack on the Avicennian notion that species cannot be transmuted. A variant of this argument is found in the *Quodlibetal Questions* of the late-thirteenth-century scholastic Giles of Rome, who rejected the transmutation of metals. One of the arguments that Giles rejects is that "true gold could be made through art because glass can be made through art."[35] An even closer parallel to Boyle's example, however, is found in the

---

[33]Robert Boyle, in *The Works of the Honourable Robert Boyle*, vol. 3, ed. Thomas Birch (London, 1772), 442–443.

[34][Pseudo-?]Arnaldus de Villa Nova, *Rosarium philosophorum*, in BCC 1:665: "Et ideo dicit Aristoteles, quod Alchimistae corpora metallorum vere transmutare non possunt, nisi prius ipsa redigantur ad suam primam materiam: tunc enim in aliam formam quam prius erant, bene rediguntur. Quoniam contra hoc non stat ratio: quippe quia destructa una forma, immediate introducitur alia, ut patet ex operibus rusticorum, qui de lapidibus faciunt calcem, & de cineribus vitrum."

[35]Giles of Rome, *Quodlibeta revisa, correcta*... (Louvain, 1646), 147.

Correctio fatuorum of Richardus Anglicus, probably composed in the fourteenth century:

> In our work, art is nothing but an aid to nature, which appears in many common works, [for example] where nature first produces wood, second, the burning of the wood by fire turns it into cinder, third, art makes glass out of the cinder, and all this must be understood in the following way: if this prime matter of the glass were not hidden in the cinders, art would by no means be able to make glass from it....[36]

Just as in Boyle's *Usefulness*, Richardus Anglicus argues that in glassmaking, art *aids* nature by performing operations that allow nature to run its course. Both authors use the manufacture of glass to show, as the *Book of Hermes* said, that "art does [not] make all these things; rather it helps nature to make them." In sum, I see no reason why one should doubt that Boyle was here drawing on stock examples from the vast apologetic literature of alchemy aimed at debunking the Avicennian *sciant artifices*.

In conclusion I would like to say three things. First, it is clear that Rossi and his followers have seriously underestimated the role of traditional alchemical literature in leading Francis Bacon to the denial of an essential distinction between art and nature. In fact, the examples that I have adduced above should make us reconsider the very premise underlying such historical claims—that art and nature were uniformly considered distinct and mutually inviolable categories in the Middle Ages. The second point is, once again, that the alchemical writers whom we have considered were deeply Aristotelian in their assumptions about nature and matter. Their counterexample should cast serious doubt on the appropriateness of viewing Aristotelianism as inimical to experiment. Third, one can find numerous instances where alchemical authors do make hard claims about nature on the basis of "contrived experience." Although I have not been able to treat these examples here, they provide still further grounds for disputing the view that natural philosophy had to wait for Francis Bacon before it could accommodate experiment.

---

[36][Richardus Anglicus,] *Correctio fatuorum*, in Manget, *BCC* 2:166: "Quare in nostro opere, ars non est aliud, quam adjumen naturae, quod patet in multis artium operibus laicorum, ubi natura primo producit lignum: secundo ustio ligni per ignem vertitur in cinerem: tertio, ars de cinere facit vitrum, & hoc taliter est intelligendum. Si in cineribus ista prima materia vitri occultata non fuisset, ars nequaquam vitrum ex eo fecisset...."

Stephen A. McKnight

THE WISDOM OF THE ANCIENTS AND FRANCIS BACON'S *NEW ATLANTIS*

THIS ESSAY ANALYZES FRANCIS BACON'S WRITINGS in order to demonstrate that his vision of a great instauration of society through the advancement of learning draws upon and integrates Judaeo-Christian apocalyptic/millenarian themes with elements of the *prisca theologia* or Ancient Wisdom tradition.[1] By demonstrating that Bacon's work combines science, religion, and esoteric wisdom, I am, of course, abandoning the long-standing positivist paradigm that groups Bacon and other major seventeenth-century figures into either the modern camp of science and technology or the ancient camp of religion and philosophy.[2] Recent work in Renaissance cultural history and the history of science is making it increasingly clear that this Comtean construction is responsible for creating polarities and juxtapositions that did not actually exist. Bacon, Newton, and many leading figures of the age often blended "science," religion, and esoteric knowledge in the search for a holistic, organic

---

[1] The phrases "great instauration" and "advancement of learning" are, of course, taken from two of Bacon's seminal works, *Instauratio Magna* and *The Advancement of Learning*. The term *prisca theologia* or Ancient Wisdom refers to a tradition of esoteric religion (Hermeticism, Orphism, Cabala) and occult knowledge (magic and alchemy) recovered by Ficino and the Platonic Academy as part of the Renaissance revival of ancient learning.

[2] The classic example is Richard F. Jones, *Ancients and Moderns: A Study of the Rise of the Scientific Movement in Seventeenth-Century England,* 2d ed. (Saint Louis: Washington University Press, 1961); a more recent example is the widely discussed book by Hans Blumenberg, *The Legitimacy of the Modern Age,* trans. Robert M. Wallace (Cambridge: Mass.: MIT Press, 1983); originally published as *Die Legitimität der Neuzeit* (Frankfurt: Suhrkamp Verlag, 1976).

understanding of human nature, the natural order, and God.[3]

The analysis will begin with an examination of Bacon's concept of instauration. The Latin terms *instauro* and *instauratio* were used in the ancient and Renaissance periods to denote a move away from a state of religious, political, and/or intellectual disorder. It is, therefore, altogether appropriate to associate instauration with progress and advancement. The prefix *in*, however, indicates that this progress depends upon renewal and recovery. This twofold meaning is crucial to understanding Bacon's vision of a great social and political renewal through (re)edification. The first part of the examination of Bacon's concept of instauration will draw upon the work of Charles Whitney and Charles Webster who link the concept to Judaeo-Christian apocalypticism and millenarianism. The second part will examine the influence of the *prisca theologia* on Bacon's vision of a great instauration by demonstrating that his writings contain references to a primeval golden age when humanity lived in harmony with God and had dominion over nature. Textual analysis will show that Bacon considered this to be humanity's true condition and believed it could be restored through the recovery and advancement of ancient wisdom. After developing the connection between the Ancient Wisdom and Bacon's instauration, the analysis will turn to the *New Atlantis* in order to demonstrate that it contains Bacon's fullest articulation of his vision of the great instauration of learning and the consequent restoration of humanity to its condition before original sin. This analysis will verify that the apocalyptic and millenarian themes identified by Whitney and Webster are indeed integral to Bacon's vision. At the same time, it will show that these Judaeo-Christian symbols are augmented by the myths and symbols of the Ancient Wisdom tradition, and will thereby demonstrate that full and complete instauration entails both recovery of religious purity and recovery of esoteric wisdom.

BACON'S CONCEPT OF INSTAURATION

Charles Whitney's analysis of Bacon's concept of instauration has provided the most detailed demonstration that renewal and recovery are preconditions for progress and advancement, and he has added substantial insight into the apocalyptic and millenarian elements of the term.[4] In Bacon's time, the primary

---

[3]See, for example, the work of B.J.T. Dobbs, which proves that Newton's interests in the Apocalypse and in alchemy were not separate from or marginal to his "scientific work." All three were components in Newton's search for an organic, holistic understanding of God, nature, and human history; see esp. *The Foundations of Newton's Alchemy* (Cambridge: Cambridge University Press, 1975), and *The Janus Face of Genius* (Cambridge: Cambridge University Press, 1991).

[4]See Charles Whitney, *Francis Bacon and Modernity* (New Haven: Yale University Press, 1986), and idem, "Bacon's *Instauratio*," *Journal of the History of Ideas* 50 (1989): 371–390.

connotation of the term *instauratio* derived from the Vulgate edition of the Bible, where it occurs in more than two dozen passages alluding to the apocalyptic restoration of Jerusalem and the golden age of the Davidic-Solomonic kingship. This apocalyptic or millenarian theme was particularly significant in Bacon's time because James I was heralded as the new Solomon, who would restore Jerusalem and make England the New Zion. The term is also used with a broader apocalyptic meaning in several passages of the Vulgate which refer to Christ's redemption and the restoration of humanity to its condition prior to original sin.[5] This latter theme has been explored in Charles Webster's important book, *The Great Instauration: Science, Medicine and Reform 1626–1660*. Webster examines the distinctive form of Puritan eschatology and millenarianism which linked scientific progress to the reversal of the intellectual decline that plagued humanity since the Fall of Adam. The advancement of learning was, therefore, considered essential to the restoration of humanity's dominion over nature and to the recovery of paradisiacal existence prior to original sin. To quote Webster, "The Puritan Revolution was therefore seen as a period of promise, when God would allow science to become the means to bring about a new paradise on earth …."[6] Francis Bacon, of course, lived and wrote prior to the period Webster investigates. His significance for the period is attested to, however, by Webster's title, *The Great Instauration*, which is borrowed from Bacon. Moreover, according to Webster, Bacon's term *instauratio* and the project it describes are emblematic of the Puritan millenarian expectation. That is, it presents the advancement of science and technology as a necessary means to usher in the religious millennium of peace, harmony, and prosperity.

Webster's and Whitney's studies have played important roles in clarifying the importance of Bacon's root concept, in placing the development of science in its intellectual and cultural context, and in pointing to the deficiencies of narrative histories that have selectively read Bacon in order to create a positivistic account of the steady march of science as it triumphs over religion and other quaint vestiges of classical philosophy and medieval theology. This important work now needs to be augmented by a demonstration of the influence of the *prisca theologia* or Ancient Wisdom. A careful reading of Bacon's

---

[5]This typological connection does not exist in the Hebrew and Greek originals. According to Whitney, "Bacon's *Instauratio*," 377, "the Vulgate in effect creates a typology or symbolism of *instauration* by lexically connecting the architectural instauration of Solomon's Temple both to a prophetic 'rebuilding' of Israel and to a Christian instauration of all things in the apocalypse."

[6]Charles Webster, *The Great Instauration: Science, Medicine and Reform 1626–1660* (New York: Holmes and Meier Publishers, 1975), xvi.

writings reveals that this ancient wisdom tradition of esoteric religion (Hermeticism, Cabala) and occult knowledge (magic, alchemy) played a complementary role to Judaeo-Christian millenarianism in shaping Bacon's concept of a great instauration through the recovery and advancement of learning. More specifically, careful textual analysis will show that Bacon made frequent reference to the *prisca theologia*'s accounts of a primordial age in which humanity lived in harmony with God, had dominion over nature, and lived in a utopian world free from want. This examination will also demonstrate that Bacon, like Ficino and the Florentine Platonists, believed that the ignorance and error of his own age could be overcome if the Ancient Wisdom could be restored.

THE WISDOM OF THE ANCIENTS AND THE CONCEPT OF INSTAURATION

Bacon's interest in and positive allusions to the Ancient Wisdom run through his writings from 1603 to 1626. These references include major texts like the *Advancement of Learning* as well as his essays and correspondence, including letters to King James I. The most useful text for our purposes is Bacon's *De sapientia veterum* (Wisdom of the Ancients) of 1609. In the preface Bacon explains that the fables of Homer and Hesiod "must be regarded as neither the invention of nor belonging to the age of the poets themselves, but as sacred relics and light airs breathing out of better times, that were caught from the traditions of most ancient nations and so received into the flutes and trumpets of the Greeks."[7] The problem is that their true meaning has been lost, obscured, or distorted over time; previous generations have been unqualified to interpret them. Bacon's purpose, therefore, is to re-present the fables and give them their proper interpretation. According to Paolo Rossi, this project is not ancillary to Bacon's efforts to promote the advancement of learning: "the explication of the true meaning of the fables is an integral part of [Bacon's] task of creating a new encyclopedia of learning."[8] Within the limited space available, our discussion must be confined to a brief examination of three fables: those of Orpheus, Prometheus, and Deucalion. For Bacon, the fable of Orpheus is the story of the decline of philosophy as it descends from

---

[7]Francis Bacon, *Wisdom of the Ancients* (trans. of the *De sapientia veterum*) in *The Philosophical Works of Francis Bacon*, ed. John M. Robinson (Freeport, N.Y.: Books for Libraries Press, 1904), 822. Robinson's text, as the title suggests, contains the "philosophical" works taken from the standard edition of Bacon's collected works, *The Works of Francis Bacon*, 7 vols., ed. James Spedding, R.L. Ellis, and D.D. Heath (1857–74). Subsequent page references to the *Wisdom of the Ancients* are cited in the text.

[8]Paolo Rossi, *Francis Bacon: From Magic to Science* (1968; reprint, Chicago: University of Chicago Press, 1978), 118.

the natural philosophy of the ancient wise men to moral and civil philosophy and finally to a state of almost total disintegration. In its pristine state, according to Bacon, "natural philosophy proposes to itself as its noblest work of all, nothing less than the restitution and renovation [*instauratio*] of things corruptible, and (what is indeed the same thing in a lower degree) the conservation of bodies in the state in which they are, and the retardation of dissolution and putrefaction" (835–836). The effort at retardation, however, means arduous labor, and failure leads to frustration and to the adoption of the easier task—the management of human affairs through moral and civil philosophy. This stage of philosophy remains stable for a while, but it too declines with the passage of time, and moral and civil laws are put to silence. And if such troubles last, Bacon warns, "it is not for long before letters also and philosophy are so torn in pieces that no traces of them can be found but a few fragments, scattered here and there...." When philosophy and civilization reach this low point, barbarism sets in and disorder prevails "until, according to the appointed vicissitude of things, they break out and issue forth again, perhaps among other nations, and not in the places where they were before" (836). Three points are worthy of emphasis. The pure, original philosophy is the magic and alchemy of the *prisca theologia*. This God-given ability is lost through the lack of human effort and will. The decline, however, is not permanent. According to "the appointed vicissitude of things," i.e., providential intervention, true philosophy will return and humanity will be restored to its primordial condition—but not necessarily in the places where it originated.

In Bacon's interpretation, "Prometheus, Or, the State of Man," is about humanity's squandering of Jupiter's gift of unfading youth, which is lost through human foolishness. For Bacon, it is also a fable about the loss and potential recovery of the regenerative power of ancient wisdom. Bacon maintains that "methods and medicines for the retardation of age and the prolongation of life were not by the ancients despaired of, but reckoned rather among those things which men once had and by sloth and negligence let slip, than among those which were wholly denied or never offered" (850). Further on, he adds that a recovery from ignorance and error is possible if the achievements of the ancients are emulated (852). A third fable, that of Deucalion, is the story of the restoration of humanity and the world after their virtual destruction by a flood. Deucalion and Pyrrha, sole survivors of the deluge, pray that they might know by what means to repair mankind (*instaurandi generis humani*). Their prayers are answered and they become the active agents for a miraculous repopulation of the world. For Bacon, this is another account of the degeneration of humanity and its subsequent restoration to its pristine state through a combination of divine and human action.

The themes developed in the *Wisdom of the Ancients* are present in other key texts of Bacon. A reference to an original, pure form of Persian magic occurs in *De ... augmentis scientiarum* (1623), an expanded Latin version of *Advancement of Learning* (1605). A similar reference is found in his "Discourse Touching the Happy Unions of the Kingdoms of England and Scotland" (1603) and in one of his masques for James I. In the latter, Bacon notes that ancient kingdoms were attended by magi and compares James I to Hermes Trismegistus. Another reference to James as Hermes Trismegistus occurs in *The Advancement of Learning* (1605). These texts cannot be examined in detail, but the brief reference to them should help demonstrate a link between the Ancient Wisdom and Bacon's concept of instauration. These references also complement the broad thematic thrust of Bacon's reinterpretations in *De sapientia*. The three fables examined describe an ideal, primordial time before corruption and decline set in. This primeval period closely resembles the mythic accounts in the *prisca theologia*, particularly the *Corpus Hermeticum*. The Hermetic account of creation depicts man as a *deus en terra*, a terrestrial god, who has full knowledge of the powers controlling nature and is an active co-creator with God of order, beauty, and harmony in the world. Hermetic accounts also lament the decline and fall of humanity from this pristine state, but the lament is followed by the reassurance that the gods will not permit the age of disorder and degeneration to persist. At the appropriate time, God will restore the world to its order, beauty, and harmony and humanity to its original state as a terrestrial god. So the delivery from an age of ignorance and disorder is a recovery of the primordial condition.[9]

While Bacon's reinterpretation of ancient Greek myths and legends clearly establishes affinities with the *prisca theologia,* his reading does not impose an interpretation that is inconsistent with themes introduced by ancient Greek authors. Bacon's *New Atlantis,* for example, alludes to two Platonic dialogues which first describe a primordial age when humanity was semidivine and had godlike knowledge and then laments the passing of this state of perfection through human degeneration and natural calamities. Before turning to the *New Atlantis*, however, a brief mention needs to be made of other works which express Bacon's interest in and use of ancient myth and legend. In addition to *De sapientia veterum*, four other works are directly

---

[9]For an analysis of these themes and their appropriation by Ficino and the Renaissance Neoplatonists, see Stephen A. McKnight, *The Modern Age and the Recovery of Ancient Wisdom* (Columbia: University of Missouri Press, 1991), esp. 27–59.

concerned with or explicitly refer to the ancient wisdom hidden in fables.[10] The *Redargutio philosophorum*, for example, refers to the secrets of antiquity which precede the learning of the Greeks which Bacon considered sacred survivals of better times. Similarly, the *Advancement of Learning* states that parables and fables are the appropriate vehicles for transmitting the secrets and mysteries of religion, policy, or philosophy, and adds that a "fable is a method of teaching by which the most difficult and unfamiliar concepts may find an easier passage to understanding.[11] I add these references not only to lend weight to the significance of the themes contained in the *De sapientia*, but also to set the context for considering the *New Atlantis* as a fable which transmits secrets and mysteries of religion, politics, and philosophy.

BACON'S NEW ATLANTIS

The *New Atlantis* begins with European sailors being blown off course by a storm and discovering the uncharted island of Bensalem. From the outset, the Europeans are struck by the charity and generosity of the people and notice that they prominently display Christian symbols. Therefore, when given an opportunity, the Europeans ask how this distant island came to be Christian. In response, one of the Bensalemite officials tells of the miraculous circumstances of the island's conversion. In a second interview, the Europeans express wonder at the order and beauty of the island and the health and well-being of people. The official responds that the source to the island's utopian condition is Solomon's House, which is dedicated to the study of God's creation and to humanity's proper use of it. In a later interview, part of the discussion centers on Bensalem's decision to remain isolated from the rest of the world. The official bluntly tells the Europeans that the choice was made long ago when the people of Bensalem realized that other civilizations were far inferior to it in knowledge and in moral conduct. The Europeans learn, however, that the current state of civilizational decline did not always exist. There was a period long ago when many great civilizations flourished, and Bensalem conducted intercourse with Atlantis and many other countries from the far-

---

[10]Francis Bacon, *Cogitationes de scientia humana* (Reflections on Human Knowledge) (1605); idem, *Of Proficience and Advancement of Learning Divine and Humane* (1605); idem, *De degnitate et augumentis scientiarum libri ix* (Nine Books of Proficience and Advancement of Learning) (1623); and idem, *De principiis atque originibus secundum fabulas Cupidinis et Coeli, sive Parmenidis et Telesii et precipue Democriti philosophia tractata in fabula de Cupidine* (On Principles and Origins according to Fables of Cupid and Coelum, or the Philosophy of Parmenides, Telesius and especially of Democritus, treated in a Fable of Cupid) (ca. 1623–24). The latter is a substantial collection of notes for a projected revision of *The Ancient Wisdom*.

[11]Bacon, *Advancement of Learning* in *Philosophical Works*, 426.

flung corners of the world. This primordial state of affairs was brought to an abrupt end by a series of calamities that completely destroyed the other civilizations or reduced them to a mere vestige of their former greatness. The destruction was so extensive that the great civilizations lost memory of their former magnificence, and records of the time virtually perished. According to the Bensalemite official, the only record of this primordial past available to the Europeans is contained in brief and incomplete references "by one of your philosophers [Plato]."

The foregoing synopsis follows the order of the narrative, which carries the discussion from the aspects of Bensalemite life most recognizable to the Europeans to those least known and understood, that is, from familiar Christian signs to Solomon's House and finally to events in the primordial past that have been virtually forgotten. In analyzing the text, the events will be treated in their chronological sequence rather than in their narrative presentation. There are five reasons for proceeding in this manner. First, setting the proper sequence of events allows the foundations of this utopian fable to become more obvious. Second, beginning with the prehistory establishes an important connection to Bacon's references to the primordial golden age in the *De sapientia*. Third, it permits a comparison of Bacon's reconstruction of Greek fables with two dialogues by Plato (the philosopher to whom the Bensalemite official refers) which describe a wondrous, primordial age when the great civilizations of Athens and Atlantis flourished. Fourth, arranging the events in chronological order casts new light on the relation of Solomon's House to the miraculous conversion to Christianity. Finally, following this chronological sequence sets the context for examining the *New Atlantis*'s integration of Judaeo-Christian apocalyptic/millenarian symbols with the *prisca theologia*'s myths of recovery of a pristine, primordial condition.

THE ANCIENT HISTORY OF THE WORLD.

The *New Atlantis*'s discussion of the great civilizational achievements of antiquity is fairly brief. As noted in the synopsis above, the Europeans are told that in the distant past Bensalem was well known and carried out travel and trade with Atlantis and other civilizations throughout the world. But a series of cataclysms destroyed the other great civilizations and left most nations in an infantile state, having lost all records of their previous greatness and all ability to restore themselves to their former condition. Not only are the other civilizations reduced to infancy and the memory of their past greatness eclipsed; they forget about the other great civilizations as well. Consequently, Bensalem, the only civilization to be spared, chooses to remain obscure because, as the Bensalemite official indicates, the country has nothing to be gained and much to be lost by making itself known in the rest of the world.[12] In recounting these remarkable events, the Bensalemite official notes that the only records of the great primeval age available to the Europeans are brief references in the work of "one of your philosophers." Surprisingly, this tantalizing reference by the Bensalemite official to the two dialogues by Plato has not stimulated much interest among Bacon scholars. There appears to be no detailed comparison of Bacon's and Plato's accounts of the primordial age of Athenian and Atlantan civilizational splendor, certainly not one that examines the two Platonic dialogues in relation to Bacon's concept of instauration.

Examination of the two Platonic accounts proves to be quite productive and reveals interesting formal and thematic affinities with Bacon's *New Atlantis*, *De sapientia veterum*, and the root concept of instauration. The first of the two dialogues, the *Timaeus*, takes up a discussion Socrates had begun the previous day with three philosopher statesmen. The topic has been the attributes of the best form of society. At the beginning of the *Timeaus*, Socrates specifically requests that the discussion move from speculation on the nature of the ideal society to accounts of the best societies to have actually existed. In response, the three agree that recounting the ancient, virtually unknown history of Athens will meet Socrates' request because it was a state that actually existed. Critias, who relates the story, explains that it originated with Solon, who had learned it from a priest during a visit to Egypt. It is important that Solon is the source of the story because he is, of course, the great Athenian lawgiver. He was also a poet, and Critias claims that Solon's recounting of the episode was as great and memorable as the stories of Hesiod and Homer, and had Solon finished his poetic account, he would have joined the ranks of the greatest poets of Greece.[13] That the story comes from the ancient Egyptian civilization is significant because the Greeks believed that the Egyptians were the most ancient civilization and the only one to survive the floods and other natural catastrophes that had decimated other civilizations. The account Solon is given by the Egyptian priest concerns the most remarkable period in Athenian history, one that deserved to be the most renowned of all, and yet it is one that was virtually lost. According to the priest, Athens and other coun-

[12]The island does monitor developments in other countries throughout the world and brings back any information that can be used by Bensalem. These expeditions are carried out in secret, however, by the most learned and incorruptible inhabitants of Bensalem, the members of Solomon's House.

[13]This remark is intriguing in light of Bacon's statement in the preface to *De sapientia veterum* that the fables of Hesiod and Homer are not products of their own age but "sacred relics ... caught from the traditions of the most ancient nations."

tries suffer the same fate: "with you and other peoples again and again life has only lately been enriched with letters and all the other necessities of civilization when once more, after the usual period of years, the torrents from the heavens sweep down like a pestilence leaving only the rude and unlettered among you. And so you start again like children, knowing nothing of what existed in ancient times."[14]

The priest tells Solon that Athens was once the most valiant in war and in all respects the best governed, and was actually a millennium older than Egypt. In its primordial golden age, Athens was "a land whose inhabitants were born of gods and nurtured by them." The wisdom inspired by the goddess Athena informed "all arts applied to human affairs, including the practice of *divination* and *medicine*, and acquiring all other branches of learning connected therewith" (17, emphasis added). The reason Athens holds a special place in the memory of the Egyptians is that it defeated the invading Atlantans, who attempted to enslave Greece, Egypt, and the rest of the world. Though Athens repels the Atlantans, Solon is told that "there came one terrible night and day in which all [the Athenian] men of war were swallowed bodily by the earth, and the island Atlantis also sank beneath the sea and vanished. Hence, to this day that outer ocean cannot be crossed or explored, the way being blocked by mud, just below the surface, left by the settling down of the island" (18). Socrates accepts this "true history" as an admirable response to his request. Critias then outlines subsequent topics to be discussed. Timeaus will speak first because he knows astronomy and can give an explanation of the formation of the cosmos and an account of humanity's original and true nature. Critias is to then give an account of the lost history of humanity, which will fill in the events from the beginning of the cosmos to the commonly known recent history.

In the *Critias* Athens and Atlantis are both portrayed as paradisiacal countries prospering from their respective patron deities, Athena and Poseidon. The preamble states that order and harmony existed among the gods, and there was complete accord regarding the division of the world among them. Critias first turns to the creation of Athens by Athena and Hephaestus, and indicates that accounts of the founding of Athens have been lost or exist in fragments. As a result, the laws and forms of government of the original great civilization have passed from memory. Critias then provides a fuller account of the founding of Atlantis. Poseidon creates the island, giving it a topography

---

[14]F. M. Cornford, *Plato's Cosmology: The Timaeus of Plato* (New York: Bobbs-Merrill, 1937), 16; subsequent pages cited in the text.

that produces an abundance of food and other natural comforts, and also protects the island from invasion. Poseidon then mates with mortal women to create a race of demigods to inhabit the land. (The firstborn is Atlas; hence the name of the country.) These people were industrious and created great feats of engineering and of navigation. "For many generations, as long as the divine nature lasted in them, they were obedient to the laws, well-affectionate toward the god, whose seed they were; for they possessed true and great spirits, uniting gentleness with wisdom" and their nobility of character made them immune to the desire for vast wealth because they valued virtue and honor over material things. But this idyllic condition did not last "when the divine portion began to fade away and become diluted too often and too much with the mortal admixture, and the human nature got the upper hand, they then, being unable to bear their fortune, behave unseemly ... and they grew visibly debased ... and became full of avarice and unrighteous power."[15] The last important episode recorded in the *Critias* occurs when Zeus, the minister of justice and order in the cosmos and on earth, convenes a council of the gods to take corrective action to chasten and improve an honorable race that was in a woeful plight. The unfinished text of the *Critias* breaks off just as Zeus is about to address the assembled deities. From these brief accounts, it is apparent that the themes presented in the Platonic dialogues parallel themes Bacon reads from/into the fables in the *Wisdom of the Ancients*. The Platonic dialogues purport to present *real* history that has been virtually lost and, as a consequence, has left humanity in a state of infancy, not knowing what has been achieved in the past and, therefore, not capable of realizing its own potential. The dialogues also state that Athenian knowledge included divinization and medicine. Similarly, the Atlantians create a paradisiacal world through feats of engineering, agriculture, and navigation.

SOLOMON'S HOUSE

From the outset, the Europeans marvel at the utopian existence of Bensalem and when they have the opportunity, they ask the Bensalemite official if he will tell them the secret of the island's prosperity and well-being. In response, they are told that the source of Bensalem's success is Solomon's House founded 1,900 years before by King Salomon. Solomon's House was created to find "the true nature of all things (whereby God might have the more glory in the workmanship of them and men the more fruit in the use of them)."[16] The

---

[15]Plato, *Critias* in *Plato*, trans. R. G. Bury, Loeb Classical Library, vol. 9 (Cambridge: Harvard University Press, 1925), 92.

[16]Bacon, *New Atlantis* in *Philosophical Works*, 722; subsequent citations will be in the text.

Bensalemite official further explains that the name Solomon's House was inspired by the Solomonic reputation for wisdom, which is known in Europe, but also because Bensalem had possession of Solomon's *Natural History*, a text that had been lost to the Europeans. This text held special knowledge of the workings of nature which Solomon's House used as the guide for its own remarkable work. Sometime later, the Europeans have an audience with an elder of Solomon's House, and they are told: "The end of our Foundation is the knowledge of causes and secret motions of things, and the enlarging of the bounds of the Human Empire, to the effecting of all things possible" (727). A detailed description of the investigation of the natural world then follows: from caves to mountain observatories to marine investigations. These investigations produce a breadth and depth of knowledge beyond anything imagined in Europe. Experiments in the Lower Region, for example, produce new artificial metals which are used for curing diseases and prolonging life. There are also a "great variety of composts, and soils, for the making of the earth fruitful," and blended mineral waters, including one called Water of Paradise which was created by the brethren "for health and the prolongation of life" (723). The elder further indicates that "we have also large and various orchards and gardens … [and] make them also by art greater much than their nature; and their fruit greater and sweeter … . And many of them we so order as they become of medicinal use"(728). Many scholars have linked this description of the activities of Solomon's House to the advancement of learning that Bacon hoped James I would have the Solomonic wisdom to support, and the *New Atlantis* is frequently referred to as a scientific utopia. But the foregoing analysis establishes parallels between the activities of Solomon's House and Bacon's accounts of Ancient Wisdom used to retard age, prolong life, and restore corruptible things to their original, pure state. While Bacon's contemporaries and later scholars rightly regard Solomon's House as an inspiration for the activities of the Royal Society, enough evidence has been supplied to also demonstrate that Solomon's House's efforts at "regeneration" are similar to the work of the *prisci magi* and alchemists of the primordial past.[17]

In addition to "pagan" sources of Ancient Wisdom, there is also a Jewish esoteric tradition suggesting close affinities between Solomon's House and Solomon's Temple. In this tradition, Solomon was not only wise in the way described in the biblical accounts; he possessed a deep understanding of the

---

[17]For example, Bacon's contemporary John Glanvill, claimed that "Solomon's House" in the *New Atlantis* was a "Prophetick Scheam of the Royal Society." Both the *Scepsis Scientifica* (1665) and the frontispiece of Thomas Sprat's *History of the Royal Society* (1667) show Bacon and the society's president supporting the bust of Charles II.

mysteries of the creation and was a magus. The reference to Solomon's "Natural History" seems to allude to this connection. Several variations of this tradition were fairly widely known in the early modern period. In one the original esoteric knowledge is given to Adam, but is lost through the Fall. Another version has the knowledge given to Moses on Mount Sinai and placed in the Ark of the Tabernacle, where it was accessible only to the high priest. The Ark and then later Solomon's Temple became an *omphalos* or center for communing with the powers and principalities governing the world, including the highest order of celestial powers, the cherubim. The close association of the cherubim with God's presence and power is inscribed on the Ark itself. Cherubim's wings are the only design permitted on the Ark of the Covenant, and they are there to symbolize God's presence. It is, therefore, intriguing that the elders of Solomon's House use cherubim's wings as their emblem.

The Conversion to Christianity

The next major event in Bensalem's history is its conversion to Christianity, which occurred shortly after the Resurrection and about 250 years after the founding of Solomon's House. As already noted, the Europeans are struck by the kindness and generosity of the people and feel that they have been delivered into a land of angels. When they ask the Bensalemite official how a country so far removed from Europe or the Middle East ever came to know about Christianity, they are told about the miraculous nature of the island's conversion. The Bensalemite official explains that shortly after the Crucifixion and Resurrection, a Pillar of Cloud appeared out over the ocean. When a member of the House of Solomon sailed out to it and asked God to reveal its meaning, the pillar transformed into an ark (small box), which contained a letter stating that the recipients had been chosen for a special blessing. The ark also contained Scriptures beyond those known in Europe. This compact episode contains references to the major symbols of Judaeo-Christian divine election, including the instrument of God's chosen people's deliverance (the Pillar of Cloud that guided them through the wilderness), the symbol of God's covenant with his *am segullah* (treasured people), which is the ark, and Christian Scriptures beyond those available to the Europeans and through which the Bensalemites maintain a pure, unadulterated Christianity. The writer of the letter contained in the ark is also worthy of note. He is Bartholomew, who, according to tradition, was the missionary to far-off lands. He is also the author of two noncanonical texts which describe the harrowing of hell and the rescue of Adam. The theme of the rescue of Adam is a key one in Bacon's work and will receive further attention later on. At this point, however, it is important to draw together the key themes presented in the *New Atlantis* and examine Bacon's integration of Judaeo-Christian apocalyptic symbols with elements of the Ancient Wisdom. After this is done, it will be possible to better understand the nature of the instauration Bacon is proposing to James I and to England.

THE GREAT INSTAURATION

Some of the Judaeo-Christian apocalyptic and millenarian symbols have already been identified. The miraculous conversion to Christianity carries the prime symbols of Judaeo-Christian divine election, including the Pillar of Cloud, the Ark, and special Christian scriptures. There is also the reference to the island's King Salomon and the island is named Bensalem. Salomon is a slight variation of Solomon and Bensalem is a neologism suggesting a New Jerusalem.[18] So, obviously these elements fit with the emphasis Whitney and Webster give to apocalyptic and millenarian themes. But the foregoing analysis makes it fairly obvious that the Bensalemite religion is significantly different from European Christianity. The narrative indicates that the Bensalemite conversion occurred shortly after the Resurrection. The island, therefore, received a pure, apostolic Christianity that had not degenerated into the kind of religious disorder, confusion, and turmoil that plagued Europe. Moreover, the Bensalemites received scriptures that were not included in the European canon (or perhaps were lost over the course of time) and these helped to keep the religion pure and unadulterated. The most obvious connection to the *prisca theologia* tradition is in the activities of Solomon's House. The Solomon revered in Bensalem is the author of an esoteric text on nature, and the work he inspires involves alchemical and magical ventures in prolonging life and adding to nature's bounty. These activities are commensurate with the *prisca theologia*'s accounts of the work done in the primordial time when humanity lived in harmony with God and was an active creator of order, beauty, peace, and prosperity.

Bacon's integration of Judaeo-Christian themes with the myths and fables of the *prisca theologia* is made more evident by reading the history of Bensalem in its proper chronological sequence. Bensalem's history then moves from the period of great civilizational achievement by semidivine men to the collapse of all civilizations but Bensalem. Bensalem escapes devastation and continues in a prelapsarian state through the work of the priests/magi of Solomon's House.

---

[18]The Hebrew *ben* means son or heir, and salem (*shalom*) is the stem of Jerusalem.

Bensalem is not only spared the destruction that befell all other civilizations; it is subsequently blessed with a miraculous conversion to Christianity through divine election. While Bacon does not explain why Bensalem is chosen for this special benediction, it seems reasonable to conclude that it was because it remained pure through the guidance of Solomon's House, while all other peoples became corrupt and all other civilizations turned toward material concerns.

This brief recapitulation is sufficient to make it clear that Bacon's utopian vision draws upon both the orthodox Judaeo-Christian tradition and the *prisca theologia*. But the exact nature of the instauration envisioned by Bacon still needs further exploration. Is it an apocalyptic instauration of the Davidic-Solomonic monarchy similar to the reform of the biblical King Josiah in 624 B.C.E. — or do the references to Ancient Wisdom and a prelapsarian golden age suggest that the instauration is to be even more fundamental? In order to put the issue in proper perspective, it is necessary to examine a recurrent theme in Bacon's writings that was briefly identified earlier — his allusions to the possibility of restoring humanity to its original state before Adam's Fall. In several writings Bacon argues that the damage done by original sin could be overcome in humanity and in nature, namely, humankind could, allegorically speaking, return to Eden. In the *Advancement of Learning*, for example, Bacon speaks of the purpose of learning as "a restitution and reinvesting (in great part) of man to sovereignty and power ... which he had in the first state of creation."[19] A similar statement occurs in the *Novum Organum*: "For man by the Fall fell at the same time from his state of innocency and from his dominion over nature. Both of these losses, however, can even in this life be in some part repaired; the former by religion and faith, the latter by the arts and sciences."[20] The notion that a restoration was possible through right knowledge also occurs in the "Proœmium" to the *Instauratio Magna*. According to Bacon, "all trial should be made, whether that commerce between the mind of man and the nature of things ... might by any means be restored to this perfect and original condition, [or at least] reduced to a better condition than that in which it now is."[21]

If we place these several references to the instauration of humanity to its prelapsarian condition in the context of the *New Atlantis*, it is apparent that Bensalem possesses both means needed to repair the ruptured union with God that was caused by original sin. For its religious instauration Bensalem

[19] Bacon, *Advancement of Learning* in *Philosophical Works*, 46.
[20] Bacon, *New Organon* in *Philosophical Works*, 257.
[21] Bacon, *Great Instauration* in *Philosophical Works*, 241.

has the benefit of a pure, apostolic form of Christianity and has both canonical and noncanonical books to guide it and keep it pure. For the instauration of the arts and sciences Bensalem has the Ancient Wisdom contained in the Solomonic *Natural History* to guide its ongoing research. Quite clearly, both elements are necessary for instauration to occur. These references and the context of the *New Atlantis,* therefore, make it clear that Bacon is proposing an instauration that goes beyond the notable religious and political instauration achieved by King Josiah. Full instauration combines pure religion with mastery of nature in order to return humanity to its original, prelapsarian condition.

Developing the full proportions of Bacon's proposed instauration perhaps helps to explain why he chooses to call his utopia the *New Atlantis*. The choice of this title is perplexing. Since the island is called Bensalem, why does Bacon not call the book *Bensalem?* While no direct response is given in any of Bacon's writings, his fables and two of his frontispieces suggest a possible explanation. And, more importantly, there is the reference to the Platonic accounts in the *New Atlantis*.

THE NEW ATLANTIS

The Platonic accounts describe a golden age that is virtually lost from memory. In its pristine state, Atlantis was a nation of great inventors, engineers, and navigators who reached the pinnacle of human excellence in the arts and sciences. This prelapsarian Atlantis should perhaps be regarded as a representation of excellence in the arts and sciences that is intended to serve as a needed complement to Bensalem's religious purity. For Bacon, complete instauration requires the religious renewal symbolized by the image of a New Jerusalem. But that religious revival must be completed by a recovery or instauration of humanity to its original state, that is, to a state of mastery over nature like that depicted in the myth of Atlantis. Since Bacon's description of the two dimensions required for humanity to overcome original sin are the religious and the scientific, perhaps Jerusalem is emblematic of the former and Atlantis emblematic of the latter. In order for England to achieve a great instauration, it must become the new Atlantis as well as the New Jerusalem. That Bacon wants James I to consider England as the New Atlantis is suggested in the frontispieces of two of Bacon's major works. The first is found in the *Instauratio Magna* (fig. 1). This image shows a ship sailing beyond the Pillars of Hercules. In Greek myth the Pillars marked the boundary of the human world. To sail beyond them was a violation of humanity's place in the cosmos and a profound act of hubris. In the frontispiece Bacon seems to make this myth part of

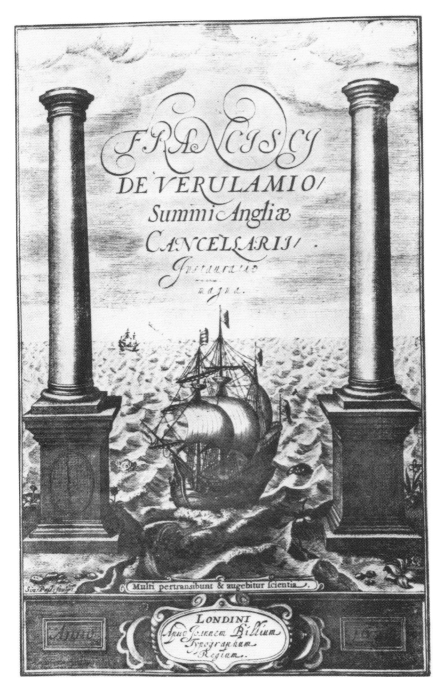

Fig. 1. Title Page, Francis Bacon, *Instauratio Magna,* title page (1620)

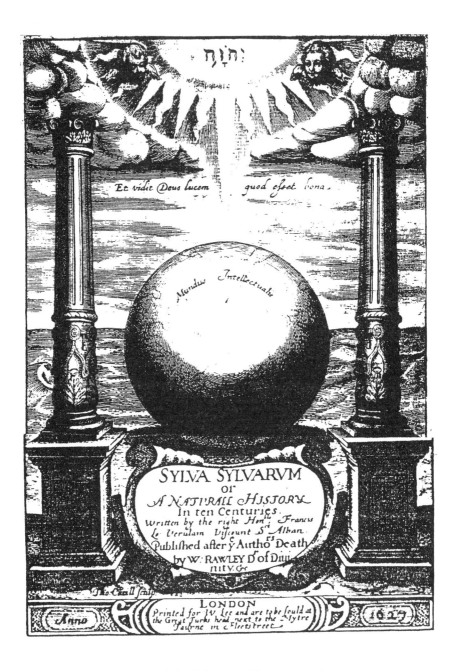

Fig. 2. Sylva Sylvarum, title page (1627)

the spurious, truncated history of Greece. The frontispiece carries an inscription taken from the apocalyptic book of Daniel, which reads "multi pertransibunt & augebitur scientia" (many shall go forth and knowledge will increase). Sailing through the Pillars, therefore, is an act of prophetic fulfillment rather than a sinful act of hubris. The second frontispiece is a modified version of the same image and theme and seems to meld the roles of Jerusalem and Atlantis. The frontispiece appearing in the *Sylva Sylvarum* also has two pillars in the foreground while the ocean expands to the far horizon (fig. 2; facing page). This image also expresses divine approval because the Hebrew name of God appears in a cloud, and cherubim watch from the heavens. But there is a significant modification. The pillars are not the Pillars of Hercules; they are the main pillars of Solomon's Temple.[22] So, the frontispieces seem to be iconographically linking the two great cities of Jerusalem and Atlantis and joining pure religion with esoteric wisdom to express the full scope of Bacon's great instauration. While these are intriguing possibilities, they are admittedly highly speculative. On the other hand, such speculation is invited by Bacon's own search for the secret truths and hidden meanings contained in fables about the pristine, primordial state of existence and the potential for its instauration. Nevertheless, the conclusion of this analysis needs to return to the main themes of the essay and the textual evidence they are based upon.

CONCLUSION

The essay has presented two principal arguments. First, Bacon uses Ancient Wisdom myths of a primordial time of human, social, and natural perfection to complement Judaeo-Christian apocalyptic images of a great instauration. For Bacon, complete instauration requires a recovery of humanity's God-given knowledge and mastery of nature as well as a recovery of religious purity. Second, Bacon's advancement of learning is also an instauration of ancient learning that had been lost or corrupted over the course of time. In making the arguments for the importance of the Ancient Wisdom in understanding Bacon's concept of instauration, no attempt has been made to deny the major role Bacon played in the advancement and institutionalization of science. Rather, the intent has been to show that the *prisca theologia* or Ancient Wisdom was an integral part of the intellectual ferment of Bacon's age and that it was reasonable for him to expect that its imagery would be recognized and understood by his intended audience.

[22]See Elizabeth McCutcheon, "Bacon and the Cherubim: An Iconographic Reading of the *New Atlantis*," *English Literary Renaissance* 2 (1972): 334–354.

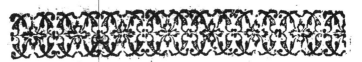

An hundred and foureteene Experi-

ments and Cures of. *Phillip Theophraſtus Paracelſus* a great Philoſopher, and a moſt excellent doctor of the one and the other *Phyſicke, written with his owne hand in the Ger*-mane tongue, which Conrad Steinberge his ſeruant found among other looſe papers and ſcrolles of Paracelſus.

Certaine Baron being diſeaſed with a wonted griefe, By drinking our *Quinta eſſentia Mercuriale*, caſt out a ſtone downeward, and became whole.

2 A certaine woman was long ſicke of the Paſsion of the heart which ſhe called *Cardiaca*, who was cured by taking twice our *Mercurial* vomit, which cauſed hir to caſt out a worme commonly called *Theniam*, that was foure cubites long.

3 One Bartholmew, had for two yeeres ſpace a paine in his ſide, whome I cured by giuing him the oyle of *Vitrial*, in a drinke comforting the ſtomacke.

4 A man that had his Nauill ſtanding out like to a mans yard, was healed with a thrid dipped in the oyle of *Vitriol*, by tying the threed hard about it euery day. After the ſame ſort I healed a great ſwelling or ouergrowing of the fleſh called *Parotis*, which grew out of a womans thigh waying fiue pound.

5 A fouldier was ſhotte through in the breaſt to the left ſhoulder with a two forked arrow, ſo that the head ſtucke faſt in the bone, the which I drewe forth with my two fingers, and powred *Kiſt* into the wound and ſo hee was healed.

6 A Phiſitian being aſtonied with a clap of thunder and Lightning, ſo that hee ſeemed to bee ſicke of the (Apo-

C   plexia)

Nicholas H. Clulee

JOHN DEE ᴬᴺᴰ ᵀᴴᴱ PARACELSIANS

JOHN DEE'S MONAS HIEROGLYPHICA is a notable example of an alchemical literature that was increasingly prone to enigmatic complexities in the later sixteenth century. Despite this, or perhaps because of it—it does seem that esoteric enigmas had something of the status of a cultural fad for some groups at this time—Dee's *Monas* became his most popular work. Originally published in 1564, it was reprinted at Frankfurt in 1591 and was included in both the 1602 and the 1659 editions of the *Theatrum Chemicum*. Besides this, there are a number of manuscript copies of the Latin text as well as manuscript translations into German and English, suggesting that the *Monas* was sought after and cherished in certain circles. The work, or more especially, Dee's unique symbol of the hieroglyphic monad, seen inside the oval form on the title page (fig. 1), was widely cited and adopted.[1] The *Monas* was perhaps the most concrete basis for Dee's European reputation, a theme developed in a recent paper on "John Dee and European Alchemy" by Urszula Szulakowska. She argues that heretofore everyone has missed the fact that Dee was a Paracelsian, and that this was the basis for his continental influence.[2] Dee's relation to Paracelsus and Paracelsianism is indeed interesting and important in helping to unravel some of the enigmas of Dee's influence. What seems to have been central in this is less any overt Paracelsianism on Dee's part than a shared interest among Dee and Paracelsians in themes inspired by Johannes Trithemius and the *Emerald Tablet*.

[1]C.H. Josten, "Introduction," in "A Translation of John Dee's *Monas Hieroglyphica* (Antwerp, 1564), with an Introduction and Annotations," *Ambix* 12 (1964): 90–99. The following list of manuscript copies and translations is not necessarily exhaustive: Milan, Ambrosiana MS S97 Sup; Florence, Biblioteca Nazionale MS Magl. XVI.65; Rome, Vatican MSS Reg. Lat. 1266 and 1344; Austria, Schlierbach MS 8; and Glasgow, Ferguson MS 21.

[2]Urszula Szulakowska, *John Dee and European Alchemy,* The Durham Thomas Harriot Seminar, Occasional Paper No. 21 (Durham, NC: University of Durham, 1996), 1–3.

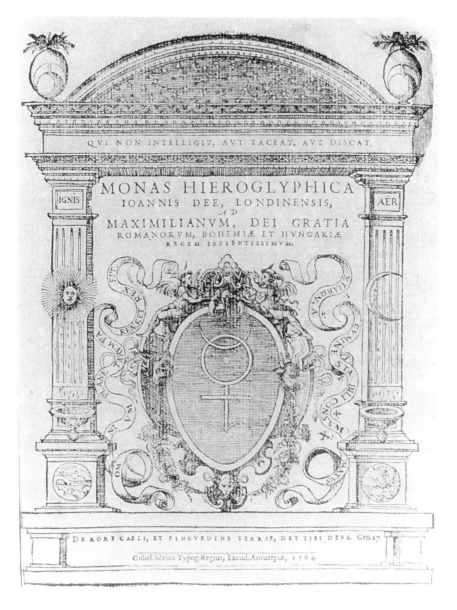

Fig. 1. Title page, John Dee, *Monas Hieroglyphica*, 1564. (By permission of the Beinecke Rare Book and Manuscript Library, Yale University).

There are two dimensions to the relation of John Dee with Paracelsianism. One is Dee's own interest in Paracelsus and Paracelsian literature. The other is the interest in Dee's works and ideas expressed by various Paracelsians. This second is potentially a very large subject, so what follows will necessarily be preliminary and sketchy, aimed only at indicating the value of this line of investigation as well as mapping out some of the necessary considerations. I will look at Dee's own interest in Paracelsus first, which is most prominently indicated by the extent of Paracelsian holdings in Dee's library.

By 1583, when Dee drew up the catalogue of his library, he had ninety-two editions of works by Paracelsus.[3] In addition to works by Paracelsus himself, Dee also had a significant number of books by Adam von Bodenstein, Alexander von Suchten, Gerhard Dorn, Leonhardt Thurneyesser zun Thurn, Joseph Duchesne, Petrus Severinus, Michael Toxites, and others who were proponents of Paracelsus and whose writings served as the vehicle for the revival and promotion of Paracelsian ideas in the late sixteenth century. Dee's catalogue is generally in no clear order; in their edition of the catalogue, Julian Roberts and Andrew G. Watson suggest that it reflects the order of books on the shelves, since the main division is between bound and unbound volumes, and within these by size. So it suggests a particular interest when some books have been grouped by subjects, such as Dee's Paracelsian books, which are clearly grouped with headings of "Paracelsici libri compacti," "Paracelsici libri latinè compacti," and "Paracelsici libri non compacti," the last of which is divided between "latini" followed by "Germanici."[4] The concordance, provided by Roberts and Watson, between the Paracelsian entries in Dee's catalogue and Karl Sudhoff's *Bibliographia Paracelsica,* provides an indication that Dee's collecting covered the whole range of Paracelsian literature.[5]

All indications suggest that Dee's interest in Paracelsus dates from the early 1560s and is related to his trip to the continent from 1561 through 1564. On April 23, 1563, during that trip, Dee visited with Konrad Gesner in Zurich. Gesner noted Dee's interest in Paracelsus in conjunction with Dee's signature in his *Liber amicorum,* suggesting one topic of their conversation.[6] Among the

---

[3]Julian Roberts and Andrew G. Watson, eds., *John Dee's Library Catalogue* (London: Bibliographical Society, 1990), 11.

[4]Ibid., nos. 1461–1501 (bound German), nos. 1502–1557 (bound Latin), nos. 2220–2240 (unbound Latin), and nos. 2241–2277 (unbound German).

[5]Ibid., 198–200.

[6]Nicholas H. Clulee, *John Dee's Natural Philosophy, Between Science and Religion* (London: Routledge, 1988), 123; Roberts and Watson, *John Dee's Library Catalogue,* 9:76; William H. Sherman, *John Dee: The Politics of Reading and Writing in the English Renaissance* (Amherst: University of Massachusetts Press, 1995), 48.

Paracelsian books in the 1583 catalogue, the earliest are 1562 imprints. Dee left earlier book lists, which show no Paracelsian titles, but these lists are known to be incomplete. However, despite the impossibility of ruling out an earlier interest, the only available indications start with a large number of 1562 imprints in the 1583 catalogue, followed by imprints from almost every year through 1582. One of the 1562 imprints, the *Baderbüchlein*, was acquired that same year since it survives and is signed and dated. Dee noted that this deals not only with ordinary baths but also with "the most secret hot springs of the philosophers."[7] The heavy annotations throughout are primarily practical; some of the notes may be later since the flyleaf notes the contents of another by Paracelsus' works, possibly the *Archidoxa,* of which the earliest edition Dee had is dated 1570. Another survivor, *Das Buch Meteororum* of 1566, with an inscription from 1567, is interesting in that it lists other works of Paracelsus, indicating that Dee was interested in the Paracelsian corpus and not just individual titles.[8]

Given the apparent extent of this interest in Paracelsus it is perhaps a puzzle that it has received relatively little notice in the literature on Dee until recently. This is perhaps because there is so little explicit reflection of Paracelsus in Dee's writings. Roberts' and Watson's publication of Dee's library catalogue, however, by calling attention to Dee's extensive Paracelsian holdings, has quite reasonably suggested to some scholars that Dee was more of a Paracelsian than previously thought. One example of this is Urszula Szulakowska's "John Dee and European Alchemy," where she posits a Paracelsian foundation to all of Dee's works in conjunction with arguing for Dee's central influence on the emergence of an "alchemical optics" in the late sixteenth century.[9] This alchemical optics involved the use of natural light in chemical procedures and is also reflected in the emergence of a new visual imagery using "optical diagrams, perspective geometry and architectural designs."[10] She finds the earliest example of this imagery in the illustrations of Heinrich Khunrath's *Amphitheatrum Sapientiae* (Hanau, 1609), where a central theme is the relation of light to the Paracelsian cosmology, astral signatures, and alchemical processes.[11] Szulakowska attributes Khunrath's expression of this alchemical optics to his meeting with Dee in Bremen in 1589 where he picked

[7] Paracelsus, *Baderbüchlein* (1562); Dee's copy is in the New York Society Library; see Roberts and Watson, *John Dee's Library Catalogue*, no. 1476; Sherman, *Politics of Reading*, 99.

[8] Paracelsus, *Das Buch Meteorum* (Cologne: Heirs of Arnold Byrckmann,1566); Roberts and Watson, *John Dee's Library Catalogue*, no. 1482.

[9] Szulakowska, *John Dee and European Alchemy*, 1.

[10] Ibid., 1

[11] Ibid., 2, 31–33.

up from Dee the unique synthesis of "medieval optics with the star-worship of neoplatonic-Hermetic mysticism and with the Paracelsian notions of 'astral signatures.'"[12]

While interesting, Szulakowska's suggestion entails a number of problems, particularly in the assumption that all of Dee's works, from the *Propaedeumata aphoristica* of 1558 through the *Monas Hieroglyphica* of 1564 to the *Mathematicall Praeface* of 1570, reflect a single body of thought and a common Paracelsian underpinning of a cosmology in which creation was a process of separation of elements from prime matter.[13] I will return to Khunrath later; at this point I'm only concerned with Dee's Paracelsianism. Despite sharing some superficial elements, Dee's *Propaedeumata* and his *Monas* are significantly different in more fundamental respects, reflecting an important shift in philosophy between the two works. While the ideas of the *Propaedeumata* were complementary to the *Monas*—Dee acknowledged this when he issued a new edition of the *Propaedeumata* in 1568 with revisions reflecting the *Monas*—the new ideas of the *Monas* should not be read back to the earlier period. It is interesting that the passages in the *Propaedeumata* usually cited to indicate a unity with the *Monas* as well as a reflection of Paracelsian ideas are all from the later edition after Dee's study of Paracelsian literature was well established.[14] The *Monas*, because of its significant alchemical dimension and composition at the beginning of Dee's interest in Paracelsus, is the more likely to reflect Paracelsian influences, but there are no clear indications of any such influence, probably because the conception of the *Monas* was well along in its development by the time Dee started to discover Paracelsus. The core ideas of the *Monas* are not uniquely Paracelsian, as we will see below, and while Dee uses two terms also used in Paracelsian texts *(Gammaaea* for talisman and *Beryllisticus* for one who has visions in crystal), these had other derivations as well and the Paracelsian source is not crucial to the core ideas of the *Monas*.[15]

---

[12]Szulakowska, *John Dee and European Alchemy*, 1–2.

[13]Ibid., 3, and passim.

[14]Ibid., 27. She refers to John Dee's *Propaedeumata aphoristica*, found in *John Dee on Astronomy: 'Propaedeumata Aphoristica'* [1558 and 1568], trans. and ed. Wayne Shumaker (Berkeley: University of California Press, 1978), 77:162–163, of which the second, alchemical portion, was added in 1568; aphorism XXVI, 134–135, with its later added reference to Gammaaeas, a term used by Paracelsus for talismans, has been used similarly. For a broader discussion of the similarities and differences of the two works, see Clulee, *John Dee's Natural Philosophy*, 116–121.

[15]Clulee, *John Dee's Natural Philosophy*, 141, 280n106; Paracelsus, *Concerning the Nature of Things*, in *Paracelsus, The Hermetic and Alchemical Writings*, ed. and trans. Arthur Edward Waite, 2 vols. (London, 1894), 1:171; Allen G. Debus, "Introduction," in John Dee, *The Mathematicall Praeface to the Elements of Geometry of Euclid of Megara* (1570), ed. Allen G. Debus (New York: Science History Publications, 1975), 7.

Dee's later writings were on subjects that did not lend themselves to clear Paracelsian references, although Paracelsian influences do manifest themselves in the "conversations with angels" that increasingly absorbed Dee's attentions after 1581.[16] We are left with a large library of Paracelsian materials with indications that they were read and studied, but no demonstrable reflection of these studies in Dee's published writings.

So, is Dee a lost chapter in Paracelsianism? Not necessarily. Dee may not have published anything that articulated or disseminated Paracelsian ideas, but as Charles Webster has suggested, he may have planted some of the earliest seeds for Paracelsian studies in England through his library and teaching.[17] Much has been made of Dee's teaching Sir Philip Sidney (which has been disputed) and the English navigators. There is also evidence that he extensively gave instruction in alchemy and Paracelsian medicine. A notable feature of his library is the large number of duplicates, and even triplicates, which very likely were used as loaners and for teaching.[18] Some of Dee's surviving copies have individuals' names inscribed and noted as "discipulus," and his diary also notes others studying with him.[19] A number of these individuals figure in the later development of English Paracelsianism. Richard Bostocke, whose *The difference betwene the auncient Phisicke … and the latter Phisicke* (1585) which Allen Debus identified as the first comprehensive English notice of Paracelsian theories, had a connection with Dee and his library.[20] Others include the surgeon John Woodall, whose *The Surgions Mate* (1617 and later editions) discusses Paracelsian principles and recommends chemical medicines. Woodall played a role in the disposition of Dee's estate and probably came into possession of large parts of Dee's alchemical and Paracelsian works as Dee's library was dispersed in the early seventeenth century.[21]

These connections are tantalizing and could use much more research and elaboration, but a couple of possibilities present themselves. First, Paracelsian medicine was filtering into England at least a decade earlier than the mid-1570s that Allen Debus has suggested, and Paracelsus' mystical universe was accessi-

---

[16]On the "conversations" and their alchemical themes, see Deborah E. Harkness, "Shows in the Showstone: A Theater of Alchemy and Apocalypse in the Angel Conversations of John Dee (1527–1608/9)," *Renaissance Quarterly* 49 (1996):707–737; and Deborah E. Harkness, *John Dee's Conversations with Angels: Practicing Natural Philosophy at the End of the World*, forthcoming.

[17]Charles Webster, "Alchemical and Paracelsian Medicine," in *Health, Medicine and Mortality in the Sixteenth Century*, ed. Charles Webster (Cambridge: Cambridge University Press, 1979), 316, 320–323.

[18]Roberts and Watson, *John Dee's Library Catalogue*, 42; Sherman, *The Politics of Reading*, 44.

[19]Roberts and Watson, *John Dee's Library Catalogue*: no. 1476, for example.

[20]Ibid., 42–43; Webster, "Alchemical and Paracelsian Medicine," 318–19.

[21]Roberts and Watson, *John Dee's Library Catalogue*, 61–68.

ble through the availability of Paracelsian books prior to Thomas Erastus' attack on it and Bostocke's defense of it.[22] While Paracelsus may have been an object of distrust and suspicion by English physicians during the Elizabethan period, among outsiders to the profession like Dee and his younger pupils, there was apparently openness and receptivity. On a practical note, it should be mentioned that Dee was sent abroad in 1578 by Leicester and Walsingham, possibly concerning Queen Elizabeth's health, and that during this trip he met with Leonhardt Thurneyesser, a major proponent of the Paracelsian analysis of urine.[23] This openness, receptiveness, and entertainment of new ideas, along with the collection of substantial published materials, constituted a foundation for the later development of Paracelsianism in England.

But it is not just later Paracelsians' interest in Dee's collections of Paracelsica that are of interest. Dee also attracted the interest of Paracelsians in his writings from an early date—in fact, almost as soon as the *Monas Hieroglyphica* was published in 1564. We get an indication of this from two of Dee's most notable characteristics. First, Dee had a particularly sharp sense of personal slights. His diaries and the several autobiographical passages and pieces he wrote are full of notes of insults and injuries both imagined and real. He was particularly sensitive to criticisms of the *Monas Hieroglyphica*. He points out that even Queen Elizabeth had to defend his credit against English academics who "dispraised it, because they understood it not."[24] In 1592, Dee projected a large work, "De Horizonte Aeternitatis," in reference to one of the mystically religious themes of the *Monas,* as a reply to Andreas Libavius' criticism of the *Monas* in the *Tractatus duo physici* (1594).[25]

In a passage attacking ideas of a cabalistic Jacob's ladder ascending from earth to heaven as "fooleries" *(ineptiae),* Libavius includes a brief, almost offhanded, reference to a Iohannes Dee, his hieroglyphic monad, and the diagram of the "Horizon Aeternitatis" (fig. 2) in which Dee tries to capture the culmination of the spiritual dimension of the *Monas.*[26] What makes this reference interesting is that it occurs in a work attacking the cure of wounds by

[22]Allen G. Debus, *The English Paracelsians* (New York: Franklin Watts, 1965), 49.

[23]John Dee, [Diary], Oxford, Bodleian Library, MS Ashmole, 487, 1578; John Dee, *The Compendious Rehearsall,* in John Dee, *Autobiographical Tracts,* ed. James Crossley, Chetham Society, Remains Historical and Literary of Lancaster and Chester Counties, 1 (1851): 21–22; Walter Pagel, *Paracelsus: An Introduction to Philosophical Medicine in the Era of the Renaissance,* 2d ed. rev. (Basel: S. Karger, 1982), 195–196.

[24]Dee, *Compendious Rehearsall,* 10, 19.

[25]Dee, *A Letter... apologeticall* (1592), in Dee, *Autobiographical Tracts,* 77–78.

[26]Andreas Libavius, *Tractatus duo physici* (Frankfurt, 1594), 41; Josten, "Introduction," 96; Frances A. Yates, *The Rosicrucian Enlightenment* (London: Routledge and Kegan Paul, 1972), 52.

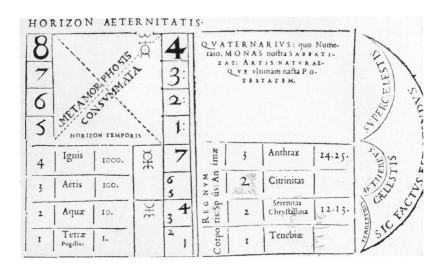

Fig. 2. "Horizon Aeternitatis," John Dee, *Monas Hieroglyphica*, fol. 27. (Rare Book and Special Collections Division, Library of Congress).

means of a weapon salve, the origin and practice of which Libavius attributes to the Paracelsians. There is no indication that Libavius is attacking Dee as a Paracelsian or the *Monas* as a whole; in his later *Alchymia* (1606) Libavius even discusses, without obvious signs of disapproval, Dee's monas symbol as an artificial language referring to the combination of constituents in chemical compounds.[27] What attracts Libavius' ire in both the *Alchymia* and in the *Tractatus duo physici* is Dee's failure to respect disciplinary boundaries by merging alchemy with theosophy. It is in this introduction into questions of medicine and physics of inappropriate considerations—including astral influences, magic, and the cabalistic interconnection of terrestrial, celestial, and supercelestial of Dee's "Horizon aeternitatis"—that Libavius finds the root of the reasoning he claims has been used to support the efficacy of a cure applied to the weapon rather than the wound.[28] It is this that bears the brunt of Libavius' attack. While the individuals Libavius attacks are a hodgepodge, not all with obvious connections to Paracelsus, the assumption of occult influences and

[27]William R. Newman, "Alchemical Symbolism and Concealment: The Chemical House of Libavius," in *The Architecture of Science*, ed. Peter Galison and Emily Thompson (Cambridge, Mass.: MIT Press, forthcoming). I wish to thank William Newman for sharing this with me before publication.
[28]Libavius, *Tractatus duo physici*, 34–43.

the interrelation of celestial and terrestrial, which Libavius sees as the foundation of the weapon salve, are attacked wherever he finds them. In this process, Libavius defined an intellectual frame that allowed him to see Paracelsians and a host of others, including Dee, in the same camp. Dee did have an explicit relationship to some in this camp; he was indebted to Pico della Mirandola and Cornelius Gemma for the cabalistic idea of the horizon of eternity. Even though Dee may have had no explicit relationship to others in this camp, including the Paracelsians, Libavius' polemic laid foundations for Dee's association with them nonetheless. There was, however, also more than this arbitrary connection, because Dee and his monas had, indeed, been taken up by Paracelsians in their own right, who also saw similarities.

We are led to the earliest example of this association by Dee's other notable trait: his particularly sharp sense of intellectual property. Dee seems to have assiduously watched for any use of his work by others, and he was quick to pounce when he noticed even the slightest unacknowledged borrowings. From the publication of his first work, the *Propaedeumata Aphoristica* of 1558, Dee maintained a campaign claiming that a Joannes Offusius had used his ideas without attribution.[29] Likewise, when Gerhard Dorn published the *Chymisticum Artificium Naturae* in 1568 with Dee's monas symbol on the title page, Dee was quick to notice. The New York Society Library, as part of its collection of remnants of John Winthrop, Jr.'s, alchemical library, has Dee's signed copy of Dorn's *Chymisticum Artificium* (fig. 3), snapped up undoubtedly as part of Dee's collection of Paracelsica.[30] Dee's monas symbol appears prominently at the center of Dorn's diagram, below which Dee notes the use of his symbol without any kind of acknowledgment or gratitude.[31]

Dorn was one of the major propagators of Paracelsianism in the later sixteenth century, so the appearance of Dee's monas on Dorn's title page promises some connection of Dee with Paracelsus in a Paracelsian's mind.[32] Before

[29]John Dee, *A Necessary Advertisement*, in John Dee, *Autobiographical Tracts*, 58–59.

[30]On John Winthrop, Jr., and his collection, see Ronald Sterne Wilkinson, "The Alchemical Library of John Winthrop, Jr. (1606–1676) and his Descendents in Colonial America," *Ambix* 9 (1963):33–51, and *Ambix* 10 (1966): 139–186. The Dorn is no. 65. This is New York Society Library no. 86.

[31]Dee's note reads, "Iste, ex nostra Monade Hieroglyphica Characteres istos novos formare didicit cum sine venia nostra, tum sine grata nostri mentione."

[32]Gerhard Dorn is less studied and consequently less well known than he ought to be as a major propagator of Paracelsian ideas in the later sixteenth century. Martha Teach Gnudi, "Dorn, Gerard," in *Dictionary of Scientific Biography*, provides a starting point. To this should be added Jean-François Marquet, "Philosophie et alchimie chez Gérard Dorn," in *Alchimie et philosophie à la renaissance*, ed. Jean-Claude Margolin and Sylvain Matton (Paris: J. Vrin, 1993), 215–221; and Didier Kahn, "Les débuts de Gérard Dorn d'après le manuscrit autographe de sa *Clavis totius Philosophiae Chymisticae* (1565)," in *Analecta Paracelsica*, ed. Joachim Telle (Stuttgart: Steiner, 1994), 59–126.

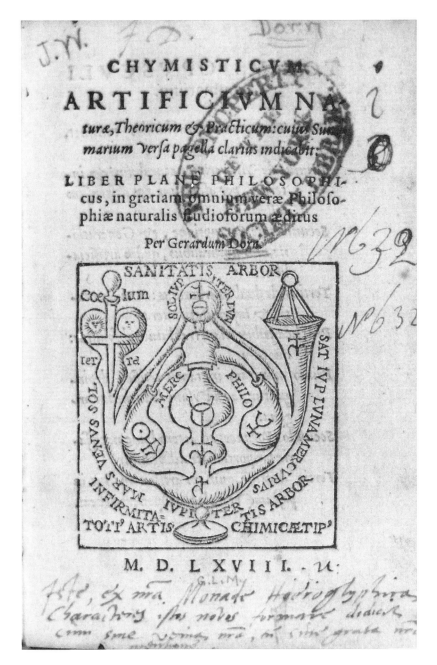

Fig. 3. Title Page, Gerhard Dorn, *Chymisticum Artificium Naturae*, 1568. (New York Society Library; Photograph by David Ortiz Photography.)

120

looking at Dorn to see what this might be, it will help to have a basic idea of Dee's *Monas Hieroglyphica,* which, for all its brevity, does not lend itself to brief synopsis.

The work centers on the diagram and symbol that is Dee's hieroglyphic monad (fig. 4). This monad, which is generated exclusively from a point, a line, and a circle (fig. 5), reveals the process of creation because "the first and most simple manifestation" of things happened by means of the straight line and the circle, but, since the line is generated by the flowing of a point and the circle by a line rotated around a point, "things first began to be by way of a point and a monad."[33] The geometrical process of the construction of the monas captures the essence of cosmogony, and the resulting symbol epitomizes all creation (fig. 6). The point represents the earth and the circle represents both the sun and the entire frame of the heavens surrounding the earth. The semicircle represents the moon, and the double semicircle at the base represents the zodiacal sign of Aries, the first sign of the zodiac and the sign under which creation took place, and suggests the entire zodiac and the fixed stars. While the circular components of the monas relate to the heavens, Dee relates the cross, composed of straight lines in four segments, to the sublunar realm of the elements.[34]

This correspondence of both the construction of the monas to divine creation and of the derived components and meanings to constituents and processes of the natural world is the key to Dee's central claim to have discovered a new and sacred art of writing or language that is an alphabet of nature and a "writing of things" because it corresponds to the "written memorial…which from the Creation has been inscribed by God's own fingers on all Creatures" and which therefore speaks of "all things visible and invisible, manifest and most occult, emanating by nature or art from God himself."[35] As a language of nature, the cabalistic techniques of *notarikon, tsiruf,* and *gematria* can be applied to the monas and its components to reveal an esoteric knowledge of creation through what Dee called the "cabala of the real" or the "cabala of that which exists."[36] So, when Dee has the point represent the earth, this is a kind of *notarikon* in which symbols represent words and concepts. As in *tsiruf,* in which individual letters of words are rearranged to find other words, the parts of the monas can be recombined to yield other symbols and meanings.[37] Thus, the monas can be disassembled into the various components shown in the center of fig. 7. These can be combined as in the figure marked α, which Dee

---

[33]John Dee, *Monas Hieroglyphica,* in C.H. Josten, "A Translation…," *Ambix* 12 (1964): 154–155.
[34]Dee, *Monas Hieroglyphica,* 154–161.
[35]Ibid., 124–125.   [36]Ibid., 132–135.   [37]Ibid., 160–165, 194–197.

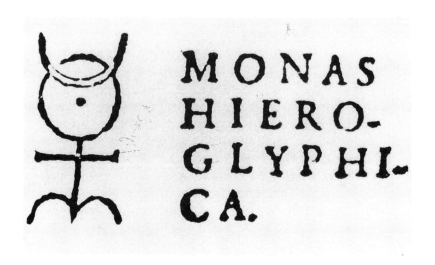

Fig. 4. Monas hieroglyphica, John Dee, *Monas Hieroglyphica,* fol. 12. (Rare Book and Special Collections Division, Library of Congress.)

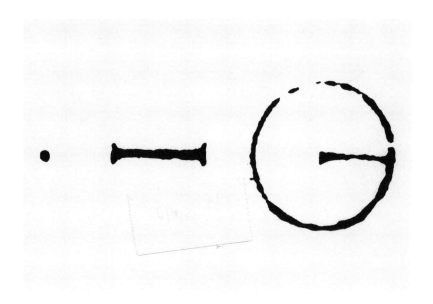

Fig. 5. Point, line, and circle, John Dee, *Monas Hieroglyphica,* fol. 12. (Rare Book and Special Collections Division, Library of Congress.)

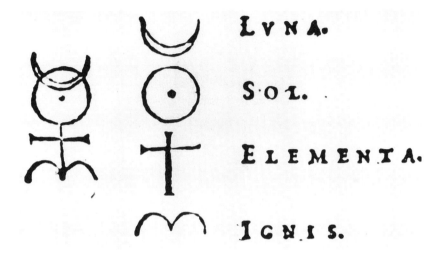

Fig. 6. Monas and cosmos, John Dee, *Monas Hieroglyphica,* fol.13v. (Rare Book and Special Collections Division, Library of Congress.)

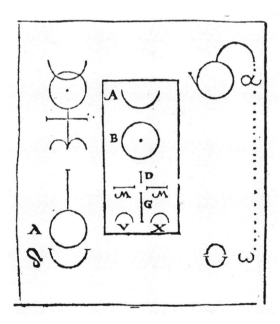

Fig. 7. Alchemical *notarikon,* John Dee, *Monas Hieroglyphica,* fol. 22. (Rare Book and Special Collections Division, Library of Congress.)

123

claims resembles a wine flask, a retort, and, with a slight alteration, the Greek letter *alpha*. Likewise, ω is another vessel and the Greek *omega*, and δ (Gk. *delta*) and λ (Gk. *lambda*) represent a mortar and pestle. These same pieces may be combined and oriented in such a fashion that symbols for all the planets in addition to the sun and the moon are contained within the monas (fig. 8). In *gematria* the numerical equivalents of letters are used, a technique Dee applies to the "cross of the elements," which yields the quaternary as well as five (V), ten (X), fifty (L), and a host of other numbers based on these.[38]

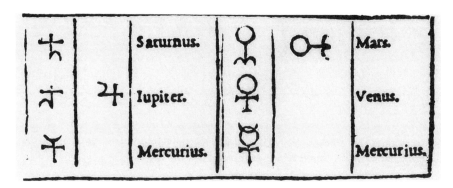

Fig. 8. Signs of the planets generated from the monas, John Dee, *Monas Hieroglyphica*, fol. 14. (Rare Book and Special Collections Division, Library of Congress.)

While this idea of a language of nature is as central to the *Monas* as is alchemy, which has often been seen as its central subject, Dee illustrates the power of this "cabala of the real" primarily by applying it to illuminating the alchemical process, which for Dee was encompassed by two themes from the *Tabula Smaragdina* or *Emerald Tablet* of Hermes Trismegistus. The first theme is the monadic character of the philosophers' stone (the *una res*) from which all things are produced similar to the creation of the universe from the unitary word of God. The second theme is the interdependence of the terrestrial and the celestial. The *una res* can accomplish miracles because "what is below is like that which is above, and what is above is like that which is below"; therefore, it is necessary "to ascend with greatest sagacity from the earth to heaven, and then again descend to the earth, and unite together the powers of things superior and things inferior."[39] Key to Dee's understanding of these themes was

[38]Ibid., 158–59,168–173.
[39]John Read, *Prelude to Chemistry: An Outline of Alchemy, Its Literature and Relationships* (London: Oldbourne, 1961), 54; Clulee, *John Dee's Natural Philosophy*, 105.

Johannes Trithemius' idea of the alchemy of the *Emerald Tablet* as a magic by which composites of the four elements are reduced to purity, simplicity, and unity by fire. For Trithemius, the essence of magic is a process by which diversity is restored to unity. All things proceed from an original creative monad, which is the source of all numbers. The order, number, and measure that establish the harmony of the universe are governed by the Pythagorean tetractys through which diversity returns to unity in the decade through the ternary and the quaternary. It is through understanding these numbers that the soul can ascend to mystical insights, gain insight into occult mysteries, and achieve the power to perform miraculous feats, one of which is the alchemical work.[40]

Dee pulls all this together by applying the cabalistic devices of his new language of nature to the symbol of the monas. As a mirror of the cosmos, the symbol yields the symbols of the planets and the alchemical metals of the lower world. Cabalistic manipulations also reveal the parallel astronomical and alchemical processes through which the elements ascend through a series of seven revolutions corresponding to the planets and are restored to unity and purity in the monad (fig. 9).[41] In developing this process, Dee evokes both themes from the *Emerald Tablet* and numerological magic of Trithemius by showing how the elements of the earth, through the separation of the sun and the moon and the elimination of impurities, are restored through the binary, ternary, and quaternary to a purified unity.[42]

Besides explicating the core alchemical process of the cosmos and thereby revealing the unity of astronomy and alchemy *(astronomia inferior),* the sacred art of writing the cabala of the real has two other consequences. The first is that the natural philosopher, by mastering this language, is given access to the innermost secrets of the cosmos, raising the philosopher to the level of "adeptship." Adeptship grants the philosopher command of a cabalistic magic that includes mastery of the "magic of the elements" (alchemy), but also a spiritual magic that opens the way to the "horizon aeternitatis."[43] The second consequence is that the new discipline of hieroglyphic writing embodied in the monas implies a radical reorganization of the traditional disciplines. Not only does this new language supersede and replace the "vulgar" linguistic disciplines of grammar and Hebrew cabala; it transcends and almost makes obsolete the traditionally legitimate disciplines of arithmetic, geometry, music, astronomy, optics, and so forth, while at the same time legitimating and elevating in status esoteric disciplines including alchemy, divination, and magic that were traditionally considered illegitimate and marginalized.[44]

---

[40]Clulee, *John Dee's Natural Philosophy,* 104.
[41]Ibid., 106–109.   [42]Ibid., 110.   [43]Ibid., 110–114.   [44]Ibid., 83–86.

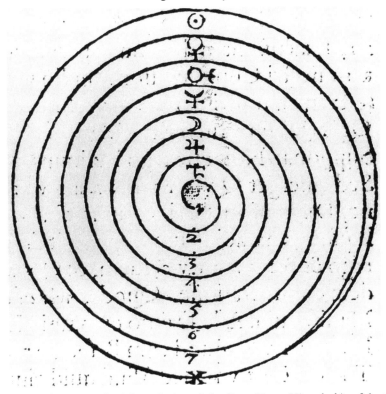

Fig. 9. The seven celestial revolutions, John Dee, *Monas Hieroglyphica,* fol. 18.
(Rare Book and Special Collections Division, Library of Congress.)

With this background, we are better prepared to turn to Dorn to see what use he made of Dee's *Monas* in conjunction with Paracelsus in his *Chymisticum Artificium Naturae.* While there are reflections of Dee's monas in a number of Dorn's works, I will confine my consideration to just the *Chymisticum* because this is the first reflection of Dorn's awareness of Dee and it reveals the central ground for Dorn's interest in the monas. On first view, however, we might be disappointed. Although Dorn's purpose in *Chymisticum Artificium Naturae* is the defense of chemical medicines, Paracelsus is not mentioned until the very end, and then only once, but quite importantly as the inventor of these medicines to whom alone gratitude is owed.[45] The *Chymisticum* of 1568 is a very early work, coming just shortly after Dorn's "conversion" to Paracelsianism sometime between 1565 and 1566, which may explain its tentativeness.[46] Other than the appearance of Dee's symbol on the title page embedded within a

45Dorn, *Chymisticum artificium naturae,* 150.
46Kahn, "Les débuts de Gérard Dorn," 93–102.

richer, more realistic, and we might say more baroque image (see fig. 3), Dorn makes no mention of Dee or the *Monas Hieroglyphica*. Perhaps all that caught Dorn's attention in the *Monas* was a clever new symbol. The only thing in the text that might point to further inspiration from Dee is a diagram of alchemical vessels derived from breaking down Dorn's title page image reminiscent of Dee's derivation of symbols of vessels from the *Monas* (fig. 10). Dorn's diagram, however, is not the central subject of his text in the way Dee's monas is to the *Monas,* nor does Dorn's text develop the diagram systematically. In Dorn there is nothing of adeptship, or of the language of nature and cabala of the real, or of the reorganization of the disciplines. If Dee's *Monas* was an inspiration, Dorn has filtered out Dee's most notable elements.

If we look at how Dorn defends chemical medicines—by placing their derivation and efficacy within a broad chemical philosophy—we can see something else which Dorn may have associated with Dee. Dorn develops the Paracelsian claim for chemical medicines as based on an ancient wisdom with roots in Egypt and the *Emerald Tablet* of Hermes Trismegistus. Chemical medicines counter corruption and illness by drawing out life with their infusion of celestial influences.[47] This is because the production of chemical medicines replicates the cosmic process, and he quotes explicitly from the *Emerald Tablet* at this point, of ascent and descent and the restoration of diversity to unity and purity through a series of chemical operations mirroring the relations of the planets.[48] Dorn also relates this process to Trithemius' concept of alchemy as a magic reducing multiplicity to unity through the quaternary, ternary, and binary.[49]

In Didier Kahn's recent study of Dorn's intellectual evolution, the discovery of Trithemius and the *Tabula Smaragdina* turns out to be an important complement to his adoption of Paracelsian medicine and alchemy.[50] In the chemical philosophy as Dorn develops it, the *Emerald Tablet* and Trithemius' numerology of alchemical magic become a major component of Paracelsian medicine and alchemy. Here we may have the deeper grounds for Dorn's adoption of Dee's symbol. It was clearly not because of any Paracelsianism on Dee's part; Dorn became a proponent of Paracelsus before he showed any awareness of Dee and his monas. Dorn was also clearly becoming interested in

---

[47]Dorn, *Chymisticum artificium naturae*, 12–21. Kahn, "Les débuts de Gérard Dorn," 93, points out that a major part of the *Chymisticum* is a commentary on the *Tabula smaragdina*. For a concise synopsis of Dorn's chemical philosophy, rooted in these key ideas, see Marquet, "Philosophie et Alchimie chez Gérard Dorn," 215–221.

[48]Dorn, *Chymisticum artificium naturae*, 69–72. [49]Ibid., 107–115.

[50]Kahn, "Les débuts de Gérard Dorn," 84–87, 93–103.

PRAXIS. 83

quæ suffecerit: cuius rei caufam poni-
mus, Spirituũ effe naturam, vt ad fubli-
mia tendant, non ad inferiora: quare fa
cilius lateraliter, quàm in decliue, pro-
filiunt. His organis A. B. defignatis,

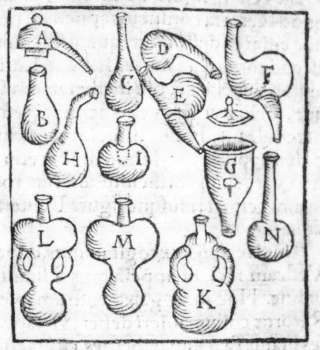

ea, quæ fucco magis abvndant, folent
deftillari: quia liberius afcendunt, &
eorũ Mercurius facilius, quàm Mars,
attollitur.
    Ad roftrum galeæ vas recipiens ap-
            F ij   plica-

Fig. 10. Alchemical vessels, Gerhard Dorn, *Chymisticum Artificium Naturae*, 83
(New York Society Library; photograph by David Ortiz Photography.)

128

Trithemius' ideas and the *Tabula Smaragdina* before he knew of Dee. Kahn suggests that the appearance of Dee's *Monas* and its appeal to Dorn were serendipitous; after synthesizing Paracelsus and Trithemius, whose philosophy involved rejecting the binary for the ternary, Dorn found in Dee's *Monas* the completion of the triad through appropriation of the monas to ornament his title page.[51] But it may also be that Dorn found in Dee confirmation of his own grounding of a chemical philosophy in Trithemius and the *Tabula Smaragdina*. At a minimum, Dorn found in the *Monas Hieroglyphica* not just a clever symbol, but one that Dee developed to epitomize the same key elements on which Dorn based his chemical philosophy, a philosophy that becomes a key companion of Paracelsianism from this point into the seventeenth century. Not only, as William Newman has suggested, did Trithemius' interpretation of the *Emerald Tablet* as a cosmic process, not just a veiled recipe, become a crucial but too little recognized component of alchemical thought in this period; he also experienced a reinvigorated influence in conjunction with the "Paracelsian Revival."[52] While the Paracelsian movement defended Trithemius against the critics of his magic, Trithemius' theory of alchemical magic and interpretation of the *Emerald Tablet* provided key components of the Paracelsian chemical philosophy.

Among others, Dee was significant for picking up on the importance of Trithemius' vision and giving it a particular if idiosyncratic expression, and this gave Dee's *Monas* a lasting appeal. Given the reputation of his "conversations with angels," Dee's was perhaps a name to be conjured with, but he was not one of the "big" names of his age, so he was rarely mentioned by name. Like Dorn, few understood the peculiarities of his cabala of the real or his suggestions for a reorganization of the disciplines. What Dorn indicates is that Dee's *Monas* was rich and multifaceted; he and others could read Dee selectively and adopt facets of the *Monas* without leaving indications of its more obvious features.[53] But if we look carefully, we can find the *Monas*, as symbol and as text, showing up frequently and usually in a Paracelsian, or perhaps we

[51]Ibid., 103.

[52]William Newman, "Thomas Vaughan as an Interpreter of Agrippa von Nettesheim," *Ambix* 29 (1982): 129–130; Kahn, "Les débuts de Gérard Dorn," 103; important studies of Trithemius in this context are Noel Brann, "The Shift from Mystical to Magical Theology in the Abbot Trithemius (1462–1516)," *Studies in Medieval Culture* 11(1977): 147–159; and Noel Brann, "Was Paracelsus a Disciple of Trithemius?" *Sixteenth Century Journal* 10 (1979): 71–82.

[53]For instance, Jacques Gohory (Leo Suavius I.G.P. [Iacobus Gohory Parisiensis]), *Theophrasti Paracelsi Philosophiae et Medicinae utriusque universae, Compendium* (Paris, 1567; reprinted Basel, 1568), 200–201, another agent of the "Paracelsian Revival," also incorporated elements from Dee's *Monas*.

should say within a Smaragdine/Trithemian, context. I can only hint in the following at some of the avenues that I and others are or will be pursuing in the future.

Most students of Dee know of Thomas Tymme, who left some manuscript notes in preparation for an English translation of the *Monas*. The focus of Tymme's fragmentary notes is on the *Monas* as a work of alchemy, but it was most likely the spiritual dimension of Dee's work that truly engaged Tymme. An important contributor to English Paracelsianism through his translation of Joseph Duchesne, Tymme traversed a spiritual odyssey from Anglican clergyman through Calvinist reformer that culminated in a search for God in the *prisca sapientia* of the occult sciences, which brought him to Dee and the *Monas*, whose spiritual dimension met a felt need.[54] Another English Paracelsian, John Tishbourn, who translated a number of Paracelsian works, was also the copyist of a number of alchemical manuscripts which include Dee's monas symbol. These manuscripts are associated with the circle around Dee and Edward Kelly in Prague and ended up in the Royal Library in Copenhagen.[55]

Outside of England, I've already mentioned the number of sixteenth- and seventeenth-century manuscript copies and translations of the *Monas Hieroglyphica*. We've also noted Heinrich Khunrath's interest in light and optics, which he combined with a clear sense of Dee's *Monas* and its concordance with his Paracelsianism.[56] Khunrath cites the *Monas* and as refers to Dee's discussion of cabala in Dee's "aphorisms to the Parisians."[57] Khunrath's association of optics with alchemy may well have been a result of his meeting with Dee in 1589. The unity of alchemy and astronomy/astrology, developed in the *Monas* under the inspiration of the *Emerald Tablet,* led him to modify the 1568

[54]Tymme, *A Light in Darkness,* Oxford, Bodleian MSS Ashmole 1440, pp. 170–171; and Ashmole 1459, pp. 469–481; David Harley, "Becoming a Disciple of Dee: The Spiritual Journey of Thomas Tymme" (paper presented at John Dee: An Interdisciplinary Colloquium, Birkbeck College, University of London, April 20–21, 1995).

[55]Webster, "Alchemical and Paracelsian Medicine," 324; Jan Bäcklund, "Edward Kelly's Career in the Court of Rudolph II: Some New MSS References in Copenhagen" (paper presented at John Dee: An Interdisciplinary Colloquium Birkbeck College, University of London, April 20–21, 1995).

[56]Szulakowska, *John Dee and European Alchemy,* 2, 32–33.

[57]Ibid., 32, quotes Khunrath as follows: "Huc pertinet Cabalisticum Gimetria; Teusrasche; et Neoteriken. [*sic*] Sive (ut Joannes ab Dee Londoniensis exprimit, in suis ad Parisienses Aphorismis, et in Praefatione ad Regem Maximilianum Monadi Hieroglyphicae praefixa) Geometria, Notariacon et Tzyruph ...." Szulakowska takes the reference to the "Parisienses Aphorismis" to be to the *Propaedeumata Aphoristica,* but this is impossible. The *Propaedeumata* was not addressed to the Parisians. The "Parisienses Aphorismis" are mentioned by Dee in the *Monas* as dealing with cabala, as Khunrath is aware, and are most likely the unpublished and now lost *Cabbalae Hebraicae compendium tabella* of 1562. See Dee, *Monas,* 134-137; Clulee, *John Dee's Natural Philosophy,* 83.

edition of the *Propaedeumata* to suggest the concordance of the two works. By the time of his meeting with Khunrath, Dee's study of Paracelsian literature may have resulted in his discussing these two works with Khunrath in a Paracelsian framework, but, as we have seen with Dorn, there were elements in Dee's work that a Paracelsian could relate to without Dee's providing any explicit Paracelsian associations.

The reflections of Dee's *Monas* in the Rosicrucian texts, again in a Paracelsian context, have also been noted often. Khunrath's association of light and optics with the *Monas* looks forward to one of the most interesting of these, the *Consideratio brevis* of Philipp à Gabella that accompanies the *Confessio fraternitatis R.C.* Structured on the *Emerald Tablet,* this not only quotes extensively from Dee's *Monas,* as some have noted, but also develops the connection of astral optics with alchemy with quotations from his *Propaedeumata aphoristica,* something I will explore further in the future.[58] We do not need Yates' intimations of Dee's hidden connections in eastern Europe to explain Dee's reflection in the Rosicrucian texts; all we need is the perception, discovered by a number of people, of the consonance of the *Monas* with the Smaragdine/Trithemian elements in the chemical philosophy.

At this preliminary stage, in conclusion, Dee's relation to Paracelsus and the Paracelsians seems fundamentally ambiguous. Dee collected and read widely in the Paracelsian literature; he may have taught Paracelsian alchemy and medicine, or at least been a center for their diffusion in England, and he may have even practiced Paracelsian medicine. A good deal more research on Dee's students and associates might yield clearer results on this score. On the other hand, his published works and writings do not indicate that he "became" a Paracelsian, and besides some possible reflections of his Paracelsian readings, they do not embody a distinctly Paracelsian message. The paradox is that it was among Paracelsians that Dee's writings had their greatest audience and that Dee had his greatest future influence, primarily through the *Monas Hieroglyphica.* This text, for all its brevity, is extremely rich. As we have seen, it could be read selectively to meet a variety of interests, but the core of its appeal among Paracelsians was Dee's embodiment in the clever symbol of the monas of a Smaragdine/Trithemian alchemical cosmology that was an important component of the "Paracelsian Revival."

---

[58] T. M. Luhrmann, "An Interpretation of the *Fama fraternitatis* with respect to Dee's *Monas Hieroglyphica,*" *Ambix* 33 (1986): 1–10. Philipp à Gabella, *Secretioris Philosophiae Consideratio brevis* (Kassel, 1615).

SVPERCAELESTES ✳   ET TERRA FRVCTVM
RORETIS AQVAE.   DABIT SVVM.

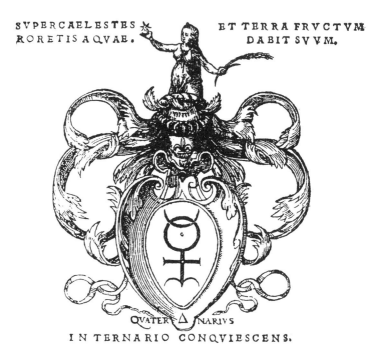

QVATER △ NARIVS
IN TERNARIO CONQVIESCENS.

Excufum Londini apud Re‑
ginaldum Vuolfium, Regiæ Maieft.
in Latinis Typographum.
ANNO DOMINI M.D.LXVIII.
Ianuarij.9.

Ana Maria Alfonso-Goldfarb

AN "OLDER" VIEW ABOUT MATTER IN JOHN WILKINS' "MODERN" MATHEMATICAL MAGICK

THERE WOULD APPEAR TO BE NOTHING MORE to be said about John Wilkins and his role in seventeenth-century British science. Acclaimed by his contemporaries as one of the leading scholars to introduce into Britain the scientific novelties of the time, he was often mentioned in the first chronicles of the Royal Society, of which he had been not only an active member, but also one of its founders—after engaging himself in the establishment of other scientific groups in Cambridge, Oxford, and London. "Thank God, that Dr. Wilkins was an Englishmen, for wherever he had lived, there had been the chief Seat of generous knowledge and true Philosophy," commented Robert Hooke, a close associate of Wilkins who also upheld the new science in contemporary controversies.[1] It is hardly necessary to detail further why Wilkins is always

---

[1] In the complete version of this quotation, Hooke also considers that most of the British "inventions" of the time somehow were "set forward with his assistance," according to the "Introduction" in his *Micrographia* (London: Martyn & Allestry, 1665); regarding the same issue, see for instance Boyle's opinions in his *Works,* ed. T. Birch, vol. 5 (London: A. Millar, 1744), 630; J. Evelyn, *Diary,* rev. ed., E. de Beer, vol. 1 (Oxford: Clarendon Press, 1955), 403; T. Sprat, *History of the Royal Society,* ed. J. Cope and H. Jones (Saint Louis: Washington University Studies, 1958), particularly 94, in which Sprat suggests that even his text would be under Wilkins' orientation. Regarding the above-mentioned controversies in which he was involved, see A. Ross, *The New Planet no Planet, Or, The Earth no Wandring Star* (London: J. Young, 1646); H. Stubbe, *A Censure upon Certain Passages Contained in the History of the Royal Society,* 2d ed. (Oxford: R. Davis, 1671); moreover, about the Ward/Wilkins *vs.* Webster debate, see A. Debus, *Science and Education in the Seventeenth Century* (London/New York: Macdonald/American Elsevier, 1970), which contains reproductions of J. Webster's *Academiarum examen* and Wilkins and Ward's *Vindiciae academiarum.*

mentioned among the major English virtuosi even though he did not author a paramount scientific theory.[2]

Likewise, it would be superfluous to explain why most scholars interested in the ancients versus moderns debate consider Wilkins the perfect example of a "modern." Regarded as crucial for the transference and the adaptation of the new cosmology to the British Isles, his work has been studied in that spirit. Particularly his *Mathematical Magick*—beyond doubt Wilkins' most mature writing—has been closely scrutinized, largely because it may have been one of the most influential sources of the so-called mechanical philosophy in the new, golden generation of British "natural philosophers."[3] Consequently, analyses of this work have overrated the clear and direct way Wilkins discusses obscure or polemical issues, to such an extent that it has become a cliché. According to such studies, the *Mathematical Magick* rids bizarre *automata,* magnetic effects, and other magical references to the burden of secrecy, and rationally explains them in conformity with the objective canons of the new "mechanical science." Such a characteristic is taken to thoroughly account for the success attained by this work, which fascinated the British public and attracted youngsters to the cause of the new science until it became obsolete and lost its relevance after the eighteenth century.[4] Could there be more to say

---

[2]See for instance the long references to Wilkins in traditional works about British science such as J. G. Crowther, *Founders of British Science* (reprint, Westport: Greenwood Press, 1982), 16–50; D. Stimson, *Scientist and Amateurs* (New York: H. Schuman, 1948), 33 ff., 78 ff., 105 ff.; M. Purver, *The Royal Society: Concept and Creation* (London: Routledge & Kegan Paul, 1967), 64 ff., 102 ff., 154 ff.; there are also various articles depicting Wilkins only as a symbol of modern British science, as W. T. Stearn, "J. Wilkins, J. Ray and C. Linnaeus,"*Notes and Records of Royal Society of London*, 40, no. 2 (1986): 101–123.

[3]Naturally Wilkins is stressed as "modern" particularly by R. F. Jones in his*Ancient and Moderns* (reprint, New York: Dover, 1982), esp. 120–121; but this idea also occurs in more extensive and recent studies on Wilkins such as M. H. Nicolson,*Voyages to the Moon* (New York: Macmillan, 1948); and mainly in B. Shapiro,*J. Wilkins: An Intellectual Biography* (Berkeley: University of California Press, 1969); this idea persists even nowadays, in studies in which he is mentioned as an example, as in W. Eamon, *Science and the Secrets of Nature* (Princeton: Princeton University Press, 1994), 309.

[4]This work was certainly well received for already in 1648, the year when it was first published, it was reprinted a second time. Next came the 1680 edition, which was reprinted in 1691. Finally, there was another reprint in 1708, together with the reedition of Wilkins' complete scientific work. The edition used here is *The Mathematical and Philosophical Works of J. Wilkins* (London: J. Nicholson, 1708). For more information about the various editions of this work, see Shapiro,*J. Wilkins*, 45. In 1802 this set of Wilkins' scientific works was simply reprinted in two volumes. Two decades ago, it had a one-volume exact facsimile reproduction in the Library of Science Classics, no. 11 (London: F. Cass, 1970), with no apparatus or additions, except for a brief presentation note by L. L. Laudan, general editor of this collection. However, a closer look at nineteenth-century accounts about the Royal Society and the origins of modern British science makes clear that works

about the *Mathematical Magick,* which today hardly seems to demand new studies since it seems to have been entirely probed? Nothing else, indeed, if one intends to stick to its traditional interpretation, which has transformed this book into a work foretelling of the Enlightenment and definitely modern. However, there is still a lot to be said about it should one consider it an early "mechanistic" and "modern" work, penned in the first half of the seventeenth century, when these concepts were taking shape. If seen as such, the *Mathematical Magick* appears to have two distinct sides, each demanding a different reading.

The first one is outlined in book 1, meaningfully titled "Archimedes, Or, Mechanical Powers," since it relies on many conceptions of the great Syracusan geometer.[5] In this book, the so-called simple machines are presented as elements capable of being mathematized and constituting the basis of the new mechanical theory. Although the teleological arguments developed in the Aristotelian treatise *On Mechanics* are discarded—after having been the main source of this subject for centuries—enough ideas from this work are preserved to establish an interplay with classical works by geometers such as Archimedes. Consequently, the book on "Archimedes, Or, Mechanical Powers" is a combination of *noeutica* and *doxa,* in compliance with the "modern" style of doing science.[6] Moreover, since he is borrowing from machinery the model to interpret each and every phenomenon of motion, Wilkins would be inserting a conspicuous mechanist bias in this part of his work. Up to this point, traditional studies about the *Mathematical Magick* could be considered accurate, were it not for the fact that its second book does not continue the procedures set up in the first one. In other words, the mechanical principles established on a nonteleological basis in book 1 are not necessarily implicit in the phenomena described in book 2, in which Wilkins seems to be resuming ancient conceptions about matter and motion.

---

such as Wilkins' had already been neglected by that time. See for instance T. Thompson, *History of the Royal Society* (London: R. Baldwin, 1812). This study does not even mention Wilkins' name in the section dedicated to "mechanical philosophy" (book 3, p. 311 and passim). See also H. B. Wheatley, *The Early History of the Royal Society* (Hertford: Stephen Austin & Sons, 1905—text read in 1894), in which Wilkins' name is included in an unorthodox list of presidents of the Royal Society (pp. 10–11); this happens once again in a list of those belonging to the anatomical committee of this Society (p. 35).

[5]Book 1, "Archimedes or Mechanical Powers," occupies the first eighty-four pages of the *Mathematical Magick,* which is the fourth work in the above-mentioned 1708 reedition. Pagination resumes at each work.

[6]It was called "mixed mathematics," an expression explicitly used by Wilkins, *Mathematical Magick,* 7, after a long explanation beginning on p. 2.

On closer inspection, book 2, titled "Daedalus, Or, Mechanical Motions,"[7] bears legends, prodigious facts, and sui generis explanations mingled with marvelous but practically unfeasible equipment and effects. Akin to ancient polygraphs such as Pliny's *Naturalis Historiae* or the so-called Renaissance *miscellanea curiosa,* the second book of Wilkins' *Mathematical Magick* sometimes even resembles more recent works, but all of them far from "mechanist" and little "modern."[8] "Daedalus" seems to bear another side of Wilkins' thought. Even though mainly written in a modern language, it is still turned to the ancient framework, requiring an adequate interpretation all anew. Among other things, traditional studies of this work have overlooked its concern with alchemy and ancient chemistry.

Strategically discussed in four short chapters, this comprehensive subject opens a very relevant section about the *perpetuum mobile.*[9] Nevertheless, it can be easily missed. For one thing, it has been discretely veiled by stories about eternal lamps that had shone in ancient mausoleums. Who would have thought that in these passages rested an interesting discussion about alchemy? After all, was not Wilkins supposed to be a champion against alchemy?[10] For that matter, Wilkins seems to begin this discussion exhibiting more doubts

[7]Wilkins, *Mathematical Magick,* 85–167.

[8]Although the content of book 2 of the *Mathematical Magick* resembles a work such as H. van Etten, *Mathematicall Recreations* (London: T. Cores, 1633), its argumentative structure is closer to a work such as A. Kircher, *Mundus subterraneus* (Amsterdam: J. Jansson & E. Weyerstraten, 1665); about the structure of the so-called Renaissance "miscellanea curiosa," see W. Shumaker, *Renaissance Curiosa,* vol. 8 (Binghamton: Medieval & Renaissance Texts & Studies, 1982); a more general commentary about this kind of literature is found in A. Grafton, "The World of the Polyhistors: Humanism and Encyclopedism," *Central European History* 18 (1985): 31–47; regarding the structure of ancient polygraphs, see for instance N. Howe, "In Defense of the Encyclopedic Mode: On Pliny's Preface to the Natural History," *Latomus* 44: 2 (1985): 561–576; or Pliny's own preface in Pliny, *Natural History,* Loeb Classical Library, reimpression (Cambridge, Mass.: Harvard University Press, 1991).

[9]Wilkins, *Mathematical Magick,* book 2, chaps. 9–12, pp. 129 and passim, mentions the notable equipment "wherein was represented the constant Revolution of the Sun and Moone" (132–133), built by C. Drebble for King James I. This is a good example of the enormous interest and the numerous and continuous speculations about the *perpetuum mobile* in that century. About this, see for instance G. Tierie, *Cornelius Drebble,* English translation (Amsterdam: H. J. Paris, 1932), 37–42; also, C. Drebelii, *Epistola ad Sapientissimum Britanniae Monarcham Iacobum, De perpetui mobilis inventione in Tractatus duo* (Geneva: Tournes, 1628). Yet, scholars like Galileo had warned that, in principle, this kind of instrument was unfeasible; cf. G. Galilei, *On Motion & On Mechanics,* trans. and ed. S. Drake (Madison: University of Wisconsin Press, 1960), 148.

[10]Such criticism in Wilkins' work has already been investigated by Shapiro, *J. Wilkins,* 45 and note. See also the *Vindiciae Academiarum;* cf. Debus, *Debate,* 228–230, in a text penned by S. Ward, but which certainly reflects Wilkins' position; the same position also occurs in T. Sprat, *History of the Royal Society,* 37, even though this time Wilkins is supposed to have been only a mentor of the text. As it shall be confirmed later, Wilkins' criticism was aimed at only a certain kind of alchemist.

than certainties about the alleged deeds of some alchemists, stating: "yet we can never see them confirmed by any real experiment." But the reason underlying his distrust soon becomes clearer:

> besides, every particular Author in that art, hath such a distinct language of his own, (all of them being so full of allegories and affected obscurities) that 'tis very hard for any one (unlesse hee bee thoroughly versed amongst them) to finde out what they mean, much more to try it.[11]

Other examples in the same chapter make clear that Wilkins does not intend to discredit the possibilities of alchemical work, but only to criticize some ways of doing it or to question the arguments used by certain alchemists.[12] Thus, in the following chapters about this subject, Wilkins makes it a point to give examples indicating that perpetual motion was possible by way of chemistry. And, since he believed that "violence and perpetuity" were not "companions," most of Wilkins' examples refer to the so-called eternal, or perpetual, lamps, which would have burned smoothly and constantly for ages.

A first-rate seventeenth-century scholar, Wilkins provides almost all the references where he found these examples. But they are so numerous, and heterogeneous, that to understand Wilkins' intentions demands an *apparatus fontium*, just like many ancient documents. On the whole, nearly thirty sources are ordered in the peculiar fashion of ancient doxographies, giving Wilkins' text an appearance far from modern. An analysis of these sources suggests that they may be classified into two basic groups.

One seems to be constituted by "authorized" or traditional sources. Works of classical authorities such as Aristotle's belonged to it, as well as those of a more recent author like Francis Bacon, referred to by Wilkins as "our learned Bacon." This group of sources also included distinguished polygraphs from all ages, ranging from Pliny's *Naturalis Historiae* to William Camden's *Britannia*. Last but not least, this group comprises Christian theological accounts. Of course preferably of a Reformed profile, these sources encompass the version of the Augustinian *De civitate Dei* which Erasmus had commissioned to Luis Vives, as well as the work of the Protestant theologian Girolamo Zanchi, called "the judicious" by Wilkins.[13]

---

[11]Wilkins, *Mathematical Magick*, 131.

[12]As it is known, these reproaches were common even in traditional works on alchemy. Although the need of secrecy was a maxim for most alchemical authors, it is unnecessary to stress that, in time, accusations of lack of clarity and minimal explanations to understand mutual texts also became traditional among these writers. Such a criticism occurs for instance in R. Bacon, *Fr. Rogeri Bacon: Opera quaedam hactinus inedita*, ed. J. S. Brewer (London: Bell & Sons, 1859), 39–41.

[13]Since the works mentioned above also occur in the present text, to avoid an unnecessary repetition, their references shall not be repeated here. The numerous sources used in the present analysis were not included here because most of them are explicit in Wilkins' writing.

The second group of sources related to this subject comprised assorted works, including treatises about curious natural phenomena and wonders fostered by technique, as well as "books of secrets"—which might seem unexpected in a book supposedly modern such as Wilkins' *Mathematical Magick*. In this group of *opera*, popular works such as Joannes Wecker's *De secretis* or Della Porta's *Magiae naturalis* are given equal treatment with the *Confession* of the Rosicrucian fraternity,[14] and a hermetic treatise. This comprehensive group seems to embrace less "authorized" sources—some of them only implicitly alluded to.

While analyzing the articulation of these two groups of sources is not a simple task, explaining why Wilkins strategically resorted to them is far easier. Possibly realizing that he was going too far in his speculations when referring to the "perpetual lamps," this scholar explains:

> Though it be not so proper to the chief purpose of this discourse, which concerns *Mechanical Geometry*, yet the subtlety and curiosity of it, may abundantly require the impertinency.

And, to better justify such boldness, Wilkins subsequently announces that:

> There are sundry Authors, who treat of this subject … out of whom I shall borrow many of those relations and opinions, which may most naturally conduce to the present enquiry.[15]

Consequently, authorized testimonies about the perpetual lamps found in ancient mausoleums or secret chambers precede or involve less authorized ones. For instance, after initially referring to a lamp that "continued burning for 1,050 years" mentioned by Saint Augustine, Wilkins alludes to the lamp "related to … the sepulchre of Francis Rosicrosse, as is more largely expressed in the confession of that fraternity."[16] Likewise, Wilkins speaks of an example given by Della Porta, carefully fitting it between an account coming from an obscure but safe fifteenth-century humanist and the report given by Fortunius

---

[14]Wilkins, *Mathematical Magick*, 136, refers to the *Confession*. However, as it shall be seen later on, the document was actually the *Fame*. Such a mistake is understandable since both works appear to have circulated together since 1633 in a British manuscript version; cf. F. N. Pryce, "Introduction" (particularly p. 3), in the 1923 facsimile edition, titled *Fame and Confession of the Fraternity of R. C.* (Margate: Societas Rosicruciana in Anglia), originally published in London in 1652.

[15]Wilkins, *Mathematical Magic*, 134.

[16]Ibid., 136; Augustine, *The Citie of God*, commented by L. Vives, 2d British ed. (London: G. Eld & M. Flesher, 1620), chap. 6, pp. 789–791; *Fama Fraternitatis or, A discovery of the Fraternity of the most laudable Order of the Rosy Cross*, 20–21.

Licetus, who according to Wilkins, is the only reliable author "that hath writ purposely any set and large discourse concerning it."[17]

Aware that he is dealing with a controversial theme, Wilkins searches for traditional theological support in books of the Old Testament, and goes as far as mentioning the occurrence of divine miracles that had renewed the ritual fire of the Jews.[18] Yet, what follows has nothing to do with the dogmatic arguments of theologians such as Saint Augustine and Zanchi, who considered these eternal fires either a divine miracle or a demoniacal or deceitful deed of human art.[19] Interestingly enough, probably due to his ideas about the so-called natural theology,[20] Wilkins trusts the data provided by other theologians, although he ignores their opinions. In the case above, for instance, he ends the array of miraculous references by immediately offering with obvious enthusiasm an interesting view of both natural and artificial possibilities of perpetual fires. To begin with, he mentions the opinion of a certain J. Gutherius, who had considered these fires neither long lasting nor eternal, but rather a phenomenon caused by new air entering into closed chambers: "As we see in those fat Earthy Vapours of divers Sorts, which are oftentimes enkindled into a Flame," adds Wilkins.[21] A believer in the benefits of technology as well as a

[17]Wilkins, *Mathematical Magick,* 135–136, J. B. Porta, *Natural Magick,* The Collector's Series in Science, ed. D. J. Price, 1658 British translation (New York: Basic Books, 1957), book 12, chap. 13; Wilkins only mentions the name of F. Maturantius and makes no reference to the work where he would have commented about the perpetual lamp found in Padua which was supposed to have been shining since Roman times. F. Maturantius, or Maturanzio, published most of his works in the fifteenth century. In the beginning of the following century, together with A. Mancinelli, he edited M. T. Cicero's *Rhetoricorum* (Paris: Paruo and Ascensio, 1508). The above-mentioned commentary occurs in the introduction, amidst many explanations about the ancient Romans. Indeed, as claimed by Wilkins, F. Liceti's book *De lucernis antiquorum reconditis* (Venice: E. Deuch, 1621) has been the only work entirely dedicated to the unique theme of perpetual lamps which we have been able to locate so far.

[18]Wilkins, *Mathematical Magick,* 139. To make such a statement, he finds support in chronicles none the less than Lev. 9:24, 2 Chron. 7:1, and 1Kgs. 18:38.

[19]In St. Augustine, *Die Civitate,* 789; and in Zanchi, *Operum theologicorum,* vol. 1, book 4 (Rome: Stephanus Gamonetus, 1605), 194.

[20]To better understand this fact concerning Wilkins' biography, see particularly B. Shapiro, "Latitudinarianism and Science in Seventeenth-Century England," in *The Intellectual Revolution of the Seventeenth Century,* Past and Present Series, ed. C. Webster (London: Routledge & Kegan Paul, 1974), 286–316; and extensive sequences in R. Westfall, *Science and Religion in Seventeenth-Century England* (Ann Arbor: University of Michigan Press, 1973), esp. chaps. 5, 7.

[21]Attractive to modern eyes at first sight, this opinion is not so "modern" in J. Gutherius' unique text, *De jure manium seu, de ritu, more, et legibus prisci funeris,* reimpression (Leipzig: H. Schurenian & J. Fritzsche, 1671). For instance, in 386 of book 2, chap. 32, he suggests that this very special phenomenon depended on "most subtle liquors." As will be seen later on, the conjecture that new air in closed chambers could cause the ignition of these lamps eventually disappears from Wilkins' text.

"natural theologian," Wilkins allowed room for unorthodox works about the wonders of art and nature, sometimes to supplement and other times to rearrange the arguments given by his classical or traditional sources. There seems to exist a coherence and a purpose underlying Wilkins' choice of sources. At first sight, analysis of their disposition is bound to bring out a structure very different from the *miscellanea curiosa* suggested by their heterogeneity. This structure is likely to share many common traits with some ancient documents, such as Isidore of Sevilles' encyclopedia, in which, underneath apparently entangled references and accounts, there is rigor in arrangement and argumentation after the fashion of classical authors.[22] As a matter of fact, Wilkins explicitly alludes to this formula when he says:

> For our fuller understanding of this [namely, accounts of perpetual lamps], there are these particulars to be explained:
>
> 1. ... *quod sit.*
> 2. ... *quomodo sit.*[23]

Thus, in accordance with the traditional convention, first comes a long survey detailing who, where, and when the existence of such lamps was given notice. Making up a second sequence, next there is a discussion of the speculations about the nature of these lamps and their *modus faciendi*. Since this last sequence constitutes an excellent place to appreciate more closely Wilkins' view about chemistry, it is worthwhile digressing at this point.

Wilkins begins this final discussion about perpetual lamps proposing two kinds of conjectures. The first was maintained by authors who thought these lamps "were not fire or flame, but only some of those bright bodies which do usually shine in dark places." Conversely, a second group of authors believed these lamps "to be fire, but yet think them to be then first enkindled by the admission of new air, when these sepulchres were opened."[24]

The second possibility was Wilkins' favorite, while the first served the classical principle of focusing on a problem from different sides, for the sake of argumentation. In fact, his preference and intent become clearer as he makes a brief *apparatus criticus* about luminescent bodies, even though resorting to authors who do not refer to perpetual lamps, as Aristotle speaking about some types of scales, stones, and the like, or Girolamo Cardano describ-

---

[22]About Isidore of Seville's encyclopedism, see for instance J. Fontaine, "Isidore de Séville et la Mutation de l'Encyclopédisme Antique," *Journal of World History* 9, no. 3 (1966): 519–538; also, in the same journal, 483–518, M. de Gandillac, "Encyclopédies pré-médiévales et médiévales"; better still, in Isidore's own work, cf. *Etymologiae* (Augsburg: G. Zainer, 1472).

[23]Wilkins, *Mathematical Magick,* 134.

[24]Ibid., 137–138.

ing the bird *Cocoyum* from New Spain. Even though briefly, he mentions the carbuncle, the legendary stone that "does shine in the dark like a burning coal, from whence it hath its name." He also provides the classical reference to this legend in Claudius Aelianus' *Historia animalium*, and mentions the recent opinion held by Anselmo de Boot, who, in his *Gemmarum et lapidum historia*, discards the existence of this fantastic stone.[25] Actually, Wilkins concluded that:

> none of these Noctiluca, or night-shining bodies, have been observed in any of the ancient sepulchres, and therefore this is a mere imaginary conjecture. And then besides, some of these lamps have been taken out burning, and continued so for a considerable space afterwards.[26]

Consequently, from then on, Wilkins concentrates his analyses on the possibility that these lamps were some form of eternal flame. Dedicating the last chapter entirely to this conjecture, he indicates in an opening gloss that he is actually discussing there, for the first time, the *quomodo* of these lamps.

It may be worth remembering that he had previously suggested the admission of new air in sepulchres as the reason why these lamps caught fire: "vapours of divers sorts, which are oftentimes enkindled into a flame." As has already been seen, following closely Gutherius' conjectures, Wilkins nearly arrives at ideas about ignition to be intensely investigated later on in his century, which gives a very modern flavor to his text. As shall be shown in more detail later on, in the last chapter about such lamps, he seems obsessed by investigating how to maintain these lamps' shining, if not eternally, at least throughout the ages, just as any ancient alchemist would tend to do.[27]

The two items which, according to Wilkins, should be considered in order to maintain this flame were the wick that keeps it burning, and the oil feeding it. He presumes that this wick could be made of some material that resisted fire and did not consume itself, like "Salamander wool," a mineral product mentioned by Bacon in his *Natural and Experimental History* as well

---

[25]Aristotle, *On the Soul* in *The Basic Works of Aristotle*, 27th reimpression, ed. R. McKeon (New York: Random House, 1941), book 2, chap. 7 (about perception of light and color); G. Cardano, *De subtilitate* (London: G. Rouillium, 1559), book 9; one notices that Wilkins relied on A. Boetius de Boot to refer to Claudius Aelianos, for de Boot used the same words about the *De historia animalium* before making his criticism; cf. A. Boetius de Boot, *Gemmarum et lapidum historia*, reedition (Leiden: Joannis Maire, 1647), chap. 8, pp. 140–141.

[26]Wilkins, *Mathematical Magick*, 138–139. By the way, this conclusion serves as an answer to the only source that raises the possibility that those eternal lamps might be luminescent bodies: F. Licetus, *De lucernis*, II.

[27]Wilkins, *Mathematical Magick*, 141 and passim; about the disappearance of Wilkins' ideas in this chapter, see n. 21.

as by other authors. Wilkins believed that it was nearly of the same nature as the *linum vivum* or *asbestinum* of the ancients, about which he tries to provide many references due to the fact that it was probably made of amianthus, a material confusedly identified and perhaps little known at his time. Since antiquity it has had a long history, both in the use of several names for the same thing and the same name encompassing several materials. In a way, Wilkins seems to realize that; whatever *linum vivus, asbestinum,* or Salamander wool was, whether it be amianthus, asbestos, or a certain plumeallum, these were just variations of the same theme.

Consequently, he says, "Some of this, or very like it, I have upon inquiry lately procured and experimented," and concludes raising the inconvenience that:

> it doth contract so much fuliginous matter from the earthy parts of the oyl (though it was tryed with some of the purest oyl…) that in a very few days it did choak and extinguish the flame.[28]

Unable to recall an account mentioning a wick in these lamps, he takes a new line of investigation to examine what made the flame perpetuate itself. Although he briefly mentions theologians' warnings against human or diabolic arts which eventually may become a means of rousing wonder and idolatry, as seen before, Wilkins is not diffident about presenting some of these possibilities. It is true that, more than ever, he blames his sources for the rather

---

[28]Wilkins, *Mathematical Magick,* 141–142; the passages quoted here are from p. 141. In a traditional source such as Dioscorides' text, which was not used by Wilkins possibly for reasons to be seen later on in this footnote, asbestos refers to quick-lime, while amianthus *(amiantos lithos)* encompasses the entire class of asbestos. In other words, to the modern eye, a portion would be naming the whole, cf. Dioscorides, *The Greek Herbal,* trans. J. Goodyer, 1655, edited and published for the first time in the English language only in 1934 by R. T. Gunther, reimpression (New York: Hafner, 1959), book 5, respectively, entries 133, 156. Pliny, in turn, according to the reference provided by Wilkins, cf. *Historia,* 19:2, seems to believe that the noncombustible material he is talking about is of vegetable origin; yet, he makes a specific reference to amianthus, or a sort of asbestos, in book 36, chapter 31, which is said to look like alum. Needless to say, myriad substances used to fall under this designation. For example, as mentioned by Wilkins, J. Wecker, s*De secretis;* cf. *Eighteen Books of the Secrets of Art & Nature,* ed. and trans. R. Read, vol. 3 (London: S. Miller, 1660), 2, 18, says that amianthus is considered an "alum stone," while on 14 of the same chapter, he considers the plumeallum, or "feathered" alum, a noncombustible material. Conversely, De Boot, *Gemarum,* vol. 2, c. 204, clearly identifies amianthus with asbestos, although he considered that the latter and plumeallum were wrongly sold as equivalent. In short, for the sake of avoiding an exhaustive revision of all the sources used by Wilkins, it should be enough to recall that, in the seventeenth century, M. Ruland, the Elder, *Lexicon of Alchemy,* trans. A. E. Waite (London: J. M. Watkins, 1612), 28, in the entry "Amianthus," makes a comparison that includes even plumeallum and Salamander wool. He claims that the latter is so called on account of the legendary animal resistant to fire; according to certain stories, such material was made from its "hairs."

peculiar ideas he is about to deal with, using such convenient formulae as "so they say," "he told so," and so forth. But the argument he comes up with after reviewing the opinion of other authors is solely Wilkins'. It expresses a view about matter and its composition that is far removed from the mechanistic and nontheological perspective held in the first book of the *Mathematical Magick*. He starts off by considering the case of lamps put in a totally empty vase which was very well sealed. If they could shine for a moment, they should shine forever, for, otherwise,

> there would be a *Vacuu,* which nature is not capable of. If you ask, how it shall be nourished, it is answered, that the oyl of it being turned into smoak & vapours, will again be converted into its former nature. For otherwise, if it should remaine rarified in so thin a substance, then there would not be room enough for that fume which must succeed it.[29]

In other words, Wilkins is echoing the long-standing *horroris vacui.* He even manages to furnish an example of such type of lamp, which, according to an account, had once been found.

As if this were not enough, he undertakes a long and final discussion about extracts that "nourish the flame of a lamp with very little or no expense of their own substance." From the start, he offers the example of gold, which can be "dissolved into an unctuous humour, or if the radical moisture of that metal were separated, it might be contrived to burne (perhaps for ever, or at least) for many ages together."[30]

His next astonishing step in this direction is commenting—without a trace of criticism or sarcasm—on none other than a hermetic treatise. Although he does not give a specific reference, it probably derives from, or even belongs to, a medieval pseudepigraphic tradition of *opera* attributing to Noah the transmission of highly important knowledge, and sometimes depicting him as the second of the three Hermeses.[31] In any case, Wilkins

[29]Wilkins, *Mathematical Magick,* 143.

[30]Ibid., 144. It is worth remembering that, as seen above, a scholar like Galileo was radically against the *perpetuum mobile,* which allowed that something could be obtained from nothing. Yet, even F. Bacon, a thinker far more conservative in his view about nature, probably would not have easily accepted this "flame nourished with no expense of its own substance." After all, one way or another he believed in the conservation of matter, for he stated, "there is no operation either from nothing or to nothing"; cf. "Historia densi et rari," *Natural and Experimental History,* in *Works of Francis Bacon,* ed. J. Spedding, R. Ellis & D. Heath, vol. 10 (Boston: Brown & Taggard, 1861), 262.

[31]Regarding this tradition, see M. Plessner, "Hermes Trismegistus and Arab Science," *Studia Islamica* 2 (1954): 53–54; about Noah as a Hermes,; see for instance J. Ruska, "Zwei Bücher De Compositione Alchemiae und ihre Vorreden," *Archiv Gesch. Math. Natur. Tech.* 11 (1929): 28-37; also L. Thorndike, *History of Magic and Experimental Science,* reimpression, vol. 2 (New York: Columbia University Press, 1923), 215, 222.

presents this treatise as "a little chymical discourse to prove that Urim and Thummim is to be made by art." Probably meaning light and truth, these words refer in the Bible to a device used as an oracle by high priests in older times. The author mentioned by Wilkins seems to have supposed that, once Urim and Thummim could be made artificially via chemistry, this knowledge could also be applied to the manufacture of another artificial light mentioned in the Bible. Namely, the light that, according to the Genesis, Noah, complying with a divine order, had kept in his ark.[32] Elated by this comparison, Wilkins asserts that the chemical preparation of light may explain subterraneous lamps. He even paraphrases the hermetic author who had considered this achievement *"the universall spirit fixed in a transparent body."*[33]

It is worth noting that Wilkins accepted this work, which probably derives from antiquity, without the usual reserve against alchemical treatises of his age. Yet, Wilkins seems to keep his readers uninvolved with the traditional symbolical difficulties inherent in each and every alchemical treatise, for he makes no comments about the explanations proposed by the hermetical author in regard to the principle, or the actual chemical preparation, of biblical luminaries. Instead, in the next paragraph, we find him overlapping Fortunio Liceto's work with Theophrastus' *De igne* to state that fire, being one of the cardinal elements, does not need any kind of nourishment to live on. Any humor or matter added to it would serve either to keep the flame "from flying upwards," or to generate a new one, but never "to foment or preserve the same fire."[34]

Actually, Theophrastus' old distinction between the element and the matter of fire, coming into view in the above argument, was continued by authors down to Herman Boerhaave. Our English scholar will make a good summary of these ancient and recurrent ideas when presenting three kinds of combinations "betwixt fire, and the humour or matter of it." In two cases, the proportions of one of them would exceed the other, and this could extinguish the flame. In the third and last one, "they may be both equall in their virtues, (as

---

[32]About Urim and Thummim, see, for example 1 Sam. 28:6; Exod. 28:15–30; and Lev. 8:8; for further references and details, see E. Frankel, B. P. Teutsch, *The Encyclopedia of Jewish Symbols,* entry 248. In Gen. 6:16, the divine order to Noah was "a window shalt thou make in the ark." According to the author of the above-mentioned treatise, who is seconded by Wilkins, the word *window* is an inadequate translation for TZOHAR, which means splendor or light.

[33]Wilkins, *Mathematical Magick,* 145.

[34]Wilkins, *Mathematical Magick,* 145. Regarding the argument about fire mentioned by Wilkins, see Liceti, *De lucernis,* chaps. 20, 21, as well as Theophrastus, *De igne,* bilingual ed. and trans. into English, V. Coutant (Assen: Royal Vangorcum, 1971), throughout the entire work, but particularly entry 4.

it is betwixt the radical moisture and naturall heat in living creatures) and then neither of them can overcome or destroy the other." Only in this case, would the flame last. Following this train of thought, Wilkins suggested that the ancients had hidden eternal lamps in closed sites because "the admission of new air unto the lamp does usually cause so great an inequality betwixt the flame and the oyle, that it is presently extinguished." At this point, the previous hypothesis, proposing the admission of new air as the cause of the ignition of these lamps, simply vanished. Now, his sole and greatest concern is the exact proportion "betwixt an unctuous humour, and such an active quality, as the heat of fire," as well as the preservation of this perfect proportion afterwards.[35]

To solve this dilemma, after Licetus' manner, Wilkins suggests that one should extract "an inflamable oyl from the stone *Asbestus, Amiantus,* or the metal gold, which being of the same pure and homogeneous nature with those bodies, shall be so proportioned unto the heat of fire." Is it or is it not a typical ending of an "ancient" sticking to the old view about matter, in which tendencies, qualities, and so on were seriously taken into consideration?

No wonder Wilkins concludes by stating that it is within the power of chemistry to achieve these strange effects, since one of its common experiments is, for instance, the so-called *aurum fulminans,* by means of which, with a small portion, one can achieve an explosion "of greater force in descent, then half a pound of ordinary gunpowder in ascent." Consequently, it would not be impossible to obtain by this same art the precious oil, "since it must needs be more difficult to make a fire which of its owne inclination shall tend downewards, then to contrive such an unctuous liquor."[36]

After these alchemical considerations, Wilkins closes his discussion seriously believing that this knowledge perished along with other ruins of time. Once again he blames the alchemists of his age, who, being the most versed in this quest, have "recovered [it] of such dark conjectures, from which a man

---

[35]Wilkins, *Mathematical Magick,* 145–146. It is worth adding that in Theophrastus, *De igne,* 23–24, which relies on a classical argumentation, the extinction of the flame in closed sites is mentioned; for further details about this ancient and recurrent theory about fire, see also the proposition offered after Wilkins by H. Boerhaave, *Traité du Feu,* in *Elemens de Chymie,* French translation (Paris: Briasson, 1754), vols. 2 and 3.

[36]Wilkins, *Mathematical Magick,* 146. The composition and the strange effects ascribed to *aurum fulminans* (gold fulminating) were much discussed by the "chymists" before and after Wilkins; J. S. Kuffler and Drebble's son presented these issues as a secret that Drebble had kept for the British Crown, cf. G. Tierie, *Drebble,* 74–75; in any case, still in the seventeenth century, Thomas Willis was able to prove that an explosion of *aurum fulminans* is not only downwards; cf. J. R. Partington, *A History of Chemistry,* reimpression, vol. 2 (London: Macmillan, 1969), 308.

cannot clearly deduce any evident principle, that may encourage him to a particular trial."[37]

Ecce our "modern" and "mechanist" author! Alas, the same one who, even before beginning a specific discussion on chemistry, had already equated the obtaining of perpetual motion with the philosophical stone of the alchemists, saying: "What one speaks wittily concerning the Philosophers Stone, may be justly applyed to this [the perpetual motion], that it is *Casta meretrix.... Quia multos invitat, neminem admittit.*"[38]

Of course this topic of Wilkins' *Mathematical Magick* demands further investigation. For the time being, one can say that it is not a simplified booklet on alchemical art of the "do-it-yourself" kind. Conversely, nothing there suggests the intention of discouraging readers from pursuing a good, old, and arduous alchemical study. After all, Wilkins seems to deem recent authors responsible for misguiding this study. For that matter, this text certainly did not discourage Boyle, who had a high esteem for the opinions of master Wilkins, or Newton, who seems to have been an assiduous reader of the *Mathematical Magick* in his younger years.[39]

Yet, it is still too early to say anything more, for its "modern" tag has just been removed. And further tags remain to be taken off this work of Wilkins', which, almost certainly—just like other *opera* of his age—did not accept categorical labels such as "ancient" or "modern." One is to hope that further investigation may enable us to better understand Wilkins—who paid an unorthodox visit to Elias Ashmole and, some time later, participated actively in the debate against the establishment of subjects such as alchemy in the curricula of British universities.[40]

---

[37]Wilkins, *Mathematical Magick*, 146.

[38]Wilkins, *Mathematical Magick*, 130–131.

[39]Boyle's high esteem for Wilkins is already commented on in a footnote above; see also R. T. Gunther, *Early Science in Oxford*, vols. 1 and 2 (Oxford: Printed for the Subscribers, 1923); Boyle's ideas about alchemy are lately being revised, for instance, by M. Hunter, *Robert Boyle Reconsidered* (Cambridge: Cambridge University Press, 1994). About Newton's interest in the *Mathematical Magick*, see, for example, E. N. da C. Andrade, "Newton's Early Notebook," *Nature* 135 (1935): 360; Shapiro, *J. Wilkins*, 45; this theme is also commented on in Eamon, *Science and the Secrets of Nature*, 309; furthermore, beginning 305, there is an excellent commentary about seventeenth-century handbooks about science.

[40]Wilkins' visit, which took place in 1652, is mentioned in *E. Ashmole (1617–1692): His Autobiografical and Historical Notes, His Correspondence, and Other Contemporary Sources Relating to His Life and Work*, ed. C. H. Josten, vol. 2 (Oxford: Clarendon Press, 1966), 615. Two years later the above-mentioned Ward/Wilkins *v.* Webster debate took place; cf. Debus, *Debate*, 43 ff., 195 ff. (*Vindiciae academiarum*).

Allen G. Debus

PARACELSUS AND THE DELAYED SCIENTIFIC REVOLUTION IN SPAIN

A LEGACY OF PHILIP II

IN RECENT DECADES, THE DEVELOPMENT OF SCIENCE in Spain during the sixteenth and seventeenth centuries has been studied intensively by José María López Piñero, his colleagues, and students.[1] Their work shows a greater awareness of contemporary scientific thought in other western countries than had been thought previously. However, it would be difficult to argue that Iberian science and medicine was innovative in the sense of the English, French, Italian, or German science of the period. This may be illustrated in part by the

---

[1]The research of early modern science and medicine in Spain is very extensive and there are several bibliographies. Of these one of the most recent in J.M. López Piñero, V. Navarro Brotóns, and E. Portela Marco, "Selección bibliográfica de estudios sobre la ciencia en la España de los siglos XVI y XVII," *Anthropos* 20 (1982): 28–36. The standard monographic study is José María López Piñero, *Ciencia y Técnica en la Sociedad Española de los Siglos XVI y XVII* (Barcelona: Editorial Labor, 1979), to which may be added his *La Introducción de la Ciencia Moderna en España* (Barcelona: Ediciones Ariel, 1969). J.M. López Piñero, V. Navarro Brotóns and E. Portela Marco have also prepared a book of source materials in their *Materiales para la Historia de las Ciencias en España: S. XVI–XVII* (Valencia: Pre-textos, 1976). Luis S. Granjel has written a four-volume history, *La Medicina Española en España* (Salamanca: University of Salamanca Press, 1978–1981), which runs from antiquity through the eighteenth century, and López Piñero, Navarro Brotóns, and Portel Marco have prepared with Thomas F. Glick an invaluable two-volume *Diccionario histórico de la ciencia moderna en España* (Barcelona: Ediciones península, 1983). For those seeking a summary of this research, see the two chapters by J.M. López Piñero on "La Ciencia en la España de los Siglos XVI y XVII" in Manuel Tuñon de Lara,ed., *Historia de España*, vol. 5, *La Frustración de un Imperio (1476–1714)* (Barcelona: Editorial Labor, 1982), 357–427, or Henry Kamen, *Spain in the Later Seventeenth Century 1665–1714* (London: Longman, 1983), 311–327.

147

Spanish reaction to the work of Paracelsus and the introduction of chemical medicine.

We need hardly be surprised to learn that the course of Spanish science was affected by the Reformation.[2] By the mid-sixteenth century, there was evidence of widespread heresy with large numbers of Protestant tracts entering the country from Geneva. For Emperor Charles V and Philip, his son, this was intolerable. The first Spanish *Index* of prohibited books was published in 1559 and at the same time there began a series of auto-da-fés that were planned to stamp out this heresy. Spain was to be separated from foreign ideas, and the Council of Castile and the Inquisition were charged with overseeing and licensing the publication of books. Those who imported books or published or circulated them without proper license were subject to death and confiscation of goods. In addition, Philip II ordered all Spanish students abroad to return home within four months except those enrolled at the theologically orthodox colleges in Bologna, Rome, Naples, and Coimbra.

These decrees were enforced and the results may be seen in the accounts of travelers decades later. Thus, in 1664 Francis Willughby was astonished to learn that the students at Valencia had not heard of the new philosophy while Lorenzo Magliotti (1668) wrote that "the whole of literature in Spain at present boils down to scholastic theology and outdated medicine as found in the works of Galen,"[3] and he added that anatomy had not been taught at Alcalá in a decade. Indeed, there is general agreement that the late sixteenth and the early seventeenth centuries constituted a period of decline for Spanish universities. Although the major universities maintained their chairs in astronomy, physics, and natural philosophy, there was a decline in the actual teaching of courses in all scientific areas. Along with this there was a sharp decline in the number of students.[4]

But how did this affect the special case of chemistry, and especially chemical medicine? In the other countries of Europe, the late sixteenth and the early seventeenth centuries saw active and often acrimonious debates relating to Paracelsus, his chemical worldview, and his belief in the chemical basis of medicine.[5] To be sure, he had argued that the search for fresh observations was essential for a new understanding of nature rather than the scholastic emphasis on disputations favored by the universities. But he also insisted that the key

[2]Henry Kamen, *Spain 1469–1714: A Society of Conflict* (London and New York: Longman, 1983), 118–120.
[3]Kamen, *Spain in the Later Seventeenth Century*, 313, 319.
[4]López Piñero, *Introducción de la Ciencia Moderna*, 38–44.

to this new learning should be chemistry, which would reveal God's hidden secrets to man. The Paracelsian worldview was set in a mystical-religious context of concern to the Church. The 1583 and 1584 issues of the Spanish *Index* called for the expurgation of two chapters and five shorter passages of Paracelsus' lesser work on surgery, the *Bertheonea*, but by the 1632 edition, Paracelsus was classed as a Lutheran and most of his work was forbidden.[6] Indeed, he was placed in the "first class of authors of damned memory" whose work is prohibited. We need only be reminded of the action of the Spanish Inquisition against Helmont at this time to realize the serious nature of being considered a Paracelsian.[7] With the attempt to prevent the importation of suspected foreign literature, the decline of the universities, and an inherent resistance to innovation, it is not surprising that there were few Spanish followers of Paracelsus in this period.

It would of course be incorrect to suggest that all chemists considered themselves to be Paracelsians. Diego de Santiago was in charge of a chemical laboratory at the Escorial established by Philip II. He wrote a practical work, the *Arte separatoria,* in 1598 in which he referred to Paracelsus along with Arnold of Villanova, Raymond Lull, and John of Repescissa, who along with many others, had followed this art and brought light to previously hidden parts of nature.[8] He wrote of the four Aristotelian elements, but asserted also that all things were composed of salt, sulphur, mercury, and earth. Nevertheless, the greater part of this text is centered on separation techniques—primarily through distillation.[9]

But it is necessary to separate the practical works on the chemistry of mining or the processes of the laboratory from the broader claims of the Paracel-

[5]The literature on Paracelsus and the Paracelsians is very extensive. Here I refer only to Walter Pagel, *Paracelsus: An Introduction to Philosophical Medicine in the Era of the Renaissance* (Basel: Karger, 1958); reprinted with "Addenda and Errata" (Basel: Karger, 1982). Allen G. Debus, *The Chemical Philosophy: Paracelsian Science and Medicine in the Sixteenth and Seventeenth Centuries,* 2 vols. (New York: Science History Publications, 1977).

[6]The problems of Paracelsus and the Spanish *Index* are discussed in anon., "La Historia de la Ciencia en España como Realidad Marginal en su Organización y Contexto Social," *Anthropos* 20 (1982): 2–15, here 4. See also J. M. Bujanda, *Index de L'Inquisition Espagnole (1583, 1584)* (Quebec: Centre d'Études de la Renaissance: Édition de l'Université de Sherbrooke/Librairie Droz, 1993), 546–547 (1583), 868–869 (1584).

[7]Debus, *Chemical philosophy,* 2:306–311.

[8]Diego de Sanctiago, Destilador de su Magistad, Vezino de Sevilla, *Arte Separatoria y Modo de Apartar Todos los Licores, que se sacan por via de Destilacion: Para que las Medicinas obren con mayor virtud, y presteza* (Seville: Francisco Perez, 1598), part 2, fol. 21v.

[9]Ibid., fol. 77r.

sian physicians. Here we find only one sixteenth-century figure, Llorenç Coçar, who became the professor of chemical medicine at Valencia in 1591 and gave a course on this subject in 1591–1592.[10] His prominence was due in part to a very short work published in 1589, the *Dialogus veros medicinae fontes indicans.* This rare work—only one copy survives—contains an attack on the ancient physicians.[11] Dissatisfied with Galen and the Arabic authors, Coçar understood that the hidden virtues of substances could only be revealed through experience. "I learned the art of preparing chemical medicines through many experiments and by listening to experts."[12] He studied the extraction of liquors and the preparation of balsams and salts. All of this seemed to confirm the truth of the work of Paracelsus. Indeed, Coçar insisted that fire divided all things into the three Paracelsian principles, and he cited the *Paragranum* to the effect that the four bases of medicine were natural philosophy, astrology, alchemy, and the art of curing.[13] Above all, he wrote, "alchemy offers the physician a clear and complete method to philosophize about the parts of animals, plants, and minerals and to investigate the nature and properties of all mixts."[14]

Coçar's *Dialogus* is short, hardly a major contribution to the corpus of Paracelsian texts, and the fact that it is the only Spanish Paracelsian apology of this period is indicative of the relative lack of interest in chemical medicine in Spain. Nor is there further reference to him or to the chair in chemical medicine after January 1592. He simply disappears from all records.

The works of Diego de Santiago and Llorenç Coçar hardly reflect the spirited debates that divided the Paracelsians and the Galenists in the other countries of western Europe at this time. In Spain the work of Paracelsus and his followers was relatively unknown. Where we do find early references they are generally antagonistic. An example is the satirist and minister of finance Francisco Gómez de Quevedo y Villégas (1580–1645), who in his *España defendida* (1609)rejoiced that there was no Paracelsian movement in Spain.[15] Indeed, Paracelsus had been a sorcerer and fabulist who attacked the medicine

---

[10]José Mariá López Piñero has touched on the work of Coçar in many of his publications. He has also reprinted the *Dialogus veros medicinae fontes indicans* in *El "Dialogus" (1589) del Paracelsista Llorenç Coçar y la Cátedra de Medicamentos Químicos de la Universidad de Valencia (1591)* (Valencia: Cátedra e Instituto de Historia de la Medicina, 1977). Here he has added a lengthy introduction on Coçar and his work. In his *Clásicos Médicos Valencianos del Siglo XVI* (Valencia: Generalitat Valenciana, 1990), López Piñero has translated a lengthy passage from the *Dialogus,* 129–134.

[11]Piñero, *Clásicos Médicos,* 129.

[12]Ibid., 129.   [13]Ibid., 130.   [14]Ibid., 131.

[15]López Piñero, *Ciencia y Técnica,* 378; Francisco de Quevedo, *Sueños y Discursos,* 2 vols. (Madrid: Editorial Castalia, 1993), 186.

of Hippocrates and Galen with his own, which was founded on the tales of old women and learned from the superstitions of sluts and vagabond knaves.[16] Others who had an interest in practical chemical processes, such as Francisco Valles, simply avoided any reference to Paracelsus.

Nevertheless, as we progress toward the middle decades of the new century, we find an increasing interest in chemical medicine. Thus Gaspar Bravo de Sobremonte (1610–1683), professor of medicine at Valladolid, referred to numerous chemical authorities and their opponents in his large *Resolutiones Medicae* (1654, 1662, 1674). Among others he read Sennert, Severinus, Seton, Dorn, Duchesne, Libavius, and Erastus.[17] He was aware that the spagyric sect emphasized the medical use of chemistry and that it placed great stress upon the separation of pure from impure.[18] Fire was for them the ultimate analyst resulting in the three Paracelsian principles.[19] Bravo was not concerned about the use of chemistry in pharmacy, but he strongly disapproved of iatrochemistry as a medical sect which, he felt, rested on false foundations that led to false conclusions. As for Paracelsus, he had used not only legitimate chemical remedies, but also magical remedies learned from the Cacodemon. The man had been a drunkard and he was both audacious and impious.[20] Nor was Helmont much better. Although he had started as an honest chemist, a true spagyrist, he had turned to the work of Paracelsus and had sought to overturn Aristotle and Galen.[21] Bravo added a section on the Harveyan circulation in the 1662 edition of the *Resolutiones*. He accepted this innovation, but felt that it was best understood as a modification or correction of true Galenic medicine. Other Spanish physicians of this period reflect Bravo's views, accepting specific chemical medicines while either ignoring or damning Paracelsus and those Paracelsian authors who insisted on a total chemical and religious interpretation of the creation and nature.

The situation changed markedly after the accession of Charles II in 1665. Although decisions during the regency were made principally by Queen Mariana, the natural son of the late king, Don Juan José, exercised increasing power until his death in 1679.[22] The influence of Don Juan was important for

---

[16]Quevedo, *Sueños y Discursos*, 2:1286–1287.   [17]López Piñero, *Ciencia y Técnica*, 379.

[18]Gaspar Bravo de Sobremonte, *Resolutiones medicae in quatuor partes tributae...* (Lugduni: Sumpt. Philippi Borde, Laurentii Arnaud et Claudii Rigaud, 1654), 4.

[19]Ibid., 5.

[20]Sobremonte, *Resolutiones medicae*, 5.

[21]Ibid., 414 ff. See also Bravo de Sobremonte, *Resolutionum et consultationum medicarum...*, 3 vols. (Coloniae Agrippinae: Sumptibus Joannis Wilhelmi Friessem, 1674), 1:11.

[22]On the importance of Don Juan see Kamen, *Spain in the Late Seventeenth Century*, 320,323; López Piñero, *Introducción de la Ciencia Moderna*, 37.

the acceptance of the new science in Spain. He had an interest in all aspects of science and technology, and we find his influence on the rapidly growing interest in these areas in the closing decades of the century.

The result of this is particularly interesting in chemical medicine. Texts that had been forbidden and at best imperfectly known earlier were now widely available. Thus sixteenth-century Paracelsian texts—many of which were already considered outdated in the other countries of western Europe— were now being read along with the very recent iatrochemical works of Thomas Willis (1621–1675) and Franciscus de la Boë Sylvius (1614–1672). Many Spanish physicians of the last two decades of the seventeenth century who were interested in chemistry were relatively unconcerned with the warning to be found in the *Index*. Rather, they saw in iatrochemistry a new observational and experimental basis for medicine.

Don Juan supported these medical chemists who rejected scholastic tradition, accepted the Harveyan circulation, and referred with interest to the scientific methodologies of Francis Bacon and René Descartes. Don Juan appointed an Italian, Giambattista Giovanni (1636–1691), as his surgeon. Giovanni adopted a Spanish name, Juan Bautista Juanini, and he became the first true Spanish defender of chemical medicine.[23]

Juanini's first work, the *Discurso político, y phisico* (1679), centered on an environmental problem, the pollution of the air of Madrid, which he saw as a source of epidemics. He pointed to the refuse in the streets ranging from human excrement to the decaying bodies of dead animals. All of this matter was filled with salts which were released through putrefaction, a fermenting process.[24] The fermentation itself was due to the three active principles, salt, sulphur, and mercury (16), and as the process proceeded, the resultant salts were raised to the atmosphere as atoms by the heat of the sun. The excrement then was converted to a volatile nitrous vapor on the one hand and to fixed salts on the other by a natural heat. And as the volatile vapors mixed with the atmosphere, the fixed salts mixed with the earth (21–22).

There were those, Juanini wrote, who accounted for the small number of elderly people in Madrid by the excessive consumption of chocolate, but he did not agree because the plague was due to malignant vapors rising from cadavers, which infected the air and filled it with saline and poisonous atoms.

---

[23]López Piñero, *Introducción de la Ciencia Moderna*, 64–67.

[24]Jean-Baptiste Juanini, *Dissertation Physique, ou l'on Montre les mouvements de la fermentation: Les effets des matieres nitreuses dans les corps sublunaires, & les causes que alterent la pureté de l'a ir de Madrid;* trans. from Spanish to French by Jean-Joseph Courtial (Toulouse: D. Desclasson, 1685), 2–9. The following page references in the text are to this 1685 French edition.

This air was carried by inspiration into the vessels of the lungs and heart, coagulated the blood, and caused sudden death (36–40, 55).

Juanini rejected the academic science of the scholastics and turned rather to demonstrations and mechanical experiments. Like other Spanish chemists of the period, Juanini enthusiastically supported the Harveyan circulation of the blood and explained respiration in terms of nitro-aerial particles. "These atoms," he wrote,

> are carried by inspiration to the lungs and heart, where they mix with the blood and act as a new ferment for it to restore its activity and vigor which has been lost in the long road to all parts of the body. Digby says that this salt is the food of the lungs and the nutriment of the vital spirit. This is the same air which is the cause of fecundity of plants, having the consistency needed for its circulation to all parts. (63)

How sad it is, Juanini added, that although the circulation of the blood is accepted throughout Europe, it is not yet received in the medical schools of Spain (93).

Juanini planned a three-part *Nueva Idea Physica Natural* of which only the first part appeared in 1685. Here he interpreted the first three days of creation in chemical terms.[25] And shortly before his death in 1691, he published a short work explaining the differences in the senses on the basis of the size and shape of the atoms of acid salts and alkalis as they penetrate the pores of the tubular nerves. Here he presented a union of chemical and mechanical concepts:

> [T]he atoms of acid, salt and alkali cause the distinction of colors in the visual organ and this is not the same as the result in the organ of sound producing the difference of sounds, and words, that we hear, nor is taste the same as touch, and it is for this reason, that the differences of the senses begin from within.[26]

Although Juanini was highly critical of the current academic treatment of natural philosophy and medicine, he conceded that iatrochemistry should not replace Galenic medicine, but rather be united to it.[27]

Even more influential was the *Carta filosófica, medico-chymica* (1687) of Juan de Cabriada, a son of a professor of medicine at Valencia. As a young

[25]Juan Bautista Juanini, *Nueva Idea: Physica Natural Demonstation, Origen de los Materias que mueven las cosas: Compuestas de la Porcion mas pura de los Elementos, Fraguadas en el Caos, Purificandas, y Passadas de Potencia, a acto en los tres primeros dias de la Creacion del Mundo...* (Saragoss: heirs of Domingo la Pugada, 1685), 58.

[26]Juan Bautista Juanini, *Cartas Escritas a los muy nobles doctores, el Doctor Don Francisco Redi...y al muy Noble Doctor D. Juan Mathias de Lucas...* (Madrid: en la Imprenta Real, 1691), 58.

[27]López Piñero, *Introducción de la Ciencia Moderna*, 76.

man little more than twenty, Cabriada had been involved in a debate during a consultation with Galenists at court.[28] This led to his writing the *Carta filosó-fica* in which he refuted the authority of the ancients and insisted that observation and experience be the basis of authority in the study of nature. The moderns stand on the shoulders of giants and we should turn to their work…to the work of Paracelsus, Helmont, Sylvius, and Willis as well as Sanctorius, Descartes, Redi, Sydenham, Boyle, and Harvey rather than Aristotle, Galen, and their followers.

> How sad and shameful it is that, like savages, we have to be the last to receive the innovations and knowledge that the rest of Europe already has. And when we bring this to the attention of Spaniards who should know it, they get offended and are irritated by the truth. How true it is that to try and switch people from an established opinion is the most difficult thing to attempt.

Cabriada asked why the king did not form a royal academy as there existed in France and England for the study of natural things through the promotion of physico-chemical experiments. And our eyes should be open to the wonders that the modern writers, new Columbuses and Pizarros, have discovered by means of their experiments, both in the macrocosm and the microcosm.[29] It is clear that Cabriada sought a total reform of Spanish science, but he was a physician and his interests were centered on a new medicine based on the Harveyan circulation and chemical medicine.

Although the *Carta filosófica* was Cabriada's only book, it initiated a decade of debate. Some sought to hold firmly to tradition while others followed Cabriada's call for reform. Thus, Father Buenaventura Angel Angeleres (1692) discussed the Galenic cure by contraries as well as the four elements, but at the same time he accepted the importance of fermentation and attempted to understand the process of calcination. Still, he rejected the possibility of transmutation and wrote that much of the work of the chemists was untrue.[30] Although unsure about the value of chemistry, he clearly aimed his book at Cabriada.

---

[28]Juan de Cabriada, *De Los Tiempos y Experiencias el Mejor Remedio al mal: Por la Nova-Antigua Medicina Carta Philosophica Medica Chymica* (Madrid: Lucas Antonio de Bedmar y Baldwin, 1687); López Piñero, *Introducción de la Ciencia Moderna*, 76.

[29]López Piñero, *Introducción de la Ciencia Moderna*, 101–107.

[30]Buenaventura Angel Angeleres, Real Filosófia, Vida de la Salvd Temporal Sabidvria Sophica, *Testamento Filomedico Arcanos Filochimicos Hipocratica, Galenica, Lilibetonica…* (Madrid: D. Mariana del Valle, 1692), I, 157, 159, 166, 179, 268.

Christoval Tixedas, a practicing physician in the University of Barcelona, wrote a *Verdad Defendida, y Respuesta* against Cabriada in 1688. Here he noted that Spaniards had always been opposed to sects and that this should hold true no less in medicine than it did in religion.[31] But Cabriada would destroy the medicine of the ancients, asserting that all the Galenists have done is in error and that the only way to a true medicine is through chemistry. Indeed, he treats Galenic medicine as if it were heretical and he loves chemistry as if it were Catholic (sig. a1r). In short, Cabriada believes that chemistry is the true natural philosophy (32).

Tixedas sought to take a more moderate course. Traditional bleeding and purging should be allowed while some chemical medicines were to be accepted, but always according to the rules of Galen and Hippocrates. The physician should know that chemical medicines are valuable only in part. In their preparation they pick up an acrimony from the fire that results too often in internal inflammation, anxieties, cold sweats, and vomiting. These effects occur only rarely with Galenic purges. Therefore, "although these remedies are said to be more efficacious than Galenicals, they are more dangerous and the physician ought to know this..." (38).

> The chemists say that Galenic purges include poisons and are inimical to nature while chemicals separate the purgative part alone and are more effective than Galenicals...But this is not proven...and if chemistry separates poisonous parts, it also produces new poisons because fire produces a more biting and acrimonious violence in them. (41)

Cabriada believes, Tixedas continued, that the king should found a chemical school where students would study chemistry and learn to despise Galen (46). But if it is true that physicians should know something about chemistry, they must not turn to it as the foundation of medicine. Spain has remained true to divine law and the Catholic faith without accepting other sects (50). We would stand with Hippocratic and Galenic medicine as well as with true sacred theology.

In 1690 José Gazola wrote an *Entusiasmos medicos, políticos y astronomicos* in which he supported Cabriada and attacked the Galenists. He was attacked in turn by Diego Mateo Zapata in his *Verdadera Apologia en Defensa de la Medicina Racional Philosophica* (1690). Although still a defender of much of tradi-

---

[31]Christoval Tixedas, *Verdad Defendida, y Respuesta de Fileatro, a la Carta Medico-Chymica, que contra los Medicos de la Iunta, de la Corte, y contra todos los Galenicos, le escrivió el Doctor Medico-Chymico D. Juan Cabriada* (Barcelona: En casa de Antonio Ferrer y Balthasar Ferrer, 1688), fol. §§2r.

tional medicine at this time, Zapata distinguished between the "Chemicos, ó Modernos" and others

> incapable of reason, witches, sorcerers, magicians and sycophants, who supplement with their illicit diabolical treatises and trade that which they lack in wisdom, as is seen in the infamous heresy of the chemists Paracelsus and his followers, whose infamous writings have justly been prohibited by the very just decision of the Holy Inquisition, to all those who follow, aid and profess these false and diabolical doctrines as stated in the Expurgation of 1640.[32]

Clearly by the final decade of the century, Spanish readers were aware of many of the Paracelsian authors that had been forbidden in the Spanish *Index* of forbidden books. And if there was not yet any agreement regarding the value of medicinal chemistry, the call for a royal academy by Cabriada bore fruit in the establishment of the Regia Sociedad de Medicina y otras Ciencias in Seville in 1700.

It would be incorrect to suggest that the newly founded Royal Society sought as its fellows only the proponents of the new medicine and science. One of them, Dr. Miguel Marcelino Boix y Moliner (c. 1633), produced a *Hippocrates defendido* (1711) that was to become a center of debate.[33] Here he painted a scene in which physicians from each major sect sought to cure a patient. One by one they came before Hippocrates, who presided over the contest. They proceeded chronologically according to the antiquity of their sects. First came the Galenist, who suggested bloodletting alone as a cure.[34] He was dismissed shortly by Hippocrates. A Paracelsian and an Helmontian approached the patient next (239). The latter spoke for the two not only because the two systems were similar, but because the Helmontian was more penetrating in his analysis. He began by stating that chemistry had been undervalued in medicine — clearly the wrong statement to make since it enraged Hippocrates, who said that he had spent much time on it and its philosophy. However, after all his study he remained convinced that diet is

---

[32]Diego Mateo Zapata, *Verdadera Apologia en Defensa de la Medicina Racional Philosophica…* (Madrid: Antonio de Zafra, 1690), 46. On Zapata see also José Guillhermo Merck Luengo, *La Quimiatria en España* (Madrid: Istituto "Arnaldo de Vilanova," 1959).

[33]Miguel Marcelino Boix y Moliner, *Hippocrates Defendido, de las imposturas, y Calumnias, que algunos Medicos poco cautos le imputan: En particular en la Curacion de las enfermedades agudas: pues hasta aora todavia se ignora como las curava; con sola la Exposicion, ò comento del primer Aphorismo: Vita brevis, Ars vero longa, &c.* (Madrid, 1711; reprint, Mexico, D. F.: Imp. del Sagrado Corazón de Jesús, 1893). Here the "Junta de Médicos" appears on 236–262. On Boix y Moliner see José F. Prieto Aguirre, "La Obra de Boix y Moliner: Historia de una Polemica," *Estudios de Historia de la Medicina Española*, n.s. 1[1959–1960], no. 6 (441 pp. plus illustrations).

[34]Boix y Moliner, *Hipócrates Defendido* (1893), 238.

more effective than the nonsense of the chemists' arcanas, corallines, and alkahests. The Helmontian remained adamant, insisting that Hippocrates could not successfully treat incurable diseases without his arcanas and secrets. Hippocrates replied that Helmont himself had been killed with the application of one of his secrets. Thoroughly angered at this point, he refused to let the Helmontian reply because the chemists had not taken into account the days or times of illnesses and without this it would be impossible to cure an acute fever.

The follower of Thomas Willis was a learned man who believed in the light of reason, but his reasoning was too subtle for a practical physician (240–241). As for Franciscus de la Boë Sylvius, there was little doubt that he was a successful doctor, but he did not have the answer for this illness either (242). Nor was Descartes helpful since his presentation did not distinguish between medicine and philosophy (243–244). Finally, Baglivi approached Hippocrates and presented his mechanical system of medicine in which the body could be viewed as a clock or a hydraulic machine (250–252). Baglivi rejected the consideration of times and days in illness as unimportant, a statement that infuriated Hippocrates, who called him a "tarantula physician" who incorporated in his system bad theory and practice and had put all medicine into confusion when he had entangled it with mathematics (259).

Finally, all of the sectarians went with Hippocrates to the bed of the sick person with the exception of the Cartesian, who did not have time to wait. It then became apparent that the only correct procedure to take would be to follow the method of Hippocrates (260).

Boix y Moliner's *Hippocrates defendido* led to a widespread debate.[35] Among the resultant works was a *Hippocrates Desagraviado* (1713) and a *Hippocrates Entendido* (1719) by Antonio Diaz del Castillo and a defense by Boix y Moliner, his *Hippocrates Aclarado* (1716). Here, Boix states that Hippocrates had been misunderstood by modern physicians and he tried to prove that scientists from other countries were taking the credit for discoveries by Spaniards. Had not Juan de Pineda, a Jesuit from Seville, stated the circulation of the blood correctly in his commentary on the twelfth chapter of Ecclesiastes in 1620(?)…and had not Gomez Pereira anticipated Descartes in 1554?[36]

---

[35]Aguirre (see n. 34) lists eight tracts related to this debate, 51–52.

[36]Miguel Marcelino Boix y Moliner, *Hippocrates Aclarado: Y Sistema de Galeno Impugnado, por estar Fundado sobre dos Aphorismos de Hippocrates no bien Entendidos…* (Madrid: Blas de Villanueva, 1716), sig. ¶¶¶¶¶¶¶ 2r, 4r.

More interesting is the *Hippocrates Vindicato* (1713) of Dr. Don Antonio Alvarez del Corral, which included a defense of chemistry. For Alvarez it appeared that Boix thought that chemistry was unnecessary because the work of Hippocrates was so excellent.[37] But, Alvarez argued, chemistry analyzes mixed bodies to give five principles, salt, sulphur, mercury, earth, and water (583–589). The separation of pure from impure is essential for medicine, and surely no one can be a true physician if he ignores chemistry (643). Beyond this, physiology had benefited from chemistry (644–647). Willis had discussed digestion in terms of fermentation and scholars had learned much of the properties and parts of human blood through its distillation. The bodily organs themselves had been compared to chemical vessels. Dr. Boix y Moliner had stressed the fact that physicians must study anatomy, but to understand this subject the student must also know chemistry (648).

Among the works attacking the *Hippocrates defendido* was *La Pharmacopea Trivnfante de Las Calvmnias y imposturas, que en el Hipocrates Defendido ha publicado el Doctor Don Miguel Boix* (1713) written by Felix Palacios. A chemist himself, Palacios rejected his opponent's views on Helmont as well as Willis and Sylvius.[38] Indeed, Palacios' main authority was Robert Boyle, whose work Palacios knew well.[39] Like Boix y Moliner, Palacios was a member of the Royal Society of Seville, and in 1706 he published his *Palestra Pharmacevtica, Chymico-Galenica…*, a work which went through seven editions by 1792.[40] In this practical work of more than seven hundred pages, Palacios sought to present his material clearly since the medicine of the Spaniards and Portuguese had been compared to the semibarbaric Moscovites in a work by Pedro de Regís, a doctor of Montpellier — and this had been repeated by an authority of no less stature than Malpighi.[41] Accordingly, Palacios described and illustrated chemical equipment as well as chemical characters in use prior to going on to discuss chemical processes such as fermentation, distillation,

[37]Antonio Alvarez de Corral, *Hippocrates Vindicato y Reflexiones medicas, sobre el Hippocrates Defendido* (Madrid: Por la Viuda de Juan Garcia Infançon, 1713), 578.

[38]Felix Palacios, *La Pharmacopea Trivnfante de Las Calvmnias y imposturas, que en el Hipocrates Defendido ha publicado el Doctor Don Miguel Boix, Medico honorario, y de la Regia Sociedad Medica de Sevilla* (Madrid: Francisco Martinez Abad, 1713), 35–36. After discussing Boix's attack on the chemists, Palacios went on to attack Boix for his views on Descartes, Gassendi, the atomists, Baglivi, and the mechanical philosophy, 38–66, passim.

[39]For example, see his reference to the *Sceptical Chymist*, 70.

[40]For a recent estimate of the work of Palacios see Patricia Aceves Pastrana, *Química, Botánica y Farmacia en la Nueva España a Finales del Siglo XVIII* (Xochimilco, Mexico: Universidad Autónoma Metropolitana, 1993), 95–101.

[41]Felix Palacios, *Palestra Pharmacevtica, Chymico-Galenica, en qval se Trata de la Elección de los Simples, sus Preparaciones Chymicas, y Galenicas* (Barcelona: Rafael Figuero, 1716), 1–2.

putrefaction, effervescence, digestion, coction, aromatization, crystallization, and calcination. Similarly, he described the preparation of extractions, tinctures, unguents, pills, elixirs, enemas, perfumes, and distilled waters. However, as in most pharmacopoeias, the great bulk of this work was devoted to the preparation of specific medicaments. And although Palacios had a special interest in chemical preparations, he also included traditional Galenicals.

Although we are now well into the eighteenth century, we may turn to Francisco Suarez de Rivera (c. 1680–1754) as a final example.[42] Trained at Salamanca, he received his doctorate in medicine in 1711. He then practiced in Seville and other cities in Spain prior to moving to Madrid, where he became a physician to the nobility and the royal family. He published more than forty books between 1718 and 1751, some fifteen thousand pages. These works are all medically oriented and range from clinical observations to botanical texts and observations on anatomy. Suarez de Rivera's medicine still reflected Galen, but he was an avid reader and his work was influenced by all medical sects. He did, however, refer to Spanish authors whenever possible,[43] and he proudly referred to his membership in the Royal Society of Seville.

Even at this late date we find a major figure defending the use of Paracelsian texts. Suarez wrote that it was of no concern to him whether or not Paracelsus was superstitious and employed remedies invented by the Cacodemon or learned from black magic. These were matters for the sacred tribunal of the Inquisition. For Suarez the main concern was simply whether or not the work of Paracelsus was useful for the public health.[44]

Pay no attention to the attacks of the Galenists, he added. Chemistry is essential for the physician. How else could the circulation of the blood be explained than as an imitation of the chemical operation termed circulation?[45] Similarly, surgery was more than the cutting of the body. There is also

---

[42]On the life of Suarez de Rivera see the short biography (with references) by J.M. López Piñero in the *Diccionario histórico de la ciencia moderna en España*, 2:339–341, and the two monographs by Luis S. Granjel, *Francisco Suarez de Rivera: Médico salamantino del siglo XVIII* (Salamanca: University of Salamanca Press: Cuadernos de Historia de la Medicina Española, Monografías IV), 1967, and José Luis Valverde, *La Farmacia y las Ciencias Farmaceuticas en la Obra de Suarez de Rivera*, Monografías, no. 13 (Salamanca: University of Salamanca Press: Cuadernos de Historia de la Medicina Española, 1970).

[43]This is done frequently, but see, for example, Suarez de Ribera, *Medicina Invencible Legal, O Theatro de Fiebres Intermitentes Complicadas* (Madrid: Francisco del Hierro, 1726), 280.

[44]Suarez de Ribera, *Anatomica Chymica, Inviolable, y Memorable* (Madrid: Manuel de Moya, 1743), 21–22.

[45]Suarez de Ribera, *Medicina Invencible*, 262–263. On page 298 he goes on to give a lengthy discussion of a Dr. Botoni on the circulation of the blood.

a true surgery in which cure occurs only with a knowledge of chemistry.[46] Thus, the physician-chemist must know the three Paracelsian principles and the use of the chemical knife, fire, which separate pure from impure and bring about new pharmaceutical preparations.[47]

Suarez still reflected the Renaissance interest in natural magic. "We rightly affirm that magic is the most subtle science of physics which consists in the investigation of phenomena which we observe in natural as well as celestial bodies."[48] For Suarez, Paracelsus was the "grande Medico Magico."[49] With this understood we need hardly be surprised to find Suarez seeking the formula of Helmont's alkahest,[50] Paracelsus' magnetic or sympathetic powder,[51] and the true preparation of *aurum potabile*. With Suarez de Rivera, surely one of the most prominent Spanish physicians of the first half of the eighteenth century, we still see an interest and concern for sixteenth- and early-seventeenth-century topics. In regard to chemical medicine, it is as if he were living a century earlier.

*　　　*　　　*

In conclusion, it seems certain the Philip II's effort to maintain Spain as a Roman Catholic country affected the development of Spanish science. From about 1560 to the early years of the reign of Charles II the new science—then flourishing in other countries of western Europe—was relatively unknown in Spain. This is not to say that the borders were completely shut to new ideas. The spread of thought cannot be managed legally as Philip would have had it. The case of Bravo de Sobremonte shows the wide extent of his knowledge of recent literature in the mid-seventeenth century. Still, there was relatively little scientific activity during this period compared to France, England, or Italy, and this was at the same time a period of decline for Spanish universities.

---

[46]Suarez de Ribera, *Canones Particulares de Cirugia, con que se Libertan Muchos Desahuciados, si al Sagrado de sus fuentes se Refugian* (Madrid: Manuel de Moya, 1751), 73; idem, *Cirugia Methodica Chymica Reformada* (Madrid: Francisco Laso, 1722), 8.

[47]F. Soares da Ribeyra, *Cirurgia Methodicae Chymica Reformada*, traduzida de Castelhano em Portuguez, Joseph Gomes Claro (Lisboa Occidental: Na Officina Ferreyrenciana, 1721), 128. Suarez de Ribera, *Anatomia Chymica*, 19–27.

[48]Suarez de Ribera, *Amenidades de la Magia Chyrurgica y Medica, Natural* (Madrid: Fernandez de Arroyo 1736), 38.

[49]Ibid., 75.

[50]Suarez de Ribera, *Illustracion, y Publicacion de los diez y Siete Secretos del Doctor Juan Curvo Semmedo, confirmadas sus virtudes con maravillosas observaciones* (Madrid: Domingo Fernandez de Arroyo, 1732).

[51]Suarez de Ribera, *Escrutinio Medico ò Medicina Experimentada* (John Crerar Library copy missing title page; introductory letter dated 1723), 271; idem, *Amedidades de la Magia*, 73.

The effect of Philip's action may be seen clearly in the case of medical chemistry and in reference to Paracelsus and his followers. Throughout most of western Europe the century from 1560 to 1660 witnessed active debate between Paracelsians on the one hand and Galenists and Aristotelians on the other. In sixteenth-century Spain we find little more than the short work of Llorenç Coçar in 1589 and the practical work on chemical preparations by Diego de Santiago a decade later. And while a limited use of chemicals seems to have been gradually accepted by the medical establishment, there was an almost uniform rejection of Paracelsus due to a large extent to the ever increasing references to his work in the Spanish *Index* of prohibited books after 1583.

Only after the accession of Charles II and during the period of the regency do we find a real interest in chemical medicine and its authorities ranging from Paracelsus to Willis and Sylvius. The works of Juanini tell of the need for a knowledge of chemistry, while Cabriada repeated this along with an attack on traditional natural philosophy and medicine. The debate that followed had as one result the founding of the Royal Society of Medicine and Other Sciences in Seville in 1700.

The story could end at this century mark, but as we have seen in the works of Boix y Moliner, Palacios, and Suarez de Rivera, there was a continued debate. Suarez even rejected the judgment of the Inquisition, stating that a physician's decision regarding Paracelsus had to be based on the usefulness of his work for public health rather than the authority of the *Index*.

Thus, Paracelsus and his work remained a subject of discussion in Spain long after it had been abandoned elsewhere in Europe. The reason for this surely is related to Philip's attempt to maintain religious orthodoxy, which gave Spain a late start as a participant in the Scientific Revolution.

ACKNOWLEDGMENTS

The present paper was completed with the aid of a research grant from the National Institutes of Health (5-RO1-LM05407). The author, who is the Morris Fishbein Professor Emeritus of the History of Science and Medicine, University of Chicago, wishes to thank the staffs at the Department of Special Collections at the University of Wisconsin-Madison, the Division of the History of Medicine at the National Library of Medicine, Bethesda, and the History of Medicine Library at the Wellcome Institute, London, for their aid in my research.

SECRETS

OF PHISICKE

AND PHILO-
SOPHIE.

The second Booke,

CONTAINING

The ordering and prepa-
ring of all Mettalls, Mineralls,
Allumes, Saltes, and fuch like,
for medicines both inward-
ly and outvvardly, and for
divers other ufes.

Printed at *London* by *A. M.* for
Will. Lugger, and are to be
fould at the *pofterne gate* at
Tower-Hill. 1633.

Martha Baldwin

DANISH MEDICINES FOR THE DANES AND THE DEFENSE OF INDIGENOUS MEDICINES

IN 1666, ONE OF THE MOST LEARNED PHYSICIANS of Europe issued a call for making profound changes in the traditional pharmacopeia used by physicians in his homeland. The man who yearned to reform the composition of drugs traditionally prescribed by his professional colleagues was the indefatigable author and neo-Galenist, Thomas Bartholin. For a man as learned as Bartholin to have issued a clarion call to revive neglected folk medicines seems truly incongruous and unexpected to historians of medicine who have long recognized this medical agenda as belonging to reform-minded followers of Paracelsus. Many Paracelsian reformers shared their mentor's animus against the traditional practices and teaching of the medical faculties of western Europe. Indeed historians have long recognized that Paracelsus had championed studying local flora and observing empirics and wise women in healing the sick as useful alternatives to the ineffective medical therapies of learned physicians. But Bartholin was no Paracelsian and in fact had much to lose and nothing to gain by having his name associated with Paracelsianism.[1] More-

---

[1] Thomas Bartholin (1616–1680) has long been recognized as an outstanding anatomist and physiologist of the Scientific Revolution; see C. D. O'Malley, "Thomas Bartholin" in *Dictionary of Scientific Biography*, 482–483; I. H. Porter, "The Bartholins: A seventeenth-century family study," *Dansk Medicinhistorisk Arsbok* (1964): 1–13. J. H. Skavlem, "The Scientific Life of Thomas Bartholin," *Annals of Medical History* 3 (1921): 67–81. Two excellent articles on the place of Paracelsian medicine in early modern Denmark are Jole Shackelford, "Paracelsianism and Patronage in Early Modern Denmark" in *Patronage and Institutions: Science, Technology, and Medicine at the European Court 1500–1750*, ed. Bruce T. Moran (Woodbridge, Suffolk: Boydell, 1991), 85–109, and idem., "Rosicrucianism, Lutheran Orthodoxy, and the Rejection of Paracelsianism in Early Seventeenth-Century Denmark," *Bulletin of the History of Medicine* 70 (1996): 181–204. Ole Grell presents an

over, Bartholin's literary style, in its lofty Latin, shared nothing with that of Paracelsus, who stuck to his Swiss-German vernacular. A venerator of the ancients, Bartholin stuffed his work, which called for a new evaluation of folk medicine practices in his native Denmark, with references to Galen, Hippocrates, Dioscorides, Oribasius, Pliny, Strabo, Soranus, and Celsus. Why then, would the learned Bartholin have taken a page from the book of the Paracelsians to endorse native medicines and native medical therapies in Denmark? What can Bartholin's text tell us about the defense of indigenous medicine in early modern Europe?

Bartholin issued his defense of domestic medicines and his cry to improve the health of his countrymen in his treatise *De medicina danorum domestica* (1666). Bartholin's arguments were not particularly complicated, for he merely stated that Danes and Danish physicians and pharmacists should seek to treat the ill with drugs prepared from common native plants. He argued that nature was beneficent in Denmark and endorsed the idea, prominent since the days of Hippocrates, that geography and health were closely aligned. Danes had at hand, indeed in their very backyards and barnyards, common plants potent to cure the various illnesses which afflicted the populace. "We have more need to search the rich storehouses of our own mountains and forests than to ask the night owls outside Athens" about remedies for diseases afflicting our own citizens, he argued. [2]

As a good Galenist, Bartholin eschewed metallic medicines, but he shared Paracelsus' scorn for learned men who zealously sought to learn about foreign plants while neglecting the indigenous flora. Such men would do better, Bartholin chided, to imitate the rustic, who knows he has at his doorstep a veritable pharmacy shop. Far gentler on the stomach and far more pleasing to the palate than the arsenic and antimony favored by the chemical physicians were traditional plant remedies. Medicaments brought back from the Indies and Africa and the Americas, be they metallic, animal, or botanical, he deemed suspicious and "dubious of faith."

Bartholin urged his contemporaries to venture outside their cottage gardens and into the Danish fields and forests to gather native wild herbs, grasses, shrubs, and their berries, barks, flowers, and resins. Here he relied on the

---

alternative view of Paracelsian medicine in Denmark in the early decades of the century in anarticle on Thomas Bartholin's father, Caspar Bartholin; see Ole Grell, "Caspar Bartholin and the Education of the Pious Physician" in *Medicine and the Reformation,* ed. Ole Grell and Andrew Cunningham (London: Routledge, 1993), 78–100.

[2] Thomas Bartholin, *De medicina danorum domestica dissertationes x cum ejusdem vindiciis et additamentis* (Copenhagen, 1666), 7.

botanical writings of a fellow physician and university colleague, Simon Paulli, who in 1648 had compiled a thorough catalogue of indigenous Danish plants which when correctly prepared could be turned into efficacious medicaments.[3] He also cited the contributions of another compatriot, George Fuiren, who had traveled throughout all of Denmark and to its more remote islands in the Baltic Sea in order to survey domestic plants more accurately.[4] Paulli's book had found a receptive audience among the Danes. In 1667, almost simultaneously with Bartholin's endorsement of folk remedies, Paulli's book appeared in an edition expanded to accommodate the needs of Scandinavian and Nordic physicians, botanists, and apothecaries. Paulli had arranged his botanical works by season, so that the reader might look under headings for spring, winter, summer, and autumn and there find an alphabetized list of plants. Such an arrangement allowed the reader to grasp quickly the indigenous fruits, barks, roots, seeds, resins, gums, juices, flowers, or leaves known to botanists and pharmacists as useful and appropriate in treating particular afflictions. In an attempt to stem linguistic confusion, Paulli listed the Latin, German, and Danish names by which each plant was known, and he urged the healer not to be discouraged by the almost countless names used for a single plant.[5] In his efforts to simplify the linguistic confusion over native plants, he compiled three separate indexes listing plants in each language.

While Bartholin applauded Paulli's efforts to bring the botanical wealth of Denmark to the attention of its scholarly community, he went farther than his

---

[3]Simon Paulli, *Quadripartitum botanicum de simplicium medicamentorum facultatibus* (Rostock, 1639). Subsequent editions appeared in 1640, 1667, 1668, 1674, and 1708. Two closely related botanical works by Paulli are *Icones florae Danicae cum explicationibus* (Copenhagen, 1647); and *Viridaria varia regia et academica publica in usum magnatum ac collecta ac recognita* (Copenhagen, 1653), to which he added a catalog of plants cultivated in the gardens of the king and medical academy of Copenhagen, as well as plants grown in the botanical gardens of Paris, Warsaw, Oxford, Padua, Leyden, and Groningen.

[4]Bartholin refers to "Georgius" (Jorgen) Fuiren (1581–1628). Georgius Fuiren was the father of two physicians who were contemporaries of Thomas Bartholin, Henrik Fuiren and Thomas Fuiren. On Georgius Fuiren see Bartholin, *Cista medica hafniensis* (Copenhagen, 1662), 272–277. Bartholin lists indigenous plants observed and collected by Fuiren on his journeys to Blekinge and Skaania (now provinces in southern Sweden) and on expeditions to northern Germany. A modern abridged version and Danish translation of Bartholin's *Cista* is available under its original title, ed. Neils W. Bruun and Hans-Otto Loldrup (Dansk Farmaceutforenings Forlag, 1982). Bartholin cites Fuiren's travels to the Baltic islands in *De medicina danorum*, 2:37–38, and speaks of further botanical expeditions undertaken by other compatriots in order to expand the Danish pharmacopeia in ibid., 2:39–60.

[5]Paulli, *Quadripartitum botanicum de simplicium medicamentorum facultatibus usus medicinae candidatorum, praxim medicam* (Strasburg, 1667), "Prooemium ad lectores," 52.

fellow physician in endorsing widely available animal products for medicaments as well. The patriotic Bartholin pointed to the Danish dairy herd as a neglected source of medical ingredients. Milk, he said, cured ulcers of the lungs, mitigated stomach pain, stopped fluxions of the eyes, extinguished sores in the mouth, and healed intestinal wounds. When injected in an enema, milk lubricated the intestinal tract, destroyed poisons lodged in the digestive system, and helped arthritic pain. Moreover, whey tempered sharp humors in the body and quenched thirst. Butter and animal fat, on the testimony of those worthy ancients Strabo and Galen, were known to aid in healing wounds and abrasions and were efficacious topical medicines. The Danish barnyard supplied further medicinal ingredients in the form of various kinds of manure and urines, commended by Bartholin and widely used by peasants and folk healers as cures for jaundice and asthma.[6]

Bartholin ventured even further to include the riches of the ocean waters off the coasts of Denmark as fruitful sources of efficacious medicaments. He noted that whale sperm was a most effective ingredient in numerous pharmaceutical preparations and that narwhal horn was especially beneficial in curing fevers and pestilence. In sum, Bartholin argued, in a metaphor that was not lost on his learned audience, the Danes "have no need to seek a temple of Aesculapius outside their own kingdom."[7] Their health and well-being lay within easy reach.

Bartholin's 1666 endorsement of native plants and animal substances as remedies for native diseases marked a sharp departure from his earlier stance as author of the first official Danish pharmacopeia in 1658. Here, Bartholin had endorsed prescribing the exotic ingredients commonly used by learned physicians throughout Europe.[8] Indeed, Bartholin appeared to be a committed medical traditionalist in this 1658 publication, for he had included numerous ingredients such as ginger, pepper, cardamom, cinnamon, lemon rind, senna, guaiac wood, and tobacco, all of which had to be imported into Denmark at great expense from the Indies, Americas, or Africa. Bartholin himself

---

[6]Bartholin, *De medicina danorum*, 2:19–25.

[7]Ibid., 2:61.

[8]Bartholin, *Dispensatorium Hafniense, jussu superiorum a medicis Hafniensibus adornatum: Thom. Bartholinus publici juris fecit* (Copenhagen, 1658). On the history of this first official Danish pharmacopeia and on the history of pharmacy in early modern Denmark, see Gauno Jensen and Aage Schaeffer, "The History of Pharmacy in Denmark: A Survey," *Theriaca, Samlinger til farmaciens og medicinens historie* (Copenhagen: J. Jorgensen and Co., 1960), 1–42; Aage Schaeffer, "Studier til dansk Apotekervaesens Historie: Hofapotekere og Hofkemikere I Denmark ca. 1540–1660," *Theriaca* (Copenhagen: J. Jorgensen and Co., 1963); Poul Reinhardt Kruse, "Laegemiddelpriserne I Danmark indtil 1645," *Theriaca* (Copenhagen: J. Jorgensen and Co, 1991), 234–254.

was quite conscious that his new call for domestic medicines represented a *volte-face* from his earlier works that urged Danish physicians to imitate the pharmaceutical preparations and medical therapies of Italian, French, German, and Dutch physicians. Having studied for more than a decade at the finest centers of medicine in Italy, the Netherlands, and France, Bartholin had returned to his native country in 1646, and had spent the next decade urging his fellow Danish physicians to take part in the advances of continental medicine. In addition to editing and updating his father's well-known volume on human anatomy, Bartholin had been at the forefront of anatomical investigations and had established Copenhagen's reputation as a center for anatomical research by his own outstanding work on the lymph glands and thoracic ducts.[9]

But by 1666 something fundamental had changed in Bartholin's thinking about medical practice and about medicinal ingredients, for now Bartholin even went so far as to give his reader directions for substituting local plants for the exotic substances he had called for in his earlier pharmaceutical recipes. For example, he pointed out in his later work exactly which local plants, namely, watercress, chicory, and cabbage, might be substituted for the exotic ginger and lemon rinds in his earlier recipes for scurvy medicines.[10]

While Bartholin exempted certain diseases from his reform agenda of domestic medicines, he did so only if he believed the disease was "imported" and foreign to Denmark. Thus, he followed the thinking of all contemporary physicians in deeming syphilis a foreign disease; therefore, he approved prescribing an American remedy, guaiac wood, for a disease whose infection he deemed had originated in the Americas. Similarly, he blamed imported French wines for many digestive afflictions of the Danes and he turned to the French pharmaceutical traditions for curing these. But Bartholin was especially insistent that two diseases he deemed indigenous, namely scurvy and "fever," be treated only with native medicaments, and he candidly pointed out

---

[9]On Thomas Bartholin's reputation as an anatomist see C. D. O'Malley, "Thomas Bartholin", in *Dictionary of Scientific Biography*; Edvard Gotfredsen, "Some Relations between British and Danish Medicine in the Seventeenth and Eighteenth Centuries," *Journal of the History of Medicine* 7 (1953): 46–55. More recently Roger French, *William Harvey's Natural Philosophy* (Cambridge: Cambridge University Press, 1994), 153–168, 239–250, has discussed Thomas Bartholin's reaction to Harveian circulation. The best biographical and bibliographical study of Bartholin is Axel Garboe, "Thomas Bartholin: Et Bidrag til dansk Natur- og Laegevidenskabs Historie i det 17. Aarhundrede," *Acta historica scientiarum naturalium et medicinalium*, vols. 5–6 (Copenhagen, 1949–50), with a useful English summary in 6 (1950): 188–196.

[10]Bartholin, *De medicina danorum*, 2:98–105.

his earlier mistaken treatments using exotic medicaments which he had gleaned from foreign books and foreign medical traditions.[11]

Although Bartholin articulated sound medical reasons to justify his reform of Danish medical practices, his motives are not to be found exclusively within a changed philosophy of healing. A closer examination of the context of his polemic on domestic medicine reveals that Bartholin was responding to a wider cultural debate taking place inside Denmark and that his medical profession had high stakes in this debate. Bartholin transparently linked his praise for indigenous medical practices to a praise for the kingdom of Denmark and for all things Danish. Nature had so endowed the kingdom, he argued, with all things necessary for her welfare and for the happiness of her citizens that she could be self-sufficient. Had not generous nature supplied her own remedy for cold winters, by endowing the native forests with furry animals such as lynx, wolves, goats, bears, and warm-feathered birds such as eider, animals whose skins and feathers the clever inhabitants so wisely used for warm clothing and bedding? And was not wise nature equally munificent in her lavish provision of wild berries and fruits whose juices relieved the natives from the heat of the summer sun? Was not the kingdom generously provided with pure spring waters and with soils fit for growing hops and barley, which native farmers used to brew Danish beer? Indeed native beer provided a means to nourish the peasant, to slake the thirst of those suffering from dysentery, to cleanse the viscera of the healthy citizen, and to improve the complexion of beautiful Danish women.[12]

Similar to Bartholin's paean on the beauties of the Danish people, climate, and natural resources was a philippic launched against imported luxuries. Here, Bartholin did not confine himself to medicinal substances and ingredients, but launched a harsh attack on imported food and drink of every description. He merely imported medicine into his argument to justify his disdain for the modern Danish fashion for consuming foreign foods. He bewailed the contemporary custom of wealthier citizens' serving roasted meats at banquets in place of the more traditional — and healthier — salted fish. While modern Danes were increasingly afflicted with gout and were dying at younger ages, he insisted that the *prisci Dani* who satisfied their hunger and thirst with local rye bread, fish, vegetables, beer, and milk were far more robust than their modern counterparts. Aping the cuisine of the French and feasting on expensive foreign meats and wines was destroying the national

---

[11]Ibid., 2:97–98.

[12]Bartholin, *De medicina danorum*, 2:8–15, 317–323 on the virtues of Danish beer; 2:61–66 on natural provisions against harsh winters; 2:160–164 on beer as a useful treatment for dysentery.

moral character and wrecking the physique of the Danish citizen. French wines were disastrous on Danish stomachs, he argued, for this foreign drink was full of tartar and accelerated diseases of the kidney stones and the joints. Why not instead drink Danish beer, which averted gout from the joints, expelled kidney stones, and cleared obstructions of the viscera? And when made with absinth or lupulin (a resinous powder derived from the seed-bearing cones of hops), beer worked like an internal balsam and cured even external afflictions. So deleterious was imported wine for the Danish physique, he protested, that Danish physicians would be wise to substitute the traditional native mead prepared from local apples and pears for the wine specified in foreign pharmaceutical recipes. Moreover, mead was in every way superior to the wines of the Italians, French, Greeks, and Spanish, since mead did not offend the lungs and acted more softly on the stomach. Only rarely, Bartholin claimed, had a Dane suffered from gout or stone before the importation of foreign wines. And to support his contention that Danish beer was a superb medicament, he quoted Olaus Magnus, the great authority on the customs of the Scandinavians, on the ease with which northern people pass stones. He also invoked Hippocrates on the beneficent effects of barley for fevers, coughs, and diseases of the kidney.[13]

Joined to Bartholin's polemic against French wines was his polemic against sugar. Bartholin despised the replacement of native Danish honey with American sugar. Although he believed it beneath his dignity as a learned physician to offer recipes to housewives, he felt so passionately about the evils of sugar, that he let down his professional guard. Thus, he gave recipes on how to make honey more fit for making jam so that Danish matrons might resist the temptation to use imported sugar. Honey had, after all, been sufficient for the Israelites, whom God had promised a land of milk and honey; if the patriarchs had not needed sugar, could not the modern Danes also live without this foreign evil?

Bartholin's tirades against replacing native medicaments and native foods with exotic pharmaceuticals and imported foodstuffs drew heavily from arguments set forth a few years earlier by his colleague Paulli, who commanded considerable respect among Danish physicians for his fundamental role in bringing anatomical demonstrations into the medical curriculum of the University in Copenhagen. When Paulli died in 1680, however, he was best known among his fellow physicians as a teacher of botany and medical chem-

---

[13]Bartholin, *De medicina danorum*, 2:10–11; for Bartholin's discussion of the Danish fashion for eating meats and neglecting fish, see 2:239–280.

istry. Five years before Bartholin first published his treatise on indigenous medicine, Paulli had issued his *Commentarius de abusu tabaci et herbae theae,* which went through several editions. Here, Paulli stated forcefully his opposition to the use of coffee, tea, chocolate, and sugar by his fellow Danes. He argued that each of these four substances, originally imported into Europe for medicinal purposes, was addictive and noxious to the health of his countrymen.

Paulli did not deny that tobacco was ever an efficacious medicament; indeed, he admitted that he had himself used it successfully every spring and autumn when he was customarily afflicted with catarrhous defluxions. However, he advocated the smoking of milder, native substances, such as marjoram, betony, and rosemary, which eliminated phlegm more safely. Moreover, these native herbs had none of tobacco's narcotic sulphur which corrupted the temperature of the brain and adhered to the membranes of the brain and lungs.[14]

Paulli spent much of his treatise reviewing the dangers of Chinese tea and American coffee, which he deemed responsible for corrupting national health and impoverishing the Danish family. Again, he admitted that when used in small quantities, tea might be a good medicament, but Danes would do far better, he argued, to drink an infusion made from the leaves of native chamaelegnus (myrtle) and betony, which were well endowed with a salutary sulfur and had all the medicinal virtues of imported tea.[15]

Bartholin and Paulli agreed in promoting native botanicals over imported spices. Far better adapted to the northern constitution were native herbal medicines such as wild radishes and watercress, conserve of roses, rob (fruit-syrup) of elderberry, electuaries of rapeseed and other indigenous plants. Moreover, Paulli associated exotic beverages with the moral depravities of the natives in whose lands they were grown. Thus, coffee suggested to him all the evils of the heretical Turks. Well versed in the extensive travel literature of his age, Paulli was aware that many claimed that coffee and tobacco were potent stimuli to venery. But Paulli retorted that salacity did not promote procreation, but only produced sterility. He agreed with his fellow Scandinavian

---

[14]Simon Paulli, *Commentarius de abusu tabaci, chavae, chocolatae et herbae theae* (Strasburg, 1665). I have consulted the English translation, *A Treatise on Tobacco, Tea, Coffee and Chocolate* (London, 1746), 21–38. For a fine scholarly discussion of medical debates on imported tobacco, coffee, chocolate, and tea in early modern Europe see Rudi Mathee, "Exotic Substances: The Introduction and Global Spread of Tobacco, Coffee, Cocoa, Tea, and Distilled Liquor, Sixteenth to Eighteenth Centuries" in *Drugs and Narcotics in History,* ed. Roy Porter and Mikulas Teich (Cambridge: Cambridge University Press, 1995), 24–51.

[15]Paulli, *Treatise on Tobacco,* 14:65–70.

Olearius that coffee emasculated the salacious Persians and he warned that such would be the fate of modern Danes who took up the custom of the coffeehouse.[16]

In their opposition to the importation of exotic pharmaceuticals, Paulli and Bartholin were consciously challenging a major source of income to pharmacists and apothecaries. Their works reveal a general hostility towards the apothecaries and a conviction that this rival healing profession was making keen profits on inefficacious and fraudulently prepared exotic medicaments. Indeed Bartholin made his hostility towards pharmacists quite apparent in the fifth "dissertation" of his book, in which he championed the wisdom of folk medicine over the quackery foisted upon unsuspecting citizens by pharmacists. He even went so far as to proclaim the isolated rustic who was deprived of the services of the pharmacist was more fortunate than the urban dweller who could avail himself of the services of such fraudulent practitioners of healing. Pharmacists, he claimed, had little interest in serving the sick; rather, they were out to "accommodate medicine to their maw and to fill their own moneybags with the sweat and coin of the sick."[17] Bartholin openly applauded the policy of the Danish crown in regulating and licensing the kingdom's apothecaries, a policy begun in 1619. He urged that even stricter controls be placed upon the profession, and he found especially irritatingthe practice of pharmacists to pass themselves off as learned physicians. "No trust should be placed in their exterior appearances,"[18] Bartholin warned, for he knew many who illicitly wore the *bulla* and robes of university-trained physicians. He referred the reader to his earlier work written to record the progress of medicine in Denmark, the *Cista medica hafniensis*. Here, Bartholin had published with pride the full royal edicts which regulated apothecaries and monitored their sales.

Bartholin was well aware that the recent proliferation of pharmacists could threaten the patient base and income of the learned physicians. Zealous to guard the doors of his profession, he noted that the number of licensed and privileged pharmacists in the nation's capital had been recently expanding from two in 1619 to seven in 1666. In addition to these official pharmacies in Copenhagen, countless other shops sold medicinal substances to the public and dozens of unskilled empirics called themselves pharmacists. The duty of the pharmacist, Bartholin wrote, lies in collecting herbs and simple medicaments, in mixing and preparing them, and in injecting enemas. Complicated

[16]Ibid., 2:163–169.
[17]Bartholin, *De medicina danorum*, 2:78.
[18]Ibid., 2:443; dditional caveats are found on 2:447–461.

compounded medicines, he proclaimed, were not to be prescribed by anyone except physicians—thus pharmacists, barbers, distillers, oculists, cutters of stone, and empirics stood beneath learned physicians and by law were properly prohibited from treading in the domain of the physician. In his treatise on domestic medicine Bartholin trotted out all the lawful ways in which the Faculty of Medicine exercised power over the lowly pharmacists, including making frequent and unannounced visits to pharmaceutical shops, reviewing their account books, and inspecting their shelves for adulterated ingredients and improperly fabricated chemical vessels. His praise for the wisdom of Danish kings in using university-trained physicians to regulate the other healing professions was patent.[19]

Bartholin did not stop at boasting over the legal control of pharmacists by physicians; he even went so far as to suggest that folk remedies prepared in the kitchens of farmers were superior to the medicines handed out in the chemical laboratories of the pharmacists. Although in Denmark the administration of enemas fell within the professional purview of the pharmacist, and not, as in France, within the realm of the barber, Bartholin suggested that this praiseworthy therapy did not require the presence of a licensed pharmacist. Moreover, the Danes were far wiser to employ the services of women or to self-administer the remedy with a homemade apparatus fashioned out of an animal bladder and sheep's intestine. Despite the pharmacists' resentment over this intrusion on their professional turf, Bartholin argued, the sick justifiably preferred the lighter touch of the wisewoman.

Bartholin also berated the fees charged by pharmacists and noted that pharmacists frequently defrauded their customers by substituting common ingredients for exotic ones without lowering their prices. How many times had a suffering soul believed himself to have purchased foreign spa waters when in fact he had merely paid an exorbitant price for local mountain spring waters? An intelligent housewife, he argued, could adapt her own kitchen to perform basic chemical operations and avoid the troublesome expenses of the apothecary. Many pharmaceutical operations were not the exclusive province of trained chemists, but were known even to rustics. Did not the good Danish wife know how to extract salt from marine algae to use as a table condiment, how to put up medicinal conserves, and how to prepare medicated drinks from beer? Had she not learned from her mother how to rid her household of lice and fleas by preparing fumigants from native woods and roots? Could she not prepare a good purgative out of milk, decocted grasses, and animal excre-

[19]Bartholin, *De medicina danorum*, 2:184–197.

ments which was every bit as effective as any purchased from a licensed pharmacist?[20]

Paulli fully shared Bartholin's animus against the pharmacists. In his enlarged edition of his popular textbook on medicinal plants, the *Quadripartitum botanicum*, Paulli included a Latin oration he had given to the Copenhagen medical faculty in 1665. Here he lambasted empirics and unskilled pharmacists. Such men, he reminded his readers, had no knowledge of the body or the theory of Galenic temperaments; furthermore, they resisted being policed by the committee from the Faculty of Medicine, on which Paulli served.[21] "Pharmacists are indignant when we warn them of their responsibility; they sell sublimed arsenic, cantharides, euphorbium, drops of gum resins for the sake of filthy lucre,"[22] he complained. Paulli was swift to cite evidence of a recent fatality of one Petrus Kiertemgyn, whose death was directly attributable to the bungling of a licensed pharmacist. The victim, a habitual taker of snuff, had died after his pharmacist had prescribed the dangerous euphorbium for a noxious discharge from his head. Only learned physicians, Paulli argued, understood the action of drugs inside the body; pharmacists, he urged, should stop diagnosing and prescribing; instead they should confine their professional activities to concocting drugs and essences ordered by physicians. Besides reiterating the standard litany of the vices of pharmacists—immodest prices, secrecy of recipes, impersonating learned physicians, selling inappropriate drugs to the sick—Paulli added the crime of performing experiments on the dead and engendering new diseases in Danes by making them habituated to exotic medicaments.

The appearance of Paulli's and Bartholin's polemics favoring indigenous medicine in the 1660s was not merely fortuitous, but was undoubtedly influenced by their personal and professional relations with the Danish crown. Paulli, a native of Rostock, was the son of a physician who had attended the dowager queen of Denmark. After attending many of the famous Lutheran universities of Germany, he had studied anatomy in Paris and Wittemberg and traveled widely on the continent, where he visited numerous botanical gardens. While teaching medicine in the academy at Rostock, he had published his botanical catalogue on the properties of medicinal plants, with remarks on the season of flowering and on places where each species could be found growing wild. Another early work was a German translation of Caspar Bar-

---

[20]Ibid., 2:200–202.
[21]Paulli, "De Officio Medicorum Pharmacopoeorum ac Chirurgorum in inclutissima Regia Hafniensi Academia anno 1665" in *Quadripartitum botanicum*, 5:627–634.
[22]Ibid., 5:631.

tholin's anatomy and Spigelius' work on the formation of the fetus. Called to Copenhagen in 1639 to teach anatomy at the medical faculty directed by Thomas Fincke, he soon opened a popular course of medical botany and was named first physician to King Frederick III of Denmark. By relinquishing his chair of medicine and anatomy in 1648 in order to pursue his botany full time, Paulli created an opening on the faculty for the young Thomas Bartholin. In 1653 Paulli edited a catalogue of plants cultivated in the gardens of the Danish king and in the academy of Copenhagen, with additional notes on the botanical gardens of Paris, Warsaw, Oxford, Padua, Leyden, and Groningen. Five years after publishing his attack on the use of tobacco and tea, the Danish crown granted Paulli the lucrative bishopric of Aarhausen. Like Bartholin, Paulli maintained contact with learned continental physicians. He dedicated the second edition of his commentary on tobacco to Guy Patin and Jean Baptiste Moreau, professors of medicine at Paris, where he had once been a medical student. Paulli's high standing among his compatriots and fellow physicians is evidenced by the appearance of a full fifty pages of congratulatory letters and poems inserted at the beginning of the 1667 edition of his *Quadripartitum botanicum*. Additional evidence of his high prestige with the crown is seen in his ability to win for his son, Jacob Henrik Paulli, a coveted chair of anatomy at the University of Copenhagen in 1662.[23]

Bartholin's ties to the Danish king were even tighter than those of Paulli. Born into the most prominent medical family in the kingdom, the young Bartholin followed his father, Caspar Bartholin (1585–1629), and grandfather, Thomas Fincke (1561–1656), in the choice of their profession. After spending more than a decade on the continent studying medicine at various universities, Bartholin returned to his native country in 1646, at the age of thirty-two; within a few years, aided by family connections and his well-established reputation as an anatomist, he took up a position on the faculty at the University of Copenhagen, first as a substitute for his aging grandfather and then holding the chair of medicine by 1648. Conducting anatomical dissections in the Domus Anatomica for eight years, Bartholin was clearly indulging not only his own intellectual interests but also providing entertainment for the king, Frederick III (1609–1670), who frequently attended, along with other wealthy

---

[23]The congratulatory prefaces appearing in Paulli's books offer valuable information on his life. Thomas Bartholin spoke of Paulli in his *Cista medica*, 4:5–6, and *Domus Anatomica* (Copenhagen, 1662), 6–33. Further biographical information appears in Troels Kardel, "Steno. Life, Science. Philosophy," *Acta Historica Scientiarum Naturalium et Medicinalium* 42 (1994): 10, 22, 60. Also see S. Andersen, "Simon Paulli: Betaekning over en kongelig ridehest," *Dansk Medicinhistorisk Arbok* (1979): 9–97.

citizens. By 1655, Bartholin began his service as the chancellor of the university and soon retired completely from his work as an anatomist. By 1658, having completed his service to the crown by publishing and editing the country's first official pharmacopeia, Bartholin requested relief from his teaching duties in order to have more time for writing. The crown did not grant Bartholin this exemption for several years, but when Bartholin's health began to decline in February 1661 as a result of renal calculus, the king finally granted him the long-sought exemption. At the age of forty-five, Bartholin was incontestably the foremost physician in the kingdom. Almost immediately Bartholin made good on his promise to devote his time to his publications, for he published that same year the *Cista medica hafniensis,* in which he chronicled the accomplishments of Copenhagen University's faculty of medicine and also included an impressive treatise on the king's prized anatomical theater, started in 1642 under the inspiration of Paulli and King Christian IV and completed in 1645 with an inaugural public dissection of a beheaded woman performed by Paulli.

Despite worries over his personal finances, Bartholin purchased a country farmhouse in 1663, Hagestedgaard, near Holbaek, while continuing to serve as dean of the faculty of medicine in Copenhagen. With the publication of his work on domestic medicine, Bartholin sufficiently ingratiated himself to the crown to be awarded a cash payment of 4,000 rix-dollars and in the following year a subsequent gift of income-producing land near his country retreat. When his house, library, and numerous farm buildings burned to the ground in 1670, the new king, Christian V, exempted him from taxes and provided him with building materials to help him recoup his losses.[24]

In 1672 Bartholin, beholden yet further to the crown, took up new administrative duties reorganizing the university library. He also accepted with alacrity the crown's request that he prepare the new royal ordinance to regulate the apothecaries, surgeons, and midwives. His recommendations became law on December 4, 1672. Bartholin's regulations, in effect for more than a century, laid down the basis for the examination and organization of Danish physicians, surgeons, pharmacists, and midwives by the medical faculty of the University of Copenhagen. In the following year Bartholin began the publication of the first medical and scientific journal in Denmark. Modeled on the *Philosophical Transactions* of the Royal Society of London, his *Acta medica & philosophica Hafniensa* appeared in only five volumes (1673, 1675, 1677, and

---

[24]Bartholin's description of the tragedy of the fire at Hagestedgaard is available in English translation; see *Thomas Bartholin on the Burning of His Library and on Medical Travel,* ed. Charles D. O'Malley (Lawrence: University of Kansas Libraries, 1961).

1680). However, the journal did much to boost the international reputation of Danish medicine, botany, and surgery in particular as well as the more general reputation of the kingdom in the eyes of learned men in Europe. Like Paulli, Bartholin also successfully used his position to win for his son, Caspar Bartholin, a chair in anatomy in the medical faculty at Copenhagen.

While it is thus clear that each of these physicians advocating indigenous medicine had been helped in large part to his personal and professional success through the patronage of the crown, it is equally important to realize that the Danish crown stood to gain much by having its two most prominent physicians championing the consumption of native medicines and native foods. It was not lost on the king or his physicians that money spent on exotic medicaments was money flowing outside the confines of the kingdom and into the coffers of foreigners. Indeed Bartholin pointed out in his work that Denmark had no native sources of silver or gold and that coinage had arrived in the kingdom relatively late (that is in the ninth century) and had only recently been introduced in the Faeroe Islands. Furthermore, as the crown's coffers were repeatedly emptied by the heavy expenses of wars with Sweden during the mid-seventeenth century, the need to conserve wealth within the kingdom was obvious to Kings Christian IV (1577–1648), Frederick III (1609–1670), and Christian V (1646–1699). Bartholin's and Paulli's medical philosophy had a political logic. Stung by heavy losses in its most recent war against Sweden (completed in 1660), the Danish monarchy faced a seriously depleted treasury. The Danish fashion for drinking Chinese tea, Paulli scolded, only enriched the Chinese merchants and impoverished the local Danes. "It is certainly unaccountable, and an unpardonable folly for a man who is rich at home to go abroad and beg,"[25] he wrote. Far better for preventing intoxication and for warding off sleep, he chided, to brew the Danish myrtle than to consume the expensive and stale tea shipped to Denmark from vast distances of the Orient. Furthermore, he warned that the Chinese themselves consumed one-year old tea leaves and shipped off for foreign consumption their leftover stale two-year-old tea leaves, which had undoubtedly lost their precious sulphur during travel. Moreover, greedy merchants adulterated imported substances whereas the duly appointed inspectors of pharmaceutical shops could safeguard the purity of native medicaments. To make his case, Paulli pointed out that his colleague Olaus Worm (1588–1654) had uncovered frequent evidence of adulterated tea coming into Denmark from merchants in Amsterdam and Hamburg. And he further reported that merchants commonly diluted ground chocolate,

---

[25] Paulli, *Treatise on Tobacco*, 14:73.

coffee, and tobacco with the macerated leaves of other astringent herbs. Hence, he argued, coinage sent out of the kingdom for exotic beverages only lined the pockets of heretics and foreign merchants.[26]

Similarly, Bartholin's medical arguments about the nutritional and medicinal superiority of native foods and beverages must also have been music to the ears of the crown. Bartholin proudly noted that Danish barley and hops were so highly regarded in Germany and the Netherlands that they were actually exported and provided the nation with a small cash surplus. He railed against "foreign luxuries, foreign dishes, foreign aromatics, unknown to our ancestors," and especially against the current fashion of aping the French custom of eating recently slaughtered meats. Instead, he commended the traditional Danish practice of eating smoked fish and eels. With pride he listed the numerous marine species with which Danes could provision their tables. Forgo meats cooked in the French manner, he urged, for even the Danish and Norwegian king, he wrote, serves fresh salmon with radish sauce at his royal table. In commending native breads made from flours ground from rye, barley, oats, and chickpeas, Bartholin consciously cast his medical vote not for wheat, the favored bread of his wealthy compatriots, but for native rye, the traditional food of the good yeoman. He also noted that the peasants' custom of making a twice-cooked yeastless bread from the barks of fir trees and ground chestnuts, beechnuts, and acorns made good political sense, since natives could make provision against famines caused by crop failures or severe winters. In doing so, Bartholin recognized that political instability often followed quickly upon famine; putting aside his Hippocratic training, he realized that diet and the provision of foodstuffs was more than a medical matter. Indeed, sufficient and affordable foodstuffs lay at the very heart of political stability. "Thus not a few of us have been seduced and we have embraced new breads along with new morals; and what must be deplored, we have taken up new ways of living along with the foods themselves; we have put on new clothes and rejected those of our forefather's simplicity and integrity."[27] One need not probe Bartholin's text too deeply to find his subtext: Buy Danish, eat Danish, support the kingdom and the crown.

The rewards and favors granted Paulli and Bartholin by the Danish crown suggest that the various kings whom they served found their medical arguments pleasing. By promoting the state economy with their medical philosophy, the two physicians also were helping to consolidate the patriotism of the

---

[26]Ibid., 14:97, 161, 169.
[27]Bartholin, *De medicina danorum,* 2:307.

Danish citizenry. While undoubtedly these kings, like other early modern monarchs, respected and rewarded learning, they also appreciated the support these two learned physicians offered their monarchy. While it would be too facile to reduce the polemic of indigenous medicine to merely a stage for early modern patronage, it would not be amiss to remember that both crown and medical profession were coming to regard a healthy citizenry as a valued resource of the state. Soldiers whose limbs were weakened by scurvy were not worth much in battle; farmers whose lungs were wracked with consumption could not gather rich harvests. Moreover, Bartholin's insistence that modern Danes were less well nourished than their ancient countrymen might well have had some basis in fact. The constant appearance in the early modern Danish medical literature of remedies for scurvy, now recognized as a nutritional deficiency, suggests that Bartholin's assessment might not have been merely pure rhetoric designed to bolster the existing monarchy.[28] Indeed, medical philosophy and political reality fit well together. Both crown and physician believed it desirable to create healthier working classes at home.

CONCLUSION

While Bartholin and Paulli sought to reform the medical practices of their countrymen, they were by no means plotting to have learned medicine subsumed into popular culture. Each wrote his text in lofty Latin and each was proud of his membership in the elite learned profession of medicine. Each sought to bolster learned medicine in his fatherland rather than see it replaced by folk medicine. But singing the praises of folk medicine provided a convenient platform for attacking the less prestigious participants in the healing profession—especially empirics and apothecaries. At the same time, praising indigenous medicine also provided these learned physicians with a way to please their patrons, the Danish kings, who could derive obvious economic advantages if the new medical philosophy was put into action. Since learned physicians rarely treated poorer patients who used the services of folk healers or empirics, they did not regard indigenous medicine as jeopardizing their professional stronghold. Rather, they continued to regard themselves as

---

[28]The best historical discussion of scurvy remains Kenneth Carpenter, *The History of Scurvy and Vitamin C* (Cambridge: Cambridge University Press, 1987). While Carpenter notes that scurvy especially plagued sailors, Bartholin's and Paulli's frequent references to the disease among native farmers suggests that it was endemic among landlubbers as well. Bartholin, *Cista*, 4:494–520, cites in full the judgment of the Copenhagen medical faculty on scurvy, handed down in 1645. Here he discusses symptoms, prevention, and cures, giving recipes for liniments, pills, sudorifics, and cataplasms. He further expatiates on scurvy in his *De medicina danorum*, 2:99–115.

having the right to speak authoritatively about sound physic, while paying lip service to the ideal of folk medicine. While Paulli's and Bartholin's plea for indigenous medicine was tied closely to the specific historical and cultural context of their fatherland, similar movements were taking place in other countries in the seventeenth century. In France, the medical faculty of the Sorbonne had done battle with chemists and pharmacists who had sought to introduce new metallic medicines such as antimony.[29] In Tuscany, the grandduke actually controlled the state-owned pharmacy and appointed his own physician, the eminent Francesco Redi, to oversee its operations and its profits.[30] In England, debates between apothecaries and physicians were frequent throughout the century. By the end of the century Christopher Merrett in London was challenging the apothecaries' right to diagnose and prescribe with the same vehemence that Paulli and Bartholin had used in Copenhagen.[31]

This call by learned physicians to embrace native medicaments and folk medical practices produced no profound changes in medical therapy in early modern Europe. The case histories reported in Bartholin's *Acta medica* reveal that most physicians in Denmark remained committed Galenists and more frequently prescribed foreign rather than native pharmaceuticals for their patients. As indigenous medicine became acceptable to learned physicians, it lost its association with Paracelsianism. Moreover, the appeal of domestic medicines did not vanish overnight. In Copenhagen, Olaf Borch, writing a full generation later than Bartholin and Paulli, reissued the same plea in his 1690 treatise for using indigenous medicine and for adopting peasant knowledge.[32] And in the eighteenth century, no less distinguished a botanist than Carl Linnaeus instructed his traveling students to study indigenous medicinal herbs and cures. Indeed Linnaeus, like his seventeenth-century predecessors,

---

[29]On the French context see Allen Debus, *The French Paracelsians: the chemical challenge to medicine and scientific tradition in early modern France* (Cambridge: Cambridge University Press, 1991).

[30]On the Tuscan context see Martha Baldwin, "The Snakestone Experiments: An Early Modern Medical Debate," *Isis* 86 (1995): 394–418; Paula Findlen, "Controlling the Experiment: Rhetoric, Court Patronage, and the Experimental Method of Francesco Redi," *History of Science* 31 (1993): 35-64.

[31]On the English context see Allen Debus, *The English Paracelsians* (New York: Watts, 1966).On Christopher Merrett, subject of a forthcoming monograph by this author, see Merrett, *A Short View of the Frauds, and Abuses Committed by Apothecaries* (London, 1669).

[32]Olaf Borch (Olaus Borrichius), *De usu plantarum, indigenarum in medicina et sub finem de clyysso plantarum & thee specifico, enchiridion* (Copenhagen, 1690).

was eager to examine and record the plant lore of the Scandinavian peasantry.[33] While the ideal of indigenous medicine may not have profoundly altered the practice of early modern medicine, it continued to be have political and economic appeal.

[33]On Linnaeus' interest in medical debates and his advocacy of native medicines in Sweden see Lisbet Koerner, "Carl Linnaeus In His Time and Place," *Cultures of Natural History,* ed. N. Jardine, J. A. Secord, and E. C. Spary (Cambridge: Cambridge University Press, 1996), 145–162, esp. 158.

Lawrence M. Principe

DIVERSITY IN ALCHEMY

THE CASE OF GASTON "CLAVEUS" DUCLO, A
SCHOLASTIC MERCURIALIST CHRYSOPOEIAN

WE NEED TO KNOW MUCH MORE about alchemy as a historical phenomenon. It is now widely accepted that many alchemical practitioners were serious investigators of natural phenomena and that their theories and knowledge made important contributions to the origins of early modern science. Yet in spite of the increased appreciation of alchemy there is still a long way to go in terms of filling out our picture of alchemy in both factual and interpretative terms. Indeed, I was struck by a comment Allen Debus made a few years ago to the effect that in the history of alchemy there "still remain many primary sources waiting to be read."[1] Indeed, the historical coverage of alchemy is very thin in many areas, and there are fundamental contributions still to be made.

We need to improve the breadth and the detail of our knowledge about alchemists and their theories, for many standard portrayals of alchemy are still of the broad brush variety. I believe that progress in this regard requires the recognition of a twofold diversity within alchemy. First, a recognition of the *diversity of pursuits* falling under the rubric of "alchemy"—a word which in current usage encompasses widely divergent pursuits including gold-making or *chrysopoeia*, chemical medicine or *iatrochemistry* or *chemiatria*, chemical technology, and so forth, as well as several anachronistic accretions. Second, a recognition of the *diversity of schools* within a subdiscipline of alchemy, and the latitude of individual attitudes, beliefs, and strategies within each school. For example, within the subdiscipline of chrysopoeia there existed many schools

---

[1]Allen G. Debus, comments made upon receiving the Sarton Medal, History of Science Society Meeting, New Orleans, La., October 15, 1994.

of thought based upon differences in approach, method, starting material, and theory. The cataloguing and classification of such internal structure will serve to provide a truer portrait of alchemy as it existed, in opposition to the notion that alchemy was a fairly uniform tradition of beliefs which showed little developmental articulation and few notable internal dissensions.

One approach towards a more accurate historical view of alchemy lies in contributing to the literature a wider set of carefully executed case studies. These should elucidate the biographies, bibliographies, theories, ideas, and social and intellectual contexts of a variety of alchemical practitioners. The compilation of these profiles of historical figures will finally comprise a sufficient data set allowing reliable conclusions about alchemy *as it actually existed* to be drawn, thus supporting, refuting, or amending wider historical claims about alchemy and the history of chemistry. Indeed, the inherent difficulty of alchemical texts and the problems in accurately citing their authors temporally, intellectually, and socially have posed the chief obstacles to an accurate understanding of alchemy. Yet taking the task of historical understanding seriously demands that we confront and surmount these difficulties. The present paper is one contribution to this greater effort.[2] It concerns a now very little known French alchemist of the sixteenth century, Gaston DuClo.

DuClo's name is in itself problematic, for it has suffered ignominiously at the hands of publishers and historians. He signs the dedicatory epistles of the *editiones principes* of his three books as Gaston DuClo, which I think we may safely take as his true name, and which I shall employ henceforth.[3] In his first book, however, DuClo latinizes his name on the title page to *Claveus*—possibly to underscore a punning reference to his ability to "unlock" alchemical secrets—thus providing the name by which he was generally known in the seventeenth and eighteenth centuries. Unfortunately, his name was obscured

---

[2]There already exist many important contributions to such an effort; for example, William R. Newman, *Gehennical Fire: The Lives of George Starkey an American Alchemist in the Scientific Revolution* (Cambridge, Mass.: Harvard University Press, 1994); idem, *The Summa perfectionis of the pseudo-Geber* (Leiden: E.J. Brill, 1992); *Alchemie et Philosophie à la Renaissance,* ed. Jean-Claude Margolin and Sylvain Matton (Paris: Vrin, 1994); Chiara Crisciani, "The Concept of Alchemy as Expressed in *Preciosa margarita novella* of Petrus Bonus of Ferrara," *Ambix* 20 (1973): 165–181; Robert M. Schuler, "William Blomfild, Elizabethan Alchemist," *Ambix* 20 (1973): 75–87; Allen G. Debus, *The French Paracelsians* (Cambridge: Cambridge University Press, 1991); Robert Halleux, "Le mythe de Nicolas Flamel, ou les méchanismes de la pseudépigraphie alchimique," *Archives internationales d'histoire des sciences* 33 (1983): 234–255, etc..

[3]I have not seen the first edition of DuClo's first book, and have relied on the testimony of Nicolas Gobet, *Les anciens minéralogistes du royaume de France,* 2 vols. (Paris, 1779), 1:15–22. The dedicatory epistle of the 1692 *editio princeps* of DuClo's second publication (which I inspected at the British Library) is indeed signed Gaston DuClo.

when a typesetter's error transposed the middle consonants of *DuClo* into *Dulco* on the title page of a 1602 edition; this error was propagated in all later editions so that the original DuClo (appearing only on the very rare first editions) was entirely forgotten.[4] Finally, in a (poor) 1695 French translation, this typographical error was taken as a latinism related to *dulcis,* "retranslated" into French, and added to the author's name as the epithet *Le Doux,* while the latinized *Claveus* was refrenchified into *de Claves,* to give the lamentable "Gasto le Doux, dit de Claves."[5] (The latter attachment has occasionally provoked confusion with DuClo's later countryman and fellow chymist, Etienne De Clave.) Thus, poor Gaston DuClo has now ended up in the major bibliographical sources as "Gasto(n) Le Doux de Claves" and one is never sure under which name he or his works might be catalogued or indexed.

Although this butchery of his name is sufficient to lay upon historians a moral obligation of compensation, there are several other reasons for paying attention to him, not the least of which is the high esteem in which he was held by notables of early modern science. For example, Georg Ernst Stahl (1660–1734), in cataloguing noteworthy writers on chemistry, cites only three authors "in that part of it called Alchemy" (which he defines strictly as metallic transmutation): Eirenaeus Philalethes, Alexander von Suchten, and "Gasto Dulcon Claveus." While Stahl gives pride of place to Philalethes, he refers to DuClo as "a very ingenuous writer," no small compliment for a writer on transmutation.[6] Perhaps more impressively, Robert Boyle (1627–1691) refers to him three times by name in his 1661 *Sceptical Chymist.* Boyle was extremely reticent to cite anyone by name in either praise or blame, and so his explicit praise of DuClo stands out dramatically. In one instance Boyle hails DuClo as one who "though a Lawyer by Profession, seems to have had no small Curiosity and Experience in Chymical affairs."[7] Elsewhere he cites him as one of the "Chymists that seem more Philosophers than the rest."[8] Boyle is particularly impressed by DuClo's "memorable Experiments." One of these is the demonstration that gold loses no weight in the fire by keeping it molten in a glass fur-

---

[4]*Apologia chrysopoeiae...Authore Gastone Dulcone sive Claveo...* (Ursel: Cornelius Sutorius, 1602).

[5]*Dictionnaire hermetique,...Traite philosophique de la triple preparation de l'or et de l'argent: Par Gasto le Doux, dit De Claves,* ed. Nicholas Salomon [or, less likely, William Salmon] (Paris, 1695). The error was perpetuated by historical writers beginning with Nicolas Lenglet DuFresnoy, *Histoire de la philosophie hermetique,* 3 vols. (Paris, 1742), 1:317–319 (see also 3:153–514) although he reverses the order of the epithets to provide *"Gaston De Claves, dit le Doux."*

[6]Georg Ernst Stahl, *Philosophical Principles of Universal Chemistry,* trans. Peter Shaw (London, 1730), 2 and 396.

[7]Robert Boyle, *Sceptical Chymist* (London, 1661), 56.

[8]Ibid., 273.

nace for two months. Boyle also cites the authority of DuClo's *"experiments whereby metalline mercuries may be fixt into the nobler metals."*[9]

BIOGRAPHY AND WORKS OF DUCLO

The little we currently know of DuClo's life comes from autobiographical remarks made in his works. He was born in the Nivernois about 1530. He practiced as a lawyer in Nevers, and eventually became Lieutenant Général du Présidial of Nevers. Around 1555 he became interested in alchemy and devoted himself for the next thirty-five years to "many meditations and experiments" in regard to alchemy, as he recalls in 1590 at the age of sixty in his first publication.[10] This first publication was his *Apologia chrysopoeiae et argyropoeiae* (Apologia for Gold- and Silver-Making), which appeared at Nevers—one of the first books published in that city.[11] The *Apologia* contains the primary exposition of his alchemical theory. The book was written in response to the denial of the transmutational art by Thomas Erastus (1523–1583) in his tract entitled "Explication of that famous question whether true and natural gold can be produced out of base metals," published in 1572 as part of his attack on Paracelsianism.[12] The first half of the *Apologia* contains a tightly coherent exposition of the principles, theory, and explanation of metallic transmutation. DuClo's style is precise and logical, and his defense builds stepwise in scholastic fashion upon definitions and distinctions, and includes experimental evidence. The second half reduces Erastus' arguments into forty-three syllogisms, to each of which DuClo responds using a combination of logic, experiments, and the alchemical theory he laboriously set down in the first half.

DuClo's refutation of Erastus is civil but firm; he respects Erastus' learning and opinion, but leaves no room for doubt regarding his error, for DuClo insists that chrysopoeia is possible and natural, and the gold produced by it is true. Several later writers compliment DuClo's style, and his civil refutation of Erastus was no doubt welcome to Boyle, who was himself no friend of the

---

[9]Ibid., 274.

[10]Gaston DuClo, *Apologia chrysopoeiae et argyropoeiae*, in *Theatrum chemicum*, ed. Lazarus Zetzner, 6 vols. (1659–1661; reprint, Torino: Bottega d'Erasmo, 1981), 1:4–80; on 8. The reckoning of biographical dates assumes that this volume was published very soon after its composition—which, by the way, occurred when Erastus, the subject of its attack, had been dead for seven years.

[11]Gobet, *Les anciens minéralogistes*, 1:17–18.

[12]Thomas Erastus, *Explicatio quaestionis famosae illius, utrum ex metallis ignobilibus aurum verum et naturale arte conflari possit*, in *Disputationum de nova Philippi Paracelsi medicina pars altera* (Basel, 1572). On Erastus, see Charles D. Gunnoe, Jr., "Thomas Erastus and His Circle of Anti-Paracelsians," in *Analecta Paracelsica*, ed. Joachim Telle (Stuttgart: Franz Steiner Verlag, 1994), 127–148; and idem, "Erastus and Paracelsianism: Theological Motifs in Thomas Erastus' Rejection of Paracelsian Natural Philosophy," chap. 3 of this volume.

arrogant and shrill Erastus.[13] But not all readers were equally pleased, for DuClo's *Apologia* invoked an angry denunciation from Andreas Libavius. Libavius' nearly four-hundred-page attack (over five times the length of DuClo's concise and orderly *Apologia)*, like much of what Libavius wrote, rambles on and keeps the modern reader reaching for his glossary of vulgar and invective Latin. But why would Libavius, in a work entitled *A Clear Defense and Declaration of Transmutatory Alchemy*, attack a fellow defender of metallic transmutation? Because Libavius asserts that DuClo

> is as bad an advocate of the Chymists as he is a patron of their causes…. It would have been more satisfactory for Gaston not to have attempted such an apologia, than to have defended it so disgracefully; we do not acknowledge his protection as legitimate, but rather we repudiate it as spurious…. As for what pertains to the method of the Art, this is sufficiently declared by many others, and usually appears in clearer form. The arguments of Erastus regarding metallic conversions have been judged and refuted by us; whoever wants responses, let him seek them there.Gaston responds too lightly and coldly, nor is that remarkable, for how else could he have done, he, a shyster lawyer who builds up upon illusions the dreams of silly old women and the hallucinations of the fever-ridden?[14]

Thus, Libavius' dissatisfaction seems to be based upon DuClo's polite Gallic manners, which did not measure up to the standards of Saxon invective; I leave this dispute to the stouthearted students of Libavius, for it tells us little of DuClo.

---

[13]For example, DuFresnoy, *Histoire*, vol. 1, 317–18. DuClo chided Erastus that disputes should be carried "by the strength and vigor of demonstrations, not by shouting after the manner of petulant old women," *Apologia*, 47. Boyle's dissatisfaction is shown by placing Erastus as the chief antagonist in his *Dialogue on the Transmutation and Melioration of Metals* and there caricaturing his rude arrogance; Boyle's text and a commentary thereupon will be published for the first time in Lawrence M. Principe, *The Aspiring Adept: Robert Boyle and His Alchemical Quest* (Princeton, N.J.: Princeton University Press, 1998).

[14]Andreas Libavius, *Defensio et declaratio perspicua alchymiae transmutatoriae, opposita Nicolai Guiperti*(!) *Lotharingi Ph. Med. expugnationi virili: et Gastonis Clavei Iurisconsulti Nivernatis Apologiae, contra Erastum male sartae & pravae* (Ursel, 1604), 693; "malus Chymicorum advocatus sit ille caussarum Patronus, ne quis obiicere arti possit futilitatem illam, qua modo sic, modo aliter atque adeo in inconstantissime & perversissime de rebus dissereretur. Satius erat Gastonem non attigisse apologiam, quam tam foede defendisse, nec agnosumus eius Patrocinium pro legitimo, sed ut spurium repudiamus ut istud sibi placere prae omnibus caeteris scripsit Penotus, fons amoris quodam fervore familiarius & indulgentius pronuncians, quam delibratius. Quod ad methodum artis attinet, ea satis a pluribus est declarata, prodeuntque indies fere clariora. Argumenti Erasti a nobis in conversiis metallicis sunt perpensa refutataque, ex quibus petat, qui volet responsiones. Nimis frivole & frigide respondet Gasto, nec id mirum. Quomodo enim potest aliter Causidicus, qui figmentis superstruxit somnia anicularum, & febricitantium spectra?"

His second publication, *De recta et vera ratione progignendi lapidis philoso-phorum* (Of the Right and True Method of Generating the Philosophers' Stone) appeared at Nevers in 1592. This tract summarizes (and slightly augments) the theory of the *Apologia*, and then points toward the correct preparation of the philosophers' stone, which he also calls the *sal aurificus* or *argentificus* (aurific or argentific salt), or, more grandly, the *Argyrogonia* (when white, for making silver) or *Chrysogonia* (when red, for making gold). It contains a lengthy practical section dealing with operations on mercury and gold. His final publication, *De triplici praeparatione auri et argenti* (Of the Threefold Preparation of Gold and Silver), was published at Nevers in 1594, neatly summarizes the theory of the *Apologia*, refutes the erroneous beliefs and processes of some chrysopoeians, and then describes three preparations capable of transmuting base metals.[15]

As is the case with most other celebrated alchemical authors, there are works spuriously attributed to DuClo. One is the brief collection of *Canones seu regulae decem*, which was appended to the 1612 collected edition of DuClo's works. The style is completely unlike anything DuClo wrote, and the editor merely states that these rules come from "an old manuscript" and never claims them to be DuClo's; nonetheless, they sometimes turn up in bibliographies under DuClo's name.[16] Another spurious attribution is that of *Le filet d'Ariadne*, published in 1695, which, again, has a style wholly unlike that of the genuine DuClo, and even mentions the late seventeenth-century Philalethes in the text. Still further off, but illustrative of the morass which is alchemical bibliography, is the somewhat similarly titled *Filum Ariadnes, das ist, Neuer chymischer Discurs*, which has no connection to DuClo whatsoever save that some have considered it a German translation of *Le filet d'Ariadne;* however, it is totally unrelated to the French work, and is the composition of one Christoph Reibehand, alias Heinrich von Batsdorff.[17]

---

[15]The publication date is generally given as 1592, an assertion which seems to date from DuFresnoy, *Histoire*, 3:154. This date seems to be an error, for although I have been unable to trace a copy of the *editio princeps*, DuClo's dedicatory epistle to the work (reprinted in the *Theatrum chemicum* edition, vol. 4, 372) is dated September 1, 1594, and in the text DuClo twice (375, 382) refers the reader to *De recta et vera ratione* as already published. The *Dictionnaire de Biographie Française* gives 1595 as the publication date, but so much of the rest of the article is erroneous, I am unwilling to credit it.

[16]*Canones seu regulae decem de lapide philosophico*, in *Theatrum chemicum*, 4:414–416; on 414. They are listed as DuClo's in John Ferguson, *Bibliotheca chemica*, 2 vols. (Glasgow, 1906), 1:227.

[17]This error was first noted by Denis I. Duveen, *Bibliotheca alchemica et chemica* (London: E. Weil, 1949), 217.

MATTER AND TRANSMUTATIONAL THEORIES OF DUCLO

DuClo's corpus is brief, occupying only a litle more than a hundred pages in the *Theatrum chemicum*, and spans only a short time period of publication. But the sophistication of his theory of transmutation—despite Libavius' rantings about dreams and illusions—warrants our attention in its own right. DuClo's system is predominantly scholastic—he employs the terminology of scholastic physics in looking for matters, forms, causes, and suchlike. He begins by discussing the composition of metals in general, and then endeavors to locate the *materia proxima* of silver and gold. This proximate matter in nature remains unknown, for authorities—Aristotle, Agricola, Gilgil the Mauretanian, Albert the Great, and others—disagree.[18] While DuClo inclines towards Aristotle's twofold exhalation (as expressed in the *Meteors*), he notes that we need not know the *materia proxima* in nature to find the *materia proxima* in art. While alchemical methods are entirely natural, they need not imitate exactly the means or starting materials used in nature. This proximate material of silver and gold, which "has an aptitude and certain natural disposition towards receiving the form of silver and gold," should be identifiable "by the similarity of its whole substance to that of silver and gold" and "by the similarities of its accidents to those inherent in silver and gold."[19]

DuClo posits four accidents proper to the noble metals, demonstrates each by an experiment, and provides a cause for each. The first, their inability to be burnt, is proved by their behavior in the fire, and this fact shows their freedom from sulphuriety or oiliness. The second, their inability to be decomposed by fire, is proved by the glasshouse experiment which Boyle admired, and this property rests upon their perfect mixture and union of dry and humid which are joined with "so strict a union that they are indissoluble in even the most violent fires."[20] Third, their fineness of essence, which is shown by the thinness to which gold and silver leaf may be beaten, due to their freedom from earthy impurity. And fourth, their great density, which he measures by a clever experiment of drawing wires of standard diameter out of each of the metals, and then comparing the weights of wires of equal lengths, demonstrating gold and silver to be densest. This density is the result of "equality and

---

[18]DuClo, *Apologia*, 17.

[19]Ibid., 18: "habilitas & dispositio quaedam naturalis ad suscipiendam formam argenteam et auream"; "ex similitudine totius substantiae auri et argenti cum hac materia proxima"; "ex similitudine accidentium ejusdem materiae, quam quaerimus, cum iis, quas argento & auro insitas."

[20]Ibid., 19; "tam arctissimo foedere sunt juncta, ut etiam ignibus violentissimis indissolubilia sint." Boyle, *Sceptical Chymist*, 57, liked the experiment, but not the "Scholastick Reason, which I suppose you would be as little satisfied with, as I was when I read it."

uniformity of parts, perfect mixture and thickening." DuClo then concludes that mercury must be the *materia proxima*, for its similarity of substance with gold and silver is demonstrated by its easy amalgamation with them, and its sharing in their accidents of nonflammability, indestructibility by fire, thinness of substance, and density. This mercury may be either common quicksilver, or mercuries which exist in the metals. Of these latter, DuClo claims he can isolate these mercuries from all the metals save iron.[21]

DuClo next asserts that this *materia proxima* must be transformed into gold by an efficient cause. This efficient cause, or more specifically *vis aurifica*, resides in another body, which, says DuClo, is gold itself, for "just as we say that the efficient cause of a dog is a dog, so likewise the efficient cause of silver is silver, and of gold, gold."[22] In this he explicitly dissents from the pseudo-Geber and Albert the Great, who posit that fire alone is the efficient cause, and from those who employ cements and salts made from imperfect metals. While DuClo allows that the latter do sometimes act as *gradators*, exalting a small quantity of base metal into a noble one, the effect is not profitable—"Indeed, all these condiments are more expensive than the fish."[23] This *vis aurifica* or *argentifica* present in gold and silver "moves the *proxima materia* by its igneous qualities towards receiving the form of gold or of silver."[24] But DuClo notes that there exists an experimental problem: when gold or silver is mixed with lead or mercury, no transmutation occurs; why not?[25] To answer this problem, DuClo turns to two classical subjects: the problem of mixture and the medical doctrine of degrees of primary qualities. The solutions he forges and their synthesis form the explanatory backbone of his alchemical system.

The doctrine of mixture comes first under DuClo's careful scrutiny. While he draws heavily from Aristotle's *De generatione et corruptione*, DuClo overlays these ideas with a corpuscularian viewpoint drawn from the alchemical tradition. Further, he criticizes the alchemical system as well, thus producing his own solution to the problem of mixture. Aristotle had defined true mixture as

---

[21]DuClo, *Apologia*, 21–23.

[22]Ibid., 25. "Et veluti dicimus, canem esse causam efficientem canis, sic etiam argentum argenti, & aurum auri." Cf. DuClo, *De triplici praeparatione argenti et auri*, in *Theatrum chemicum*, vol. 4, 371–388; on 375: "Ignis est principium generandi & augendi ignis ex alio corpore. Argentum & aurum sunt principia argenti & auri generandi & augendi in proxima materia."

[23]DuClo, *De triplici*, 374–75; "Verum condimenta haec omnia piscibus sunt cariora." Cf. DuClo, *De recta et vera ratione progignendi lapidis philosophorum*, in *Theatrum chemicum*, vol. 4, 389–413; on 390–91. On the different kinds of transmutations acknowledged by chrysopoeians, see Principe, *Aspiring Adept*, chapter 3.

[24]Duclo, *Apologia*, 25; "Sic & vis argentifica aut aurifica per qualitates igneas movebit materiam nostram proximam, ad formam argenti aut auri capessendam."

[25]DuClo, *De triplici*, 376.

the "union of miscibiles that have been altered" (*miscibilium alteratorum unio*). Two mixed substances—wine and water, tin and copper fused together to make bronze—unite fully so that no part of the ingredients remains and a wholly new form is produced. The stagyrite denied that atomistic theories could allow for true mixture, for when constant indivisible particles (for example barley and wheat by analogy) are mixed together, they are merely juxtaposed and not altered; thus the composition of a tiny part differs from that of the whole. For Aristotle, a true mixture must be *homoeomerous*, that is, of uniform composition at every level; otherwise, as the Philosopher argues, one arrives at the (unacceptable) paradox that for normal men an atomist's mixture is homogeneous, but for the sharp-sighted Lynceus who could see the individual and differing atoms merely lying in contact but unchanged, it would be heterogeneous.[26]

DuClo quotes his near contemporary, the humanist Julius Caesar Scaliger (1484–1558), saying that such a system is "unworthy" of Aristotle, and provides Scaliger's own definition of mixture as "the motion of the least bodies (*minima corpora*) into mutual contact."[27] Here Scaliger's mention of the "least bodies" or "least parts" ties him to the tradition of medieval corpuscularianism, itself deriving ultimately from passages in Aristotle's *Physics* and *Meteors*. As William Newman has shown, this tradition was developed and given wide currency in alchemical thought via the pseudo-Geber's highly influential thirteenth-century alchemical treatise, the *Summa perfectionis*.[28] There a language of "least parts" (*minimae partes*) is used extensively as an explanatory system for rationalizing the chemical behavior of metals, minerals, and other substances. Much Geberian language, in fact, appears in DuClo's writing, and he cites Geber several times: "Geber teaches in many places that the cause of true union and mixture is the reduction of different bodies into their least parts." Yet DuClo is dissatisfied with Geber's system (both directly and as transmitted through Scaliger) for although "thinness of substance" is the helper (*adjutrix*) of mixture it is not the true *cause*, for it leads only to juxtaposition—no change in the ingredients can occur.[29]

Thus DuClo, having criticized both Aristotle and Geber, charts his own middle course between them by noting the equivocal nature of "mixture," and

---

[26] Aristotle, *De generatione et corruptione* I.9.327a–328b.

[27] DuClo, *Apologia*, 27: "Mistio est motus minimorum corporum ad mutuum contactum."

[28] Newman, *Summa perfectionis*, esp. 143–160.

[29] DuClo, *De triplici*, 377: "Geber etiam multis in locis docet reductionem diversorum corporum in minimas partes mistionis & verae unionis esse causam. Nos autem cum Aristotle dicimus tenuitatem substantiae corporum non esse principem causam mistionis, sed adjutricem...." See Aristotle, *De generatione* I.10.328b.1–3.

in good scholastic form he distinguishes different kinds of mixture. Most important for this discussion is the division he makes based upon the fate of the ingredients. In one kind the "least parts" mingle and come into mutual contact and retain their original natures. This parallels Geberian mixture. DuClo gives three examples of this sort of mixture—water mixed with wine, metals fused together, and dry substances reduced to *"tenuissimae partes"* and mingled. Interestingly, the first two examples were used by Aristotle himself to instance his contention that the original natures of the ingredients were wholly lost. Clearly DuClo is disagreeing with the philosopher, having adopted a corpuscularian view, and probably informed by the practical knowledge that mixtures of water and wine or alloyed metals can be separated again into their primary ingredients by distillation and assaying. Indeed, when DuClo treats "dissolution" as the opposite of mixture, he is explicit that the survival of the mixed ingredients is proved by their subsequent separation from the mixture: "for if such bodies [water mixed with wine, or silver with gold] are separated, the bodies will reappear in their own prior forms, for they were merely contiguous, not corrupted."[30]

DuClo contrasts this Geberian type of mixture to one in which "the mixed bodies lose their original form, and unite to produce a new, single form." It is this sort of mixture which is crucial for DuClo, for it is exemplified by the transmuting action of the philosophers' stone upon base metals. Transmutation for DuClo is nothing other than mixture where the mixed substances alter one another, losing their original natures to form a new homoeomerous product. Now while this notion is reminiscent of Aristotle's *miscibilium alteratorum unio*, it differs in an important way, for DuClo overlays it with an explicitly corpuscularian mechanism, noting that mixture begins with the apposition of the "least parts" which then alter one another and unite.[31] What this division of DuClo's represents is (in modern terms) the difference between physical mixture and chemical reaction.

In light of Robert Boyle's esteem for DuClo expressed in the *Sceptical Chymist*, it is interesting to note that Boyle's own lengthy excursus on the problem of mixture very closely parallels DuClo's by taking "a middle Course" between the scholastic *miscibilium alteratorum unio* and the juxtaposition of noninteracting corpuscles favored by "the Chymists."[32] Boyle, like DuClo,

[30]DuClo, *Apologia*, 30: "ut aqua mista vino, aut argentum auro. Hujusce corporis genera, si dissolvantur, in priorum formarum suarum corpora redibunt, cum tantum essent contigua, nisi corrumperentur."
[31]Ibid., 31; DuClo, *De recta*, 402.
[32]Boyle, *Sceptical Chymist*, 136–161, on 147.

notes that both types of mixture seem to occur. Perhaps most significantly, when Boyle cites how it "seems not always necessary, that the Bodies that are put together *per minima,* should each of them retain its own Nature," he adduces the very example which is the crux of DuClo's system, namely, the transmutation of lead into gold by the philosophers' stone.[33]

Now we are ready to return to the problem that gold, although it contains the *vis aurifica,* when mixed with lead provides no transmutation. To complete his chrysopoetic system, DuClo turns to the medical doctrine of the degrees of primary qualities. According to a development of Galenic medicine, pharmaceutical simples exercise their effects through their primary qualities of hot, dry, wet, or cold and these exist in certain degrees of intensity. Medicines are then to be chosen in the appropriate degree to match and thus counteract illnesses of a given degree. In the case of gold, it cannot act on another body except through its primary qualities which are its instruments of action, the active ones being the fiery qualities of hot and dry.[34] But in metallic gold these qualities are not in a high enough degree of intensity to act upon another body, since they are in perfect equilibrium with the others, which is the definition of the perfection of gold. When gold is alloyed with lead, the two mingle at the level of their least parts but do not act upon one another, and thus a "Geberian" mixture is produced, which involves no alteration of the miscibles. But if gold's fiery qualities are intensified, they are enabled to act upon the coldness and wetness of common mercury (or the mercuries contained within the metals), and then the mixture (now with alteration of the miscibles) can achieve "temperment ... as the physicians are accustomed to speak."[35] Thus DuClo argues that "the intension of the grade of qualities in gold and silver ... is the whole and key part of argyropoeia and chrysopoeia."[36] It is the action of the external fire used for the digestion of the prepared materials which acts to intensify the qualities of hot and dry.[37] This conclusion leads

---

[33]Boyle, *Sceptical Chymist,* 158; see also Principe, *Aspiring Adept,* chap. 2.

[34]DuClo, *Apologia,* 24: "Haec vis ... a forma ortum habet"; 25, "a forma eiusque viribus effectus omnes ... sine qualitatibus primis Elementorum, quae sunt in misto corpore, esset inefficax, non secus atque artifex sine instrumentis"; cf. *De triplici,* 376.

[35]DuClo, *Apologia,* 33: "Mistionem Elementorum in unoquoque corpore naturali perfectam appello, cum aequales eorundem vires in unum coierint, ut calidi, frigidi, humidi, siccique pares sunt portiones, ex justitia, ut dicere solent Medici"; cf. *De triplici,* 387: "Hoc temperamentum non ponderis sed Justitiae solent appellare medici."

[36]DuClo, *De triplici,* 378: "Haec autem intensio gradus qualitatum in argento et auro ex eorum diversa praeparatione dependet, quae tota & praecipua Argyropoeiae & Chrysopoeiae pars est"; cf. *Apologia,* 33–34.

[37]DuClo, *Apologia,* 26: "Calor igitur hic externus ... qualitates igneas utrique semini insitas dum concoquitur & producitur, intendit, & in immensum auget"; cf. ibid., 43.

naturally to DuClo's three preparations, resulting successively in a calx, an oil, and a spirit, bearing increasing grades of qualities, increasing thinness of substance (to facilitate contact at the level of least parts), and therefore, increasing powers of transmutation.

Proper understanding of "true, simple mixture" (i.e., involving alteration) is crucial, for transmutation for DuClo is nothing other than mixture. In each of his three works, DuClo proclaims "the law of mixture" magisterially: "That there is first a mutual and mathematical contact of the mixed bodies, and this in their least parts, then they mutually act and are acted upon, and that by equal and opposing powers."[38] DuClo explicitly describes how transmutation occurs when the "seed," that is, an aurific preparation, is mixed with mercury: "the hot and dry qualities of the seed act upon the cold and wet qualities of the mercury, the former are reacted upon by acting, and the latter react by being acted upon. If both contraries are of equal strengths—for example, if the seed is hot and dry in eight degrees, and the mercury cold and wet in the same number of degrees—then the mercury is led to temperment." The experienced alchemist adjusts the relative amounts of aurific powder and ignoble metal to be mixed so that perfect temperment—i.e., pure gold—results. This system allows for the great power of the stone, for this "equilibrium of qualities" or "temperment" needed for gold is measured in strength not in weight, meaning that if, for example, the transmuting calx is hot in three degrees and common mercury cold in one, then "let one ounce of powder be mixed with three ounces of mercury" and their mixture will provide perfect gold. The completed stone may have degrees of hot and dry reaching to many thousands, and thus be of stupendous virtue.[39]

DuClo provides the reader with three preparations to effect chrysopoeia. The first is a calx prepared by the decoction of mercury with common gold.

[38]DuClo, *Triplici*, 377: "Mistionis enim verae hic ordo, haec est lex. Primum ut miscibilium corporum sit mutuus, & mathematicus contactus, isque in perexiguas partes, hinc ut agant & patiantur invicem, idque aequalibus & pugnantibus viribus." Cf. *Apologia*, 31. "Mistio vera, perfecta & simplex, est diversorum minimorum corporum in communi materia motus per qualitates pugnantes aequis viribus, ut fiat unio materiae & formae futurae, & unica ex omnibus mistis forma nova exurgat, manentibus quibusdam sensilibus accidentibus prioris materiae & subjecti"; and *De recta*, 402: "haec enim lex est, & ordo omnium quae tandem verè miscentur, ut primum se tangant partes, servatis formis prioribus integris in mistione, & deinde alterentur, postremò uniantur."

[39]DuClo, *De triplici*, 386: "Quam aequibilitatem non magnitudine molis aut pondere metriri licet, sed potestatis vi efficienti"; 387: "ut calcem auri pondere unciam, caloris autem siccitatis & tenuitatis gradus hujusce unciae esse tres, patientis verò subjecti ut argenti vivi unius unciae gradum unum esse contrarium qualitatum. Miscenda erit una uncia calcis tribus unciis Argenti vivi"; cf. *Apologia*, 33–34.

But common mercury, because it is "too cold and wet," is unsuitable for the work. DuClo gives two options. One is to extract the mercury from a metal, which is "better cooked" and therefore hotter in quality, and DuClo recommends in particular the mercury extracted from silver. Boyle cites this section in DuClo as proof that not all "mercuries" have the same properties, and Boyle commends DuClo's careful distinction between "mercurii corporum," or the mercuries of metals, and common mercury, or quicksilver—a discrimination purposefully and confusingly avoided by many other writers.[40] But DuClo notes that this extraction of metalline mercuries is difficult, and suggests that it is easier in practice to purge common mercury of its excessive coldness and wetness. Gold is to be laboriously incorporated with the mercury by grinding, digestion, and distillation until the two unite inseparably; thus, the hot, dry gold corrects the cold, wet mercury. This mercury is now freed from the excessive coldness of common mercury, and DuClo calls it his "animated" mercury.

Digestion of this animated mercury with powdered gold then provides a red calx, which when fused turns entirely to gold. DuClo suggests that only half the calx be fused into gold, and the remaining half amalgamated and digested with its own weight of animated mercury to provide more calx, which upon repetition provides a steady supply of gold while preserving the original quantity of transmuting calx. This is the earliest reference known to me to what was later called the "perpetual mine."[41]

The second preparation, which is little described, converts this calx into an oil by repeated dissolution in a powerful solvent. DuClo refers the reader to (pseudo-)Raymond Lull and his quintessence of spirit of wine, and states that this oil, mixed and cooked with common quicksilver, transmutes it into gold. This oil, whose qualities are intensified over those of the calx, is both *aurum potabile* and Geber's transmuting "medicine of the second order."[42] Finally, DuClo comes to the third preparation, which is of "far more intense powers, and superior faculties," in short, the philosophers' stone itself. The choice, preparation, and coction of gold and mercury into the Stone is detailed most fully in *De recta ratione*.

[40]Boyle, *Sceptical Chymist*, 273–274.
[41]The perpetual mine is fully described in the anonymous *Coelum philosophorum* (Dresden and Leipzig, 1739), 11.
[42]Newman, *Summa perfectionis*, 162ff., 546–585, 752–767.

DuClo in the Alchemical Context

Having detailed DuClo's transmutational theory and practice, we need to resituate him in the context of the wider field of alchemy. What are his sources, and who—if any—are his followers? More broadly, how does this study of DuClo amend our views of alchemy in the late sixteenth century?

Clearly, DuClo's approach is primarily that of scholastic physics; as such it recalls the medieval alchemical tradition (indeed he draws heavily from Geber and Albert, although with some disagreement) and provides an example of the endurance of this tradition down to the close of the sixteenth century. Among other alchemists he cites only two—not counting the alchemical poet Giovanni Augurello—the pseudo-Lull and Bernard of Trier. An important contemporary source for DuClo is the humanist J. C. Scaliger, whom he calls "that most subtle philosopher," and from whose *Exotericae exercitationes* he quotes frequently.[43] As we have seen, he draws also from Galenic medical theories. What we find in DuClo then is a synthesis of diverse strands of thought into a coherent and rigorous theoretical framework. Moreover, this framework is supported at numerous points by experimental evidence, sometimes of a rather classical nature and sometimes inventively designed.

Equally enlightening is what *does not* appear in DuClo's corpus. There is no reference to Paracelsus, Paracelsian notions, spagyria, or even the *tria prima*, and this at a time when neo-Paracelsian thought was widespread and vigorous in France.[44] Similarly, DuClo has no interest in chemical medicine or any other alchemical practices outside of transmutation. The context of the contemporaneous "antimony wars" and other battles over chemical medicine make no appearance in DuClo. Only once in his corpus does he ever mention chymical medicine, when he claims that the oil made from gold is *aurum potabile*, but he refuses to endorse or deny its reputed medical efficacy because that "lies beyond the limits of our profession and our chrysopoetic art, and should be left to the judgment of physicians."[45] While this refusal to engage with medical topics may reflect not only DuClo's lack of interest but also his unwillingness to transgress professional boundaries, it is worth pointing out that contemporaneous Paracelsian chymists were notorious for vaunting their medicaments against the medical establishment.

---

[43]DuClo, *De recta,* 393.
[44]Debus, *French Paracelsians,* esp. 17–45.
[45]DuClo, *De triplici,* 381: "aurum potabile, quod multis morbis desperatis remedium est accommodatissimum, si vera sunt, quae de auro potabili referunt, quae affirmare non ausim quod nostrae professionis & Chrysopoeiae artis limites praetergrediantur & medicorum judicio relinquenda sunt."

One belief commonly associated with alchemy is vitalism or hylozoism. Many popular interpretations of alchemy claim that alchemists saw the world as alive, and believed that metals and minerals grow and reproduce by seed in the fashion of animals and plants. It is the central thesis of this study that while this view and others like it *may* have been held by *some* alchemical writers, they cannot be attributed broadly to alchemists as a whole. DuClo's physical system shows not the least trace of vitalism, and he repeatedly and insistently separates animate nature from inanimate bodies. In plants and animals changes occur by generation and corruption, but changes in inanimate substances occur only by simple mixture and dissolution. Plants and animals have an internal power of change and development, but inanimate bodies change only by being "agitated by external influence." The laws that govern animate systems are different from those that govern inanimate ones.[46] Much of DuClo's refutation of Erastus rests upon such distinctions, for Erastus (like many opponents of chrysopoeia since the Middle Ages) had used analogies from animate nature to argue against transmutation (e.g., species are immutable, for one cannot change a donkey into a man; therefore, one cannot change lead into gold). But DuClo's system rules out all similes drawn from animate nature which functions by principles different from those governing the inanimate substances under the alchemist's care.

Indeed, DuClo *explicitly* dissents from a vitalist interpretation: "I cannot agree with those," he writes, "who have said that the metals, or our aurific or argentific seed, or philosophers' stone, are alive, which perhaps they have understood metaphorically on account of the excellence of the strengths and fiery qualities of them."[47] His allowance that such notions as the "life of metals" are metaphorical allows us correctly to understand DuClo's own usage of superficially vitalistic terms such as *seed*. He states that mercury and the base metals are seeds of gold, and that gold and its proper mercury form together the seed of the philosophers' stone.[48] But how does he intend for his use of the term *semina* to be understood? A vitalist interpretation would incline us to view DuClo's *semina* as a transferal of agricultural notions and

---

[46]DuClo, *Apologia*, 39: "quaestio non est de vegetatione aut sensu, sed de mistione inanimorum corporum, quae non insita vi, sed pulsu agitantur externo"; see also 27, 28, 49, 64, 65, 68, 69, 79, and *De triplici*, 383, 388.

[47]DuClo, *Apologia*, 65: "Non enim iis subscribere possum, qui metalla aut semen nostrum aurificum aut argentificum, seu lapidem Philsophorum, vivere dixerunt, quod forsitan metaphorice intellexerunt, ob virium & qualitatum ignearum excellentiam."

[48]DuClo, *De recta*, 396: "Aurum enim & argentum vivum suum…sunt semen salis aurifici: & argentum vivum & metalla relinqua sunt semen auri: At illa salis aurifici & auri semina natura imperfecta relinquit, nec ultrà progressa est, sed ars eandem adjuvat naturam, ut perficiantur."

causation into chrysopoeia; in fact, DuClo does liken the alchemist to the farmer planting a field.[49] But this would be a serious misunderstanding. For DuClo, a *semen* represents only a specific *potentia*; the base metals are all potentially gold and, following the classical formulations of medieval alchemy, are in fact imperfect gold—substances checked from their natural course to perfection by a variety of interfering causes. Likewise, gold and its mercury have the potential to become together the *sal aurificus* or philosophers' stone. Thus, DuClo's language of *semina* is metaphorical; just as a seed can give rise to a specific plant (which represents its perfection) so the metals can give rise to gold, and a mixture of gold and its mercury can give rise to the stone. DuClo explicitly denies that the *causation* and *mechanism* of the perfection of a true plant or animal seed and a metaphorical "seed" are akin. Thus, the word *seed* for DuClo does in no way demand a vitalistic view of metallic nature; it merely represents in a metaphorical way the directed potential of a thing.

Similarly, DuClo refers in the same way to his use of the word *animated* to describe a specially prepared mercury. Though *prima facie* interpretable as a vitalistic term meaning "possessing a soul [anima]," DuClo is quick to point out that he uses the phrase "only metaphorically." Recall that this mercury was prepared by uniting hot, dry gold with cold, wet common mercury to correct its "excessive coldness." DuClo comments that the resultant mercury "is called *animated* metaphorically, for just as the *anima* is the principle and cause of heat in animal bodies, and without which they are thrown out as dead bodies, so silver or gold is the principle of heat in mercury, which otherwise would remain most cold and not altered at all."[50] It is wise to extend this observation on DuClo's terminology into a more general caveat for reading and interpreting alchemical texts—words like seed, soul, growth, and maturation do not *necessarily* imply a vitalistic or hylozoic worldview.

In addition to falling squarely in the tradition of scholastic alchemy, DuClo also identifies himself with a specific school of chrysopoeians: "I subscribe to the opinion of those who, imitating nature, take up, dissolve, and cook together gold and its mercury as the matter or subject of the argentific or

[49]DuClo, *Apologia*, 43–44; *De recta*, 400.
[50]DuClo, *Apologia*, 36–37. "Hoc argentum vivum metaphorice animatum appellant. Nam veluti in animalium corporibus anima caloris est principium, & causa, & sine qua mortua jacerent corpora: sic argentum vel aurum principium est caloris in argento vivo, quod alioqui frigidissimum nec quidquam alteratum persisteret." Cf. *De triplici*, 399.

aurific seed."[51] I refer to this school and its adherents as mercurialists, and in fact, many subsequent mercurialists acknowledged DuClo as a chief of their school. The mercurialist camp counts as members many of the major alchemists of the seventeenth century—Eirenaeus Philalethes, Johann Joachim Becher, and even Robert Boyle; Stahl claims this as the most promising of the chrysopoetic schools.[52]

Not only the choice of gold and mercury as components, but especially DuClo's purgation and animation of common mercury is key to the practice of scores of alchemical practitioners. One hundred years later, Becher's *Concordantia mercuriorum lunae* begins with DuClo's animated mercury.[53] The precious antimonial mercury which has been shown to lie at the heart of the whole highly influential seventeenth-century Philalethan corpus is in fact mentioned by DuClo where he mentions chrysopoeians who employ a "mercury drawn from the regulus of antimony." DuClo may be referring to his contemporary Alexander von Suchten, whose publications on antimony describe the antimonial mercury later used by many seventeenth-century mercurialists including philalethes.[54] Alternatively, both DuClo and Suchten may be drawing from some more widespread set of antimonial mercurialists of which we are not presently aware. In any case, these specially prepared mercuries from DuClo occupied the thoughts and laboratory operations of very many chrysopoeians until the 1720s at least.

In terms of the larger project of producing a truer, more complete view of alchemy by recognizing its internal diversities, we have in Gaston DuClo an alchemist denominable as a scholastic mercurialist chrysopoeian. With such a classification he not only provides a concrete example of a specific alchemist of noteworthy influence but also supplies a point of comparison with alchemists whose practices, goals, and styles diverge from his. We find in DuClo a purely physical, rational, and coherent system of transmutational alchemy; one which employs subtle reasoning and experience (for example, noting the difference between physical mixture and chemical change), weaves together strands of thought from several disparate sources both classical and contem-

---

[51]DuClo, *Apologia*, 59: "Illorum igitur tantum opinioni subscribo, qui naturam imitantes, aurum & suum argentum vivum pro materia aut subjecto seminis argentifici aut aurifici assumunt, solvunt & concoquunt."

[52]Newman, *Gehennical Fire*, esp. 210–227; Principe, *Aspiring Adept*, chap. 5; Stahl, *Principles*, 393–424, esp. 401 ff.

[53]Johann Joachim Becher, *Tripus hermeticus fatidicus* (Frankfurt, 1689), 150–183, on 152–513.

[54]Newman, *Gehennical Fire*, esp. 125–169: "Newton's *Clavis* as Starkey's *Key*," *Isis* 78 (1987): 564–574; DuClo, *De recta*, 410; Alexander van Suchten, *De secretis antimonii* (Strasburg, 1570); idem, *Antimonii mysteria gemina* (Leipzig, 1604).

porary, adopts a corpuscularian perspective, rejects vitalism, and adduces experimental evidence. At present, these attributes are likely to strike many readers as atypical of the alchemical enterprise as a whole, but an accurate assessment of how typical or atypical DuClo's thought really is must await further studies. At present, we can however find in DuClo a clear counter-example to many of the descriptors too casually and hastily applied to the whole of a supposedly uniform alchemy—vitalism, Paracelsianism and chemical medicine, obscurantism, and so forth—which are absent from the corpus of Gaston DuClo. Clearly, a huge amount of work remains to be done—this paper is not the last word on Gaston DuClo, and is only one small piece to the vast alchemical project I advocate.

APPENDIX

BIBLIOGRAPHY OF GASTON DUCLO

Note: I have seen all the editions listed here unless otherwise noted; the locations of rare editions are cited.

1590. *Apologia chrysopoeiae et argyropoeiae adversum Erastum.* Nevers: Pierre Roussin. Dedicated to Louis de Gonzague, Duc de Nivernois and de Rethelois, April 1, 1590. [Bibliothèque mazarine, not seen;[55] Gobet, *Minéralogistes,* 17–20.]

1592. *De recta et vera ratione progignendi lapidis philosophorum.* Nevers: Roussin. Dedicated to Prince Ernst, Elector Archbishop of Cologne, April 1592. [Brit. Lib.]

1594. *De triplici praeparatione auri et argenti.* Nevers: Roussin. Dedicated to Jacques de Laffin, Chevalier de l'Ordre du Roi, Sept. 1, 1594. [not seen, no copies located; Gobet, 21–22; DuFresnoy, *Histoire,* 3:154, gives the date 1592, and *Dict. Biog. Fr.* gives 1595.]

1598. *Apologia crysopoeiae*(!). [Geneva]: Heirs of Eustathius Vignon. Ed. Bernard Penotus, with Penotus' marginal annotations, preface, and dedicated to Moritz of Hessen-Kassel. Possibly an abortive attempt at a collected works edition, for an *Elenchus* (title-page *verso*) lists all three works, but only *Apologia* (pp. 1–216) appears. [University of Maryland]

1602. *Apologia chrysopoeiae* and *De triplici.* Ursel: Cornelius Sutorius. Printer's dedicated to J. R. Schefer, Elector Archbishop of Mainz; *Apologia:* Penotus' preface and annotations from 1598; *De triplici:* DuClo's dedication from 1592, Penotus' annotations. [DuFresnoy, 3:154, lists Frankfurt as imprint.]

1602. *Apologia.* In *Theatrum chemicum,* vol. 2, Ursel: Cornelius Sutorius. Text, annotations, preface from 1598.

1612. (Collected works) *Philosophia chymica tribus tractatus comprehensa.* Geneva: Jean Vignon. Penotus' dedication, preface, and annotations from 1598 and 1602, plus the anonymous *Canones decem.*

1612. Identical to above, but with Lyons imprint. [National Library of Medicine]

1613. *De triplici* and *De recta.* In *Theatrum chemicum,* vol. 4, Strasburg. Texts and matter from 1612.

1617. *Claveus Germanicus; das ist, Ein kostliches Büchlein von den Stein der Weisen auß den latein ins Teutsch versetzt.* Halle: Peter Schmidt and Joachim Krusicken. Trans. of *Philosophia chymica,* 1612.

1659. *Apologia, De triplici, De recta,* in *Theatrum chemicum,* 2:4–80, 4:363–88, 388–413. Reprint of 1613 *Theatrum.*

1695. *Traité philosophique de la triple preparation de l'or et de l'argent, et De la droite et vraie maniere de produire la pierre philosophique.* In [Nicolas Salomon?] *Dictionaire hermetique,* Paris: Laurent d'Houry, 1695. French translation of texts only, no front matter.

---

[55]As a result of archival research funded by the American Philosophical Society, I finally located a copy of this rare edition as this paper was going to press. Further details, including newly uncovered biographical data, will be forthcoming in a separate paper.

1981. *Apologia, De triplici, De recta*, in *Theatrum chemicum*, 2:4–80, 4:363–88, 388–413. Reprint of 1659, Torino: Bottega d'Erasmo

Spurious Attributions

1695. *Le filet d'Ariadne, pour entrer avec surete dans le labirinthe de la philosophie hermetique*. Paris: Laurent d'Houry. Reprint, edited by Sylvain Matton, Paris: Gutenberg reprints, 1984.
1718. *Filum Ariadnes, das ist, Neuer chymischer Discurs von den grausamen und verfuhrischen Irrwegen der Alchymisten*. Gotha: Jacob Mevius. [Supposed German translation of 1695 *Le Filet d'Ariadne;* actually an unrelated text by "Heinrich von Batsdorff," alias Christoph Reibehand, first published at Leipzig and Gotha, 1690].

Thomas Willard

THE MANY WORLDS OF JEAN D'ESPAGNET

THERE IS A WONDERFUL SCENE in Umberto Eco's novel about the age of discovery, *The Island of the Day Before*, where two clergymen debate, at swordpoint, the thesis that there are many worlds, many suns with many planets that can sustain life.[1] This was not a new idea; it was a doctrine of the Epicurean philosophers, which the Roman poet Lucretius voiced memorably, and Giordano Bruno wrote Latin verse in the manner of Lucretius when he revived the doctrine.[2] But Bruno was burned as a heretic in 1600, half a century before Eco's novel is set, and the notion of what William James would call a pluralistic universe seemed a dangerous *concetto*, if not an oxymoron.[3] Eco's liberal Frenchman has the upper hand in the swordplay, and has the conservative Italian worried about the providence of a world that is not the center of God's attention. But just as the Frenchman presses home his point, a stray bullet ends his life, making us wonder again about the workings of providence.

I take this as a starting point because it reminds us how much anxiety the doctrine of many worlds aroused in the late Renaissance. Even in a work on the alchemical cosmology, Jean d'Espagnet attracted the greatest attention in a section he glossed, "MVNDI PLURES IN VNIVERSO." The Latin tag *plures mundi* means "a great many worlds"—not just "many worlds," which would be *multi mundi*. I shall use it when I refer to the philosophical doctrine, for I

---

[1]Umberto Eco, *The Island of the Day Before*, trans. William Weaver (New York: Harcourt, 1994), 131–141; originally published as *L'Isola del giorno prima* (Milano: Libri & Grandi, 1994).

[2]Lucretius, *De rerum natura*, 1:951–1007; Frances A. Yates, *Giordano Bruno and the Hermetic Philosophy* (Chicago: University of Chicago Press, 1964), 318.

[3]William James, *A Pluralistic Universe: Hibbert Lectures at Manchester College on the Present Situation in Philosophy* (London: Longmans, 1909).

201

want to point out, more generally, that D'Espagnet was a typical "Renaissance man" and moved in many worlds. He was a magistrate and a mathematician, an antiquarian and an alchemist, a poet in Latin and French, and a friend of French literati. He concealed his identity behind anagrams when he published his alchemical masterpiece: *Enchiridion Physicae Restitutae* (1623), a general guide to cosmology, bound with *Arcanum Philosophiae Hermeticae Opus*, a more specific guide to alchemy.[4] In reference to his identity he said only that he was retired from public service (*curia*).[5] But the anagrams also revealed an affinity to the Paracelsian tradition and especially to Michael Sendivogius, the "noble Polonian" who concealed his identity in a "double anagram."[6] His true identity was not revealed for another generation, when his work was translated into English, French, and German and was anthologized alongside the poetic *Chrysopoeia* and his beloved Sendivogius.

D'Espagnet sees a contradiction in the traditional Western cosmology. The earth is a cesspool of all that is vile and sublunary, yet the innumerable heavenly bodies exist only to serve man on earth:

> Is it not rather more likely, that every Globe doth rather of it self make a peculiar world, and that so many worlds as feodaries to the eternal Empire of a God, are diffused through the vast range of the heaven, and there do hang as bound each to the other by the common bond of the heaven, and that the whole large Universe doth consist of those manifold natures?[7]

D'Espagnet sees no reason to think of the earth as a fixed point at the center of creation. How much more likely that the earth and its moon are two more objects in space, illuminated by the same sun? Nor does he suppose that life exists only on earth. Why not on the moon or elsewhere? He understands the appeal of the Ptolemaic cosmology, which places the sun midway between the empyrean and the earth,[8] but can also see the beauty of Copernican space, where the sun is like "an immortal Lamp, hanging up in the middle of the hall of the Great Lord, and enlightening all the corners & recesses of it."[9] He understands the beauty of man's relation to the God who took on human

---

[4]Jean D'Espagnet, *Enchiridion Physicae Restitutae; or, the Summary of Physics Discovered* with *Arcanum; or, the Grand Secret of Hermetick Philosophy*, ed. Thomas Willard (New York: Garland, forthcoming); originally published as *Enchiridion Phisicae Restitutae... Tractatus alter inscriptus Arcanum Hermeticae Philosophiae Opus* (Paris; 1623) and translated into English in *Enchyridion Physicae Restitutae. Or, the Summary of Physics Recovered*, trans. John Everard (London, 1651) and *Fasciculus Chemicus, Or, Chymicall collections... Whereunto is added the Arcanum, Or, Grand Secret of Hermetic Philosophy*, trans. James Hasolle [i.e., Elias Ashmole] (London, 1650). Subsequent references to these texts are to paragraph (¶) or aphorism (§) numbers.
[5]D'Espagnet, *Enchiridion*, ¶1.   [6]D'Espagnet, *Arcanum*, §12.
[7]D'Espagnet, *Enchiridion*, §241.   [8]Ibid., §30.   [9]Ibid., §243.

form at the incarnation; but he cannot see how man is any less honorable, or God any less honored, if other beings elsewhere praise his creation.

> Is it not more for Gods glorie, to assert the intire Fabrick of the whole Universe to be like a great Empire, graced with the various natures of many worlds, as with so many Provinces or Cities? and that the Worlds themselves are as so many habitations & tenements for innumerable Citizens of divers kinds, and all created to set forth the superlative glorie of the great Creatour.[10]

If the religious wars in France taught D'Espagnet anything, it was that a universal God has no part in local politics: as soon as he becomes partisan and sectarian he loses his omnipresence and omnipotence and becomes another idol. A universe with many worlds and many believers in the supreme being does not diminish man, in D'Espagnet's opinion, so much as it exalts God.

D'Espagnet adds the maxim "CŒLVM VNIVERSVM CONTINVVM EST" (the sky is a universal continuum).[11] He draws the line at the possibilities of "many skies" or "heavens," which would deny the existence of a universe and, with it, the unity of God's design in the creation. He elsewhere cites Aristotle's *De caelo*, the first sentence of which states that heaven neither came into being nor will be destroyed.[12] Moreover, in insisting on the continuum of the heaven, D'Espagnet rejects the "fancied Astrology" as an affront to the divine hierarchy: "fancied" because astrologers think they control events by reading the stars, when the stars only reflect the will of God. For D'Espagnet, the stars are so many "intelligences," directed by the divine power. Here he is closer to the second *libelium* of the *Corpus Hermeticum* than to the second book of Aristotle's *De caelo*. Movement need not come from outside the universe, he suggests, only from outside matter.[13]

D'Espagnet sees many worlds not only "out there" in the macrocosm or great world but "in here" as well. Traditionally, the microcosm or little world is understood to be man, and he devotes an aphorism to "HOMO MICROCOSMOS."[14] But it seems to him that the creation can be epitomized in other creatures:

> Lest man should dream fancies to himself, glory in divers priviledges, assume to himself as proper onely to him the name of *Microcosm*, or the Worlds lesser

---

[10]D'Espagnet, *Enchiridion*, §242.   [11]Ibid., §237.
[12]Ibid., §14; Aristotle, *De caelo* 268a.
[13]D'Espagnet, *Enchiridion*, §238; *Hermetica: The Greek* Corpus Hermeticum *and the Latin* Asclepius, trans. Brian Copenhaver (Cambridge: Cambridge University Press, 1992), 11 (*Corpus Hermeticum* 2.12).
[14]D'Espagnet, *Enchiridion*, §160.

draught, because there are discernable in his material workmanship, an Analogie of all the natural motions of the *Macrocosm*, or the larger Volume of the World, let him consider that every creature, even a worm, that every plant, even the weed of the Sea, is a lesser world, having in it an epitome of the greater. Therefore let man seek for a world out of himself, and he shall find it every where, for there is one and the same first Copy of all creatures, out of which were made infinite worlds of the same matter, yet in form differenced. Let therefore man share humility and lowliness of spirit, and attribute to God glory and honour.[15]

These are humbling thoughts for the elect, but inspiring for the scientist:

not onely man, but even every living creature, yea, every Plant is a *Microcosm*. So is every Grain or Seed a Chaos, in which are the seeds of the whole World compendiously bound up, out of which in its season a little World will spring.[16]

Wherever there is a perfect mixture of elements, there is "a body, spirit, and soul." D'Espagnet proceeds to identify the body with the element of earth (not any physical lump of soil), the spirit with the element of air, and the soul with the element of fire. When the elements are joined in a "perfect" or stable mixture, life is created, and each life epitomizes the whole creation. It follows that there is a whole "little world" in the alchemical vessel and that the perfect mixture is living. D'Espagnet likes especially to write about *argent vive* or quicksilver. In his companion tract on the *Arcanum: Or, the Grand Secret of Hermetick Philosophy*, he talks about the circulation of the matter in the retort on the analogy of the circulation of water in the world at large. He refers the reader back to the *Enchiridion*, saying: "Let the Philosopher therefore consider the progresse of Nature in the Physicall Tract more fully described for this very end."[17]

In the *Arcanum*, D'Espagnet notes: "The generation of the Stone is made after the patterne of the Creation of the World."[18] Moreover, "The Generation of the Philosophers Stone, is not unlike the Creation of *Adam*."[19] The alchemical work sums up the six days of creation, culminating with the breath of life into the red clay, *terra Adamica*. D'Espagnet is willing to expand the interpretation of the six days of creation to six thousand years on the principle that a day with God is as a thousand years.[20]

---

[15] D'Espagnet, *Enchiridion*, §146. [16] Ibid., §161.
[17] D'Espagnet, *Arcanum*, §83; see D'Espagnet, *Enchiridion*, §135–41.
[18] D'Espagnet, *Enchiridion*, §73. [19] Ibid., §74. [20] Ibid., §37; Ps. 90:4.

D'Espagnet recognizes that the reactions in the alchemist's laboratory must occur on a very small scale. He therefore accepts the doctrine of atomism some years before Gassendi made it fashionable:

> Experience teacheth us in the artificial resolution & composition of mixt Beings, which are tryed by distillations, that the perfect mixtion of two or more bodies, is not done but in a subtile vapour. But Nature doth make her mixtions far more subtile, and as it were spiritual, which we may safely believe was the opinion of *Democritus*: for the grosseness of bodies is an impediment to Mixtion, therefore the more any thing is attenuated, the more apt and fitted it is for mixtion.[21]

What keeps D'Espagnet so far removed from Gassendi, and in league with the alchemists rather than the new scientists, is his conviction that the old sympathies are still very much at work in a pluralistic universe. However vast the worlds, there is the theme of perfect harmony: "These, though so far severed in nature and place, yet do joyn in a mutual love, so as to make up a perfect harmonie in the Universe."[22]

The *plures mundi* above, in the astrologer's heavens, are still one world or macrocosm because they still work in unison, guided by the single intelligence, which D'Espagnet called God. Similarly, the many worlds below, in the alchemist's vessel, are a single world or microcosm as long as the work is successful and the matter is alive. The human being sets the pattern for understanding the living heavens and the living stone: to be alive is to be animated, to have a soul controlling the body. The soul of the alchemist has a special kinship with the Soul of the World, for the *anima mundi* is at work in all life processes, even in the alchemist's vessel. The soul at work animating the stone is an inner alchemist or *artifex*. After all, D'Espagnet writes about alchemy as *philosophia Hermetica*. He quotes the *Corpus Hermeticum* frequently, and his early French editor, who called himself Chymeriastes, regarded the *physica restituta* or recovered science of D'Espagnet's first tract as one and the same with the *philosophia Hermetica* of the second tract.[23]

Why the anxiety about *plures mundi*? The great modern commentator on the *Corpus Hermeticum*, Father Festugière, suggests that the cosmos became a god in the late classical world—not just an image of God, as in Plato's *Timaeus*—and that the cosmos was secularized only with the opening up of space:

> What strikes the modern is the infinity of space. In this infinite space, innumerable stars move about at immense distances from one another, so

---

[21]D'Espagnet, *Enchiridion*, §153.   [22]Ibid., §241.   [23]Ibid., appendix 1.

that it is impossible to connect them and reassemble them into a single order. Moreover, these stars are pure matter; they are not living beings, let alone divine beings. For the ancient man, on the contrary, the world is truly a *Kosmos*: it is an order. Limited, it makes up a certain number of concentric spheres, whose revolutions are in accord and make harmony. Moreover, the sky is animated; the universe is a great Being, and each of the stars that revolve in the sky is also itself a being. Finally, since the stars move in regular movements they are divine. The ancient recognized a tie between the souls of the stars and the human soul, and the idea of a communion was born. The means of this communion, in the present life, would be contemplation. After death, the human soul would go to rejoin the star that was akin to him *(synnomon astron)*.

That is not enough to explain everything. To unite itself to the cosmic Deity, it is necessary to pass through the world, and hence to contemplate the world. This contemplation requires a science. And because this science leads to God, it is very much a religion. In turn, the study requires a type of life, which, considering its goal, would be the highest life. It is here, in this conception of science, and consequently the life of science, that ancient man differs from modern man. First of all, modern man distinguishes radically between science and religion, no longer adoring the sky as a visible god and the image of the invisible God.[24]

In a later essay, Festugière points out "a direct analogy" between the Demiurge animating the cosmos and the alchemists' "perfect magistery": "for the latter consists partially of producing a tincture (or elixir, or ferment, or 'mercury') that will be the principle of life for all metals and that will then play, in that regard, the role of soul."[25]

Alexandre Koyré explains in his famous lectures on the transition *From the Closed World to the Infinite Universe* that Descartes saw as much to celebrate in the opening of space as Bruno did.[26] But Festugière has an important point. The separation of science and religion proved the crucial event in the scientific revolution, and that event occurred when the cosmos and matter itself became "inanimate" and *anima*, soul, became the exclusive concern of religion.

D'Espagnet's insistence on soul in matter and in the cosmos leaves him finally with the alchemists rather than the scientists. His French translator of 1651 wrote that the maxims of Descartes "detracted neither from the author of

[24]A. J. Festugière, *La Révélation d'Hermès Trismégiste,* 4 vols. (Paris: Gabalda, 1944–1954), 1:174–175.

[25]A. J. Festugière, *Hermétisme et mystique païenne* (Paris: Aubier-Montaigne, 1967), 233.

[26]Alexandre Koyré, *From the Closed World to the Infinite Universe* (Baltimore: Johns Hopkins University Press, 1957).

the *Enchiridion* nor from his glory of being the first in France who worked to restore the ancient philosophy."[27] A few years later, the royal historian Charles Sorel ranked D'Espagnet with the "modern innovators in science," but added a note on the *Arcanum*:

> Truly, since many rightly regard the Philosophers' Stone as a chimera, that [alchemy] could discredit the whole book, were it not so beautifully explained that it has won him a reputation. The Peripatetics condemn it entirely. Others approve some opinions, and reject those which seem full of visions, like saying that the light of the sun and all other light is spiritual and that physical fire is spiritual in this respect.[28]

Before the seventeenth century was out, the biographer Pierre Bayle described D'Espagnet as a literary man with some curious ideas about science:

> One could say that this [*Enchiridion*] is the first book to appear in France with a natural science completely contrary to Aristotle's. Although the author pretends it as simply the ancient philosophy whose claims he reestablishes, many things put in there are perhaps of his invention.[29]

The word "invention" has the old ring of "rhetorical invention" rather than the new emphasis on scientific discovery.

In the eighteenth century, D'Espagnet kept his reputation as an alchemical philosopher in the school of Sendivogius, a proponent of the aerial niter theory that preceded the discovery of oxygen. But he became known increasingly as a philosopher dedicated to the "resacralization" of nature.[30] In a recent book on *physica sacra*, Antoine Faivre suggests that the *Naturphilosophie* of the nineteenth century had its roots in the theosophy of the eighteenth century and the Paracelsian theory of the seventeenth. Faivre adds that the *philosophia sacra* worked for "the restoration, which is to say, the re-Christianization of the natural sciences."[31]

D'Espagnet names no contemporary thinkers except for alchemists; there is no evidence he knew of Bruno, but he shared with Bruno a fascination with the art of Ramon Lull. D'Espagnet was "addicted" (his son's word) to the alchemical works of pseudo-Lull, whereas Bruno mastered the mnemonic art

---

[27]Jean Bachou, trans., *La philosophie naturelle restablie en sa pureté.....Avec le traicté de l'ourvrage secret de pierre philosophie d'Hermez, qui enseigne la matiere et la façon de faire la pierre philosophale* (Paris, 1651), sig a6r.

[28] Charles Sorel, *De la perfection de l'homme* (Paris, 1655), 250.

[29]Pierre Bayle Pierre, *Dictionnaire historique et critique*, 4 vols. (Rotterdam, 1697), 1:1095.

[30]Antoine Faivre, *Philosophie de la Nature: Physique sacrée et théosophie XVIIIe–XIXe siècle* (Paris: Albin Michel, 1996), 10.

[31]Ibid., 26.

of the Mallorcan mystic.[32] But Bruno did not draw a distinction between the two groups of texts, which were published together as late as the eighteenth century. Indeed, in referring to Paracelsus as a practitioner of *medicina Lulliana* under newfangled names of his own, Bruno showed that both he and Paracelsus were familiar with the pseudo-Lullian corpus.[33] Like Paracelsus and Bruno after him, Lull drew a distinction between blind "influence" of stars on human life that D'Espagnet would call "fancied Astrology" and the genuine "correspondence" of things above and below. Lull's powers above are close to Platonic ideas; goodness (*bonitas*) is one. For Lull and even more, perhaps, for the pseudo-Lullians, the correspondences enhanced the powers of humanity, whereas the influences limited them.

The French alchemists were steeped in the theory of "Lullius": not the Majorcan mystic himself, who specifically denied the logic of transmutation, but the subsequent writers who mounted their theory and practice on his "art."[34] The *ars Lulliana* was above all a combinatorial art: it showed how almost infinite variety could emerge from the combinations of a set number of concepts. The pseudo-Lullian texts were Lullian inasmuch as they employed the wheels of letters, each letter representing a thing or state of being. D'Espagnet recognized the infinite possibilities for generating new things and beings, whereas Bruno evolved a combinatorial art which, Eco says, "positively thirsts after infinity."[35]

The major printed texts of Lullian alchemy are a pair of tracts on the theory and practice of transmutation with a codicil on the art of transmuting the soul of metals.[36] The theoretical tract begins by identifying the "dispositions" on which all practice must be based; and here by distinguishing the temperate body from the intemperate and the neutral, the natural body from the unnatural and the "contra-natural." From these it proceeds to the four principles of

---

[32]Reported in Olaf Borch, *Conspectus Scriptorum Chemicorum Illustrorum* (Copenhagen, 1697), 36–37.

[33]See Frances A. Yates, "The Art of Ramon Lull: An Approach to It through Lull's Theory of the Elements," reprinted in *Collected Essays*, vol. 1, *Lull & Bruno* (London: Routledge, 1982), 27, and the response to Yates's remarks in Walter Pagel, *Paracelsus: An Introduction to Philosophical Medicine in the Era of the Renaissance*, 2d ed. (Basel: Karger, 1982), 241–247.

[34]Jean-Claude Frère, *Raymond Lulle: Le docteur illuminé* (Paris: Grasset, 1972), 260–262; see the epilogue on seventeenth-century Lullism in J. N. Hillgarth, *Ramon Lull and Lullism in Fourteenth-Century France* (Oxford: Clarendon, 1971), 293–298.

[35]Umberto Eco, *The Search for the Perfect Language*, trans. James Fentress (Oxford: Blackwell, 1995), 137; originally published as *Ricerca della lingua perfetta nella cultura europea* (Bari: Laterza, 1993).

[36]Raymundus Lullius, *Theorica, Practica,* and *Codicilus,* in *Theatrum Chemicum*, 2d ed., 6 vols. (Strasbourg, 1659–1661), 4:1–134, 135–70, 171–98.36. D'Espagnet, *Enchiridion*, §244.

the macrocosm or *magnum mundum* (angels, heaven, world, and nature) and the four principles of the microcosm or *magisterium*, including here the four elements (fire, air, water, and earth) and the four qualities (hot, cold, moist, and dry). But it adds to this a fifth principle, which it calls "primordial and substantial" and from which the others proceed. It then juxtaposes the universal or "extreme" principles with the temporal or transient, the four elements with the vapors of the elements.[37] We are now in a world of impermanence yet of permanence, of endless variation yet of certain fixtures designated with letters of the alphabet, as in the works of the "real" Lull. The alphabets change through the *Theorica* and *Practica*. One runs to twenty-four letters, including Greek *zeta* (ζ). Here is the last table *De Significatione Literarum*[38]:

A	God, who is the first cause of this work
B	the four elements confused in metals
C	lunary rectified, in which metals are dissolved
D	the quintessence of wine, or the quintessence in its perfection
E	the soul of metals, which is called the sulphur of metals
F	sulphur
G	the residues of the elements
H	the first degree of heat, in the bath
I	the second degree of heat, in the ashes
K	the third degree of heat, for the sublimation of sulphur
L	the soul of the body, i.e., the calx dissolved in its proper menstrum
M	the spirit of the perfect body
N	water
O	air
P	fire
Q	the glass vessel
R	the stone itself

[37]Lullius, *Theorica*, in *Theatrum Chemicum*, 4:3–12 (chaps. 2–4).
[38]"De Significatione Literarum," in *Theatrum Chemicum*, 4:195.

For Lull and for the pseudo-Lullians, these magical letters seem to grow on trees. But whereas Lull's tree, popularized in France by Jacques Lefèvre d'Étaples, taught the philosophy of love,[39] the alchemists' tree taught metallic transmutation. Christopher of Paris, writing c. 1545 and described as "an imitator of the old philosopher Raymond Lull," devoted a book of his opus on transmutation to "The Practice of the Philosophical Tree."[40] Capital letters drop like apples from a tree, as they do again in a design from Michael Maier's chapter on French alchemy.[41] A treatise on the "solar tree" which comes immediately before Christopher's text in the *Theatrum Chemicum*, and which seems related, is said to be "translated from the manuscript of an anonymous French adept" and is sometimes attributed to D'Espagnet.[42] It does not use the alphabetic mnemonic, and is entirely compatible with the "mineral tree" of Paracelsians like Gerhard Dorn.[43] Although I see no reason to think that D'Espagnet wrote it, I am tempted to think that he passed his knowledge on to his real son (as the Danish alchemist Olaf Borch suspected) very much as the adept who introduces the work speaks to his alchemical "son."[44] But the little tract serves as a reminder that the Lullian and Paracelsian traditions came close together.

Of all the alchemists, Michael Sendivogius had the strongest influence on D'Espagnet, and is most often bracketed with D'Espagnet by later alchemists. Sendivogius followed Lullius and recommended his work.[45] Sendivogius even wrote a parable about the "solar" tree.[46] But he also used the ideas of Paracelsus—and occasionally used such Paracelsian terms as *archeus:* "the servant of Nature,"[47] otherwise called "the occult virtue of Nature, universal in all things, the artificer, the healer," "the dispenser and composer of all things."[48] He never mentioned Paracelsus by name, however, and gave this "artificer" figure a name of his own: the "central sun."[49] He was fascinated by the gener-

[39]Hillgarth, *Ramon Lull and Lullism*, 318.
[40]Christophorus Parisiensis, *Elucidarius…liber secundus seu Practica Scientiae Arboris Philosophalis*, in *Theatrum Chemicum*, 6:228–254; for the date and quotation see 6:288.
[41]Michael Maier, *Symbola Aureae Mensae Duodecim Nationum* (Frankfurt, 1617), 345.
[42]*De Arbore Solare*, in *Theatrum Chemicum*, 6:163–194.
[43]Gerhard Dorn, *Genealogica Metallorum*, in *Theatrum Chemicum*, 1:574.
[44]Borch, *Conspectus Scriptorum*, 36–37.
[45]Michael Sendivogius, *De Lapide Philosophico*, "Epilogus," in *Theatrum Chemicum*, 4:440.
[46]Ibid., "Parabola," in *Theatrum Chemicum*, 4:444.
[47]Ibid., tract 2, in *Theatrum Chemicum*, 4:424.
[48]Martinus Rulandus, *A Lexicon of Alchemy*, English translation [by Julius Kohn], ed. Arthur Edward Waite (London, 1893; reprint, York Beach, Maine: Weiser, 1984), 36, 37.
[49]Michael Sendivogius, *De Lapide Philosophico*, tract 11, in *Theatrum Chemicum*, 4:437. Similarly, Walter Pagel, *The Smiling Spleen: Paracelsianism in Storm and Stress* (Basel: Karger, 1984), 21,

ation of the two from the one and the regeneration of the one from the two, which he says is the work of the adept.[50] In the companion tract "Concerning Sulphur," he considers the generation of the androgynous stone from the male and female principles, and of them, in turn, from the *tria prima* (sulphur, mercury, salt) and the four elements (fire, air, water, earth):

> as the three Principles are produced out of the four, so they, in turn, must produce two, a male and a female, and these two must produce an incorruptible one, in which are exhibited the four (elements) in a highly purified and digested condition, and with their mutual strife hushed in unending peace and goodwill.[51]

The male and female are Sol and Luna, the celestial sun and moon generated by the one God. These are not gold and silver, in Sendivogius, but sulphur and mercury in the forms of niter and quicksilver. This niter is "a vital substance presumed to be present in the air and in rain," a usage common in England between the mid-seventeenth and late-eighteenth centuries.[52] Endless generation follows from them, the proliferation of all things under the sun; from them the alchemist produces the one stone of the philosophers.

D'Espagnet follows Lull and Sendivogius in regarding the four elements as principles rather than materials, to be grasped in theory rather than in practice. He emphasizes the work on sulphur and quicksilver, as they both do, and has the same interest in generation; hence the "wheels" of nature in the *Enchiridion* and the "circulation" of elements in the *Arcanum*. However, Lull and Sendivogius discuss only the generation of life in the sublunary world; over that there is the single macrocosm and its pattern in what Lull calls the angelical world and Sendivogius calls the archetype.[53] D'Espagnet takes their thought a step further and, like Bruno and the ancient Epicureans, considers the profusion of worlds beyond the earth and its moon. What saves

---

has called D'Espagnet a Paracelsian, and a strong one too—not a moderate or conservative. This seems quite an accurate assessment. For although D'Espagnet never mentions Paracelsus by name, and prefers traditional alchemical and philosophical terms to the Swiss reformer's neologisms, he belongs to the same tradition in alchemy.

[50]Michael Sendivogius, *De Lapide Philosophico*, tract 6, in *Theatrum Chemicum*, 4:430.

[51]Sendivogius, *The New Chemical Light*, in *The Hermetic Museum, Restored and Enlarged*, English translation, ed. Arthur Edward Waite, 2 vols. (London: James Elliott, 1893), 2: 143.

[52]*The New Shorter Oxford English Dictionary, s.v.* "nitre"; see Allen G. Debus, "The Paracelsian Aerial Niter," *Isis* 55 (1964): 43–61, and Zbigniew Szyldo, "The Alchemy of Michael Sendivogius: His Central Nitre Theory," *Ambix* 40, no. 3 (Nov. 1993): 129–146.

[53]Sendivogius, *New Chemical Light*, in *Hermetic Museum*, 2:138.

D'Espagnet and Bruno from despair at the endless diversity is the hermetic faith (also Christian and Platonic) that they will find the one in the all. D'Espagnet, who is more orthodox than Bruno, admits that the thirst for infinite knowledge lies behind man's fall from grace and expulsion from Eden,

> so he that would stretch himself to a sinfull desire of a forbidden knowledge, might be nipt by a just deprivement of what was given: and…might be punished with the loss of that true Knowledge, which was one of all things. That is the Cherub, the guardian of the Garden, he that hath his flaming faulcheon, striking blind the guiltie souls of men with the brightness of his light, and forcing us off from the secrets of Nature, and the truth of the Universe.[54]

He thus likens the fear of the infinite to the cherub with the flaming sword guarding the gates of Paradise.[55]

The theory of *plures mundi* raises further possibilities today. The Jungian approach to alchemy as a study of personality allows the possibility of many worlds within the personality. C. G. Jung referred to D'Espagnet's *Arcanum* mainly for its mythological references, documenting the mental and emotional powers that alchemists placed on their stone and their work.[56] Neo-Jungians have paid increasing attention to the gods and goddesses within the psyche, and to the experience of being possessed by the numinous in one form or another. In this discussion, Jung tended to be more monotheistic, while the Neo-Jungians tend to be more polytheistic, but there is talk of unity and diversity, the psyche and the archetypes, much as D'Espagnet and his contemporaries talked of a single god with many forms of worship or the representative life of the prince and the many lives of the prince's subjects.[57]

The term "many worlds" has yet another meaning in quantum mechanics, where it describes the theory that with every major event in the universe, a split occurs and a parallel world breaks off where the event never occurred.[58] The present essay has in fact broken off from a conference presentation on D'Espagnet, and the presentation, in turn, broke off from the preface to a new

---

[54]D'Espagnet, *Enchiridion*, §244.

[55]Gen. 3:24.

[56]D'Espagnet, *Enchiridion*, §135–145; *Arcanum*, §83–91. C. G. Jung, *Mysterium Coniunctionis*, trans. R. F. C. Hull, 2d ed. (Princeton: Princeton University Press, 1970), 157, 163, 302, 356; Jung cites references to Diana, Hercules, Venus, and Jove in *Arcanum*, § 42, 52, 46, 137, respectively.

[57]D'Espagnet wrote the continuation of a Renaissance tract on the training of a prince, published as the *Rozier des guerres* (Paris, 1616; facsimile reprint, Paris: Collection Zanzibar, 1994). For a Neo-Jungian approach to alchemy see "The Salt of Soul, the Sulfur of Spirit," in *A Blue Fire: Selected Writings of James Hillman*, ed. Thomas Moore (New York: Harper, 1989), 112–129.

[58]See Bryce S. DeWitt, ed., *The Many Worlds Interpretation of Quantum Mechanics*, Princeton Series in Physics (Princeton: Princeton University Press, 1973).

edition of the *Enchiridion* and *Arcanum*.[59] Inevitably, the D'Espagnet presented here is slightly different from the others, and it may be appropriate to add a few words about each of them.

One of the last things I did after annotating D'Espagnet's texts was to prepare a glossary of terms. It took only a few hours, but proved a very instructive project. To gloss a word is, etymologically, to interpret another *glossa* or tongue—that is, to translate the word—and I found it tempting to translate D'Espagnet's terminology. For example, when he wrote of metals "fitly prepared with their proper Sulphur and Arsenick,"[60] it was tempting to suggest that he meant yellow arsenic or orpiment rather than red arsenic or realgar, and tempting to explain further that he thus indicated arsenic trisulphide (As_2S_3) rather than the monoclinic sulphide of arsenic (AsS). When he referred to "a perfect fixation and permanency to endure a strong tryall, and resist searching *Saturne*," I was tempted to gloss "*Saturne*" with the "Azoqueated Vitriol of Raymund Lully,"[61] but I was also tempted to gloss "vitriol" as sulphuric acid (H_2SO_4) or possibly a sulphate. The temptations passed. (I am an English professor; the chemist is my wife.) D'Espagnet lived in a world where there were Lullian trees instead of periodic tables and where there were three gradations of heat between freezing and boiling, not one hundred degrees. He knew about realgar but knew nothing of sulphides, not knowing about valences, and what he could read about realgar would tell him there were four kinds: realgars of fire, air, water, and earth.[62] He wrote about a world that no more exists today than the horse-drawn caroches he describes,[63] a world where transmutations are said to take place.

When the papers from this volume were first presented, in shorter versions, the subsequent discussion made it clear that key words like "science" had quite distinct meanings in the late Renaissance, pointing in quite different directions. This was hardly a new proposition, of course, for during the last fifty years historians have invited us to contemplate that great cosmological break known as the Scientific Revolution. Allen Debus especially has helped us to glimpse the possibilities of a parallel world where the ideals of the alchemists and their fellow travelers—Paracelsians, Rosicrucians, cabalists—led the

---

[59]See n. 4.

[60]D'Espagnet, *Arcanum*, §29.

[61]Ibid., §33; "A Supplement to the Alchemical Lexicon of Martinus Rulandus," ed. Arthur Edward Waite, in Rulandus, 422.

[62]Rulandus, 274–275.

[63]D'Espagnet, *Enchiridion*, §72.

advancement of science.[64] In the world where Paracelsianism was next to god-liness, Jean D'Espagnet stands out as a voice of reason and order. And if the theory of many worlds seems the quintessence of relativism, Aristotelian bifurcation run amok, D'Espagnet reminds us that the splits all go back to a primal unity, which he calls God.

[64]The sense of parting ways is a regular theme of Debus' work, from "The Elizabethan Compromise" in *The English Paracelsians* (London: Oldbourne, 1965; New York: Watts, 1966), 49–85, to "the great chemical debate" in *The French Paracelsians* (Cambridge: Cambridge University Press, 1991), 46–101. A good place to begin is his chapter on "The New Philosophy—A Chemical Debate" in *Man and Nature in the Renaissance* (Cambridge: Cambridge University Press, 1978), 1116–1130.

Kathleen Wellman

Talismans, Incubi, Divination, and the *Book* of *M*✣

The Bureau d'Adresse Confronts the Occult

As the title of this chapter suggests, participants in the weekly conferences held at the *Bureau d'adresse* addressed a wide range of occult topics.
These topics, broadly construed, discussed phenomena that operated in ways
which could not be readily incorporated into an understanding of the usual
operations of nature; they demonstrated hidden rather than manifest qualities.[1] Participants raised questions about the existence or appearance of bizarre
creatures. They discussed occult phenomena like the unicorn and the philosophers' stone and assessed the merits or lack thereof of occult practices and
texts.

These conferences were one of the many intellectual and institutional
innovations sponsored by Theophraste Renaudot,[2] an influential bureaucrat
patronized by Richelieu during the reign of Louis XIII. Renaudot used his
office of intendant of the poor, to create a career of enormous influence. He

---

[1]It is important to note that "occult" is not used as a term of opprobrium to discredit certain
opinions. Instead, topics with occult ramifications are treated in the same way as more orthodox
topics although they generally posed more difficulty for discussion.

[2]Although Renaudot's career has been the subject of scholarly interest, the conferences them-
selves have been neglected. The best source on Renaudot's career is Howard Solomon, *Public Wel-
fare, Science and Propaganda in Seventeenth-Century France: The Innovations of Theophraste Renaudot*
(Princeton: Princeton University Press, 1972), 162–200. For other biographies of Renaudot, see
Gaston Bonnefont, *Un Docteur d'autrefois* (Limoges, 1893); *Un Oublié, Théophraste Renaudot:
Créateur de la Presse, de la Publicité, des Dispensaires, des Monts-de-piété* (Limoges, 1899); Gilles de la
Tourette, *Theophraste Renaudot, d'après des Documents inédits* (Paris, 1884); *La Vie et les Oeuvres de
Théophraste Renaudot* (Paris, 1892); Albin Rousselet, *Theophraste Renaudot, Fondateur de Policlin-
iques* (Paris, 1819).

215

founded government-operated pawn shops, opened his premises to free med-ical consultations, created a low-interest loan program for the poor, and oper-ated a *Bureau d'adresse* — an employment, housing, and information clearing house. Renaudot was also keenly involved in the intellectual issues of his day. Besides publishing the *Gazette de France* (for which he is still honored as a founder of the French press and repudiated as a royal propagandist), he spon-sored a series of conferences held every Monday afternoon between August 22, 1633, and September 1, 1642.

Renaudot's conferences occupy an unusual position in the history of early modern academies. He saw them as a new intellectual forum that would delib-erately undermine the typical rules of conduct of an academy; he made the gatherings public, not private, and, unlike traditional French academies, he welcomed participants who were not members of the nobility. Thus it included notable scholars and professionals such as doctors and lawyers. And, as contemporary critics often pointed out, the *Bureau* also attracted a number of dilettantes or virtuosi, as they called themselves — men of rank, leisure, and wealth.[3]

The procedures governing the conferences were as unconventional as its membership: The *Bureau* opened its doors to all, setting no limit on the num-ber of speakers and imposing no moderator to regulate opinion; all topics were to be admitted save religion and affairs of state (although political issues were frequently discussed in the later years). It used a novel forum, with unre-stricted membership and unfettered discussion to treat a vast array of topics.[4] Every Monday afternoon a room at the *Bureau,* which held at least one hun-dred people, was filled to capacity to discuss the topic proposed the week before. Proceedings of the conferences were published every week from 1634 to 1641 by Theophraste Renaudot on inexpensive paper for weekly distribu-tion; they were reprinted in folio editions in leather-bound volumes in collec-

---

[3]Most studies of Renaudot's group include Tomaso Campanella, Etienne de Claves, and Jean-Baptiste Morin as important scholars who attended the conferences. I have been unable to find any primary evidence to support those claims. The claim is also made that because the confer-ences provided such an open forum that women likely attended. But since conference participants preface their remarks by saying things like "if the ladies were here to defend themselves," it does not seem likely that women attended. It is more reasonable to assume, as most scholars have, that many of the physicians staffing Renaudot's medical clinics in the morning remained to attend the conferences in the afternoon, especially since so many medical issues were discussed.

[4]This article is a small part of a larger study of the content of the conferences which situates them into the broader context of the seventeenth century and conceives of them as a crucial link between Renaissance humanism and Enlightenment social science.

tions of one hundred conferences.[5] (The conferences of 1642 were published in 1655 as a collection by Renaudot's son, Eusèbe.) The published proceedings of these meetings can be used to canvass a range of seventeenth-century opinion on a variety of issues.

It is not surprising that the group which met at the *Bureau d'adresse* should bring occult topics under its purview. It fancied itself a gathering committed to wide-ranging discussion of intellectual issues at the cutting edge of science, and science was the specified topic of about half of the conferences. Many of the participants were physicians who also staffed Renaudot's medical clinic and chemical dispensary.[6] But regardless of their specific expertise, participants felt empowered to discuss scientific issues. They presented themselves as bound by the highest standards of skepticism and empirical judgment. This article will focus specifically on their responses to the occult topics they proposed for discussion. It is not at all unusual that such a group should dedicate a number of conferences to occult topics. Although they are perhaps foreign to our notions of science, occult topics were integral to seventeenth-century scientific discussion and lay bare some of the fundamental epistemological problems of the scientific revolution.[7]

"OF TALISMANS"

I would like to present an overview of a specific conference, "Of Talismans,"[8] April 7, 1636, in order to highlight the style, tone, and method of these conferences. This particular conference also effectively points to some recurrent themes in the treatment of the occult.

The first speaker on the topic defines talismans as nothing but "images in relief or engraved upon medals or rings, ordinarily of metal on precious

---

[5]These volumes went through several editions in the seventeenth century, sometimes without indication of their source. Individual conferences were sometimes reprinted in both French and English. A two-volume folio edition appeared in England in 1664 and 1665, perhaps to coincide with the foundation of the Royal Society. *A General Collection of Discourses of the Virtuosi of France, upon questions of all Sorts of Philosophy, and other Natural Knowledge. Made in the Assembly of the Beaux Esprits at Paris, by the Most Ingenious Persons of that Nation*, 2 vols; vol. 1 trans. G. Havers, and vol. 2 trans. J. Davies (London: Thomas Dring and John Starkey, 1664–1665).

[6]Once again, this is conjectural but it seems quite likely that physicians attended.

[7]For a discussion of the centrality of occult phenomena, see Keith Hutchison "What Happened to Occult Qualities in the Scientific Revolution?" *Isis* 73 (1982): 233–252.

[8]Conference 108, part 1, "Des Talismans," *Troisième Centurie des Questions traictées aux conférences du Bureau d'Adresse, depuis le 18 Fevrier 1636. jusques au 17 Janvier 1639* (Paris: Bureau d'Adresse, 1642), 65–70. For an overview of the role of amulets in seventeenth-century medical practice, see Martha Baldwin, "Toads and Plague: The Amulet Controversy in Seventeenth-Century Medicine," *Bulletin of the History of Medicine* 67 (1993): 227–247.

stones, in the shape of men or animals." These images, produced under specific constellations, retain the influence of that constellation. Thus this speaker assumes not only that the macrocosm/microcosm relationship is efficacious, but also that its power can be captured in objects. "These figures act, as they say, either upon men's minds, as to cause one to be loved or honored ... or upon their bodies, as to cure them."

Other speakers too find in the fundamental natural relationship of the macrocosm/microcosm the most compelling support for talismans: "For everything below is as that which is above, and the effects of inferior things proceed from the various configurations of the celestial bodies." Furthermore, a speaker insists, "the knowledge of these sympathetic correspondences is the true magic ... the highest point of human knowledge, marrying heaven with earth"; its opposite, "black magic, is detestable, shameful and ridiculous." A speaker points to "the magnetic cure of wounds, by applying the medicine to the weapon that did the hurt or to the bloody shirt"[9] as a concrete demonstration of the efficacy of talismans. In general, when speakers discuss any occult topic, they align their belief in a particular occult phenomenon with their overall understanding of nature and marshall empirical evidence to support their positions.

Another speaker insists that talismans are "natural agents ... by occult and sympathetic virtues, which cause many strange effects, which the ignorant vulgar incongruously ascribe to magic or spells." Although he is careful to distinguish his understanding of the issue from that of the vulgar, he does not doubt the efficacy of talismans. To support his belief, he cites historical evidence, such as the golden calf attested to by Marsilio Ficino, the idols of the pagans, and Paracelsus' talismans against the plague, which, for this speaker, "render their effects as common, as their existence [is] certain."[10]

---

[9]In the seventeenth century many people believed in sympathetic action in nature. Paracelsians, in particular, believed that sympathy allowed the possibility for action at a distance. This action could then explain magnetism and other natural phenomena. One of the most controversial applications of this notion of sympathetic action was the belief in weapon/salve, a practice of treating the weapon rather than the wound. For an extensive discussion of this belief and the controversy it provoked, see Allen G. Debus, "Robert Fludd and the Use of Gilbert's *De Magnete* in the Weapon-Salve Controversy," *Journal of the History of Medicine and Allied Sciences* 19 (1964): 389–417. The weapon-salve issue had become particularly controversial in the 1620s in Paris with the publication of Jean-Baptiste van Helmont's *De Magnetica vulnerum curatione* in 1621. For a discussion of this particular controversy, see Allen G. Debus, *The French Paracelsians: The Chemical Challenge to Medical and Scientific Tradition in Early Modern France* (Cambridge: Cambridge University Press, 1994), 102–115.

[10]In general, in the conferences, speakers are inclined to use the historical record to provide concrete substantiation of specific points rather than as textual authorities.

Another speaker presents an analogy which he finds so compelling that he assumes there can be no effective rebuttal. He says that "it is not necessary to seek reason and authorities to prove talismans, either in art or nature; since man himself may be seen to be *the* talisman and perfection of God's works, placed by Him at the center of the universe." His ultimate point is the query, "In fact, isn't this soul in its immortality a talisman of His divinity?" In other words, the relationship of resemblance in nature is a microcosmic reflection of God's relationship to man and therefore beyond dispute.[11]

For other speakers, the topic of talismans raises epistemological issues. Some object to what they see as too rigid an insistence on empirical demonstration; "He is too sensual who impugns the truth of things under pretext that they fall not under our reason."[12] Instead of relying on puny reason, this speaker urges one to "witness what is seen in all the admirable works of nature and art, in the magnetic cure of wounds and that of disease, by the amulet."[13]

Other speakers take more skeptical and critical stances. One speaker insists that "occult" phenomena must act in accord with our understanding of causation: "Everything acts in the world by the first or second qualities, or by its substance." But talismanic figures, he claims, "act neither by heat, cold, hardness, softness, nor any other first or second quality, any more than by their substance, which is different in talismans of copper, iron, stone, etc." Following up on this skeptical position, another speaker contends that none of the supposed connections between talismans and effects can be sustained. Remedies cure not by resemblance, but by virtue of the properties inherent to their substance. A talisman, he insists, cannot act through its own power, nor can it act on the will, nor is there any connection to the stars. Another speaker points out that because belief in talismans cannot be substantiated by our

[11]While speakers do not discuss religious topics, they sometimes use religion to shape discussion of other kinds of topics. Often they distinguish between the religious ramifications of topics and the aspects of topics which could be explored without recourse to the inexplicable. In other words, they avoid the mystical and the theological and concentrate instead on historical evidence or direct experience or, simply, more naturalistic phenomena. For example, one speaker on the topic of amulets insists that it can be decided "in the ordinary course of natural things ... without recourse to good or bad angels"; conference 173, May 17, 1638, "Des amuletes, et si l'on peut guérir les maladies par paroles, brevets, ou autres choses pendues au col, ou attachees aux corps des malades," *Troisième Centurie,* 465.

[12]*Too sensual,* in this case, is an attack on too great an appreciation of reason "which though very weak and uncertain, abusing the principality which it usurps over all the faculties, has turned its denomination into tyranny"; conference 108, "Des Talismans," *Troisième Centurie,* 66.

[13]The story of Gyges' ring is a source of great fascination for speakers, and many seem to accept it as a legitimate example of the use of magic. Perhaps the story has enhanced authority because its source is Plato, "The Republic," in *Plato: The Collected Dialogues,* ed. Edith Hamilton and Huntington Cairns, (Princeton: Princeton University Press, 1982), 2.359d.

understanding of the operations of nature, some have resorted to the argument that the relationship between talismans and ordinary natural phenomena must be one of contraries. "So to cure hot and dry diseases, they engrave their talismans under a constellation contrary to the evil, such as cold and moist." But, the speaker objects, such arguments are "an invention of Paracelsus, who fancies poles, a zenith, a nadir, an equator, a zodiac, and other fantastical figures in our bodies, answering to those of heaven, without the least proof of his sayings."

This brief overview of one specific conference gives some notion of how they were conducted, that is, how topics were raised, how speakers responded to other arguments, and how wide and diverse the response to a specific topic could be. This particular conference also casts into high relief some of the themes which reoccur in discussions of other occult topics which I will explore in greater detail. These are: (1) the particular problems of definition posed by occult topics; (2) the question of what counts as sufficient evidence to substantiate claims for occult phenomena; (3) the role religion plays in these conferences; (4) and, most generally, the grounds on which occult phenomena are understood, believed, or doubted.

DEFINING THE TERMS

Unlike more conventional topics, occult topics require clarification and definition as a way for speakers to gain control over them since they are by their very nature elusive and contentious. But even if a conference begins with a relatively clear exposition, subsequent speakers frequently offer emendations which obscure the issue.[14] (Ultimately some conferences degenerate into sessions which look like definition by committee.)

Speakers frequently put forward definitions as initial responses to a topic and, more specifically, as a way to demystify occult topics. (For example, in a conference "Of the cabala," the first speaker claims that "cabala ... signifies

---

[14]For example, in a conference on sympathy and antipathy, the first speaker defines sympathy and antipathy "as the similitude or contrariety of affection." But another speaker reveals some of the difficulties in applying or extending the definition to specific cases. "Every thing naturally affecting to become perfect seeks this perfection in all the subjects which it meets; and when the same disposition is found in two or several bodies or minds, if they would arrive at that perfection by one and the same way, this meeting serves for the means of union, which is our sympathy; and their different disposition or way, the contrary"; conference 32, part 1, "De la Sympathie & Antipathie," *Récueil Général des Questions Traittées es Conference du Bureau d'Adresse, sur toutes sortes de Matières, Par les plus beaux Esprits de ce temps* (Paris: Chez Jacques Le Gras, 1635), 257.

nothing else but tradition."[15]) Definitions allow participants to discriminate "true manifestations from delusions," to curtail the influence of practitioners of the occult as narrowly as possible, and to discuss belief in the occult in terms of human psychology. Speakers are not simply skeptical; they also conscientiously winnow out the acceptable from the unacceptable. Other speakers, who concede some legitimacy for occult practitioners, like sorcerers, then circumscribe their activities so they fit into ways of discussing the natural rather than the occult. For example, in "Of divination," a speaker insists that they are talking neither about medical diagnosis based on the reading of symptoms in the sense of Hippocrates' *Prognostics*,[16] nor about reading perfectly obvious and consistent natural signs, like the prediction of rain based on seeing a rainbow. Instead, he says, "if, not knowing a prisoner or his affairs, I foretell that he will be set free or not; that an unknown person will be married, and how many children he will have, or such other things which have no necessary, or even contingent causes known to me; this is properly to divine." He concludes, "Therefore all your soothsayers, augurs, sorcerers, fortune-tellers, and the like, are but so many impostors." For this speaker, any claim to divination that is not a reading of natural signs based on an understanding of nature is fraudulent. Another speaker classifies the "occult" out of consideration by removing two kinds of divination from discussion, those caused by God or the devil.[17] He then focuses solely on natural divining by drops of oil, looking glasses, crystal cylinders, enchanted rings, entrails of beast, amniotic fluid, and so forth.

Although definitions serve many important functions for speakers, they do not always offer satisfactory solutions to the intellectual complexities of occult topics. Some speakers, frustrated by the difficulties involved in discussing these topics, adopt strongly skeptical positions. For example, the question "of sympathy or antipathy" raises, for at least one speaker, fundamental doubts about our ability to know. As he concludes, "to speak truth, all these effects are no more known to us than their causes.... He who endowed them with forms, having annexed properties thereunto, both the one and the other, impenetrable to human wit." Another speaker goes further, suggesting that "it

---

[15]Elaboration by subsequent speakers complicates the issue. Another speaker insists that when Moses received the Ten Commandments, he also received another law not written and more mysterious; conference 37, "De la Cabbale," *Récueil Général*, 297.

[16]Because of this ability to read natural signs, according to this speaker "nothing makes physicians more resemble gods"; conference 80, part 2 "S'il y a quelque Art de Déviner," *Deuxième Centurie des Questions traitées aux conferences au Bureau d'Adresse*, 247.

[17] These, he says, are not, therefore, properly divination; ibid., 248.

is more fit to admire these secret motions…than to seek the true cause of them unprofitably."[18]

Substantiating the Occult

Speakers are well aware that arguments made in support of the occult require strong substantiation, but they demonstrate conflicting notions of what counts as compelling evidence. Some evidence is drawn from the historical record. A speaker on the topic of the philosophers' stone cites its historical witnesses, for example, Hermes Trismegistus, Johan Glauber, and Raymond Lull. Although speakers are certainly willing to discount a particular source or its application to a particular issue, some contend that it would be unwarranted hubris to dismiss the entire historical record. On the question of spirits, for instance, a speaker is unwilling to discount the ghost of Brutus or the scriptural accounts of the return of "Samuel, Moses, and Elias." As one participant put it, "it is presumption to disbelieve all antiquity."[19]

How should one evaluate evidence? What are the limits to human certitude about evidence? Although many speakers take critical positions in discussing occult topics, some speakers express concern that skepticism has perhaps gone too far. They seem to espouse the constructive skepticism associated with contemporary thinkers like Marin Mersenne and Pierre Gassendi.[20] For example, a speaker counsels moderation in either accepting or rejecting satyrs, because,

> it is as dangerous to conclude that all that we have not seen is impossible as to be credulous about everything. But when reason and the authority experience carries with it are on the same side, our incredulity has no excuse. Now the satyr is such a case; for it may be as well produced by the mixture of the seeds of two species, just as mules are. Besides, is not the imagination of the mother, of which we have daily examples, capable of imprinting this as well as any other change of figure in a child's body?[21]

Another speaker follows up on these points, advising caution in the face of growing skepticism. "It is easier to overthrow than to establish a truth, when the question is about a thing apparently repugnant to reason, which many times agrees not with our own experience."[22]

---

[18]Conference 32, part 1, "De la Sympathie & Antipathie," *Récueil Général*, 258.

[19]Conference 79, part 2, "De l'Apparition des Esprits ou Phantômes," *Deuxième Centurie*, 235.

[20]See Richard Popkin, *The History of Scepticism from Erasmus to Spinoza* (Berkeley: University of California Press, 1977), 129–156.

[21]Conference 250 "Des Satyres," *Quatrième Centurie*, 257–260.   [22]Ibid.

To discuss those phenomena which are widely believed to exist, speakers take a number of different positions. While a very few are disconcertingly credulous, most recast the topic in credible terms. The conference on "Incubi and succubi,"[23] for example, is a particularly interesting discussion of the physiology of occult phenomena. One speaker points to diseased states as the cause, that is to say, one believes in incubi and succubi because of the impeded movement of spirits through the brain.[24] Another speaker distinguishes between the "superstitious and the ignorant vulgar and the physician." He further suggests that a legitimate treatment of occult phenomena requires medical expertise,[25] because physicians are able to distinguish "what is fit to be attributed to nature and her ordinary motions from what is supernatural." A speaker explores the physiological conditions which might cause one to believe in the incubus: "When respiration (the most necessary of all the animal functions) is impeded, we imagine we have a load lying on our breasts…. And because the brain is involved in the incubus, all the animal functions are hurt; the imagination depraved, the sensation obstructed, motion impeded." He also describes the effects of disease states on the imagination and physiology.

> Though the cause of this disorder is within ourselves, nevertheless, the distempered person believes that some body is about to strangle him by outward violence, which the depraved imagination thinks about rather than about internal causes…. This has given rise to the error of the vulgar, who charge these effects to evil spirits, instead of imputing them to the malignity of a vapor or some phlegmatic and gross humor oppressing the stomach.[26]

However, as one speaker on the topic of mandrake notes, the association of certain occult phenomena with the vulgar has led to an unwarranted dismissal of them. Unfortunately, he claims, the superstitions of the vulgar have made it less likely that the mandrake, despite its beneficial medicinal proper-

---

[23]Conference 128, "Des Incubes & Succubes & Si les Demons peuvent engendrer," *Troisième Centurie*, 185–188.

[24]This speaker extends the medical analysis: "the case of it is a gross vapor, obstructing principally the hinder part of the brain, and hindering the egress of the animal spirits designated to the motion of the parts…which vapor is more easily dissipable than the humor which causes the lethargy, apoplexy, and other symptoms, which are therefore of longer duration than this; which ceases as soon as the said vapor is dissipated"; ibid., 186.

[25]"Two sorts of people err in this matter—the superstitious, and ignorant vulgar, who attribute everything to miracles, and account the same done either by saints or devils, and the atheists or libertines, who believe neither the one nor the other. Physicians take the middle way, distinguishing what is fit to be attributed to nature, and her ordinary motions, from what is supernatural"; ibid., 187.

[26]Conference 128, "Des Incubes & Succubes & Si les Demons peuvent engendrer," *Troisième Centurie,* 185–188.

ties, will be used, because "mountebanks have by their frauds and tricks brought people to believe their strange stories of it, even that it eats like a man, and performs his other natural functions." [27]

On the topic "Of the Unicorn," the first speaker assumes that because so many written sources deny the existence of the unicorn, belief in it is simply a popular error. He does not find it credible that the Romans, who "were very careful to delight their people with spectacles of the rarest beasts, would have forgot to show them unicorns, if there had been any." However, he is refuted by a speaker who claims that negative arguments are not sufficient to dismiss or discredit an occult phenomenon or an occult practitioner.

> If the verity of things were shaken by the false conceits others have of them, there would be no physicians, because there are often ignorant ones; no point of right, because many do not know it…no true religion, because the pagans and others have had false ones…. It follows not that they had no unicorn in their amphitheaters, because there is no mention made of any; an argument drawn from negative authority is not demonstrative. [28]

While it is fairly common to argue against a certain phenomenon because the vulgar believe in it, one speaker makes an argument reversing this perspective. He insists that the unicorn must have existed, because so many influential people have put unicorns to so many uses. "In short, it is not credible Clement VII, Paul III, and diverse others, would have taken this animal for their arms, if there were no such animal; nor do popes so much want understanding that Julius III would have brought a fragment of it for twelve thousand crowns which his physician used successfully in the cure of venomous diseases." [29] The appeal to social evidence, that is to say, the argument that because powerful and influential elites believe in a phenomenon, it must therefore exist, is highly unusual in these conferences. It is an interesting reversal of the much more common argument, which might be summarized as "the vulgar believe it; therefore it is not credible." Occult phenomena (more than conventional topics) require speakers to determine which authorities are appropriate as historical sources, to distinguish the uninformed beliefs of the vulgar from the educated understanding of the physician, and to determine which popular beliefs are credible. While some do insist on professional status or education as necessary criteria for discussing occult topics or performing occult prac-

---

[27]Conference 222, "De la Mandragore," *Quatrième Centurie des Questions traitées aux Conférences du Bureau d'Adresse, depuis le 24 Janvier 1639. jusques au 10 Juin 1641* (Paris: Au Bureau d'adresse, 1635), 162.

[28]Conference 248, "De la Licorne," *Quatrième Centurie,* 246.   [29]Ibid., 247.

tices, these speakers do not suggest training in arcane knowledge or apprenticeship to an occult practitioner as necessary or advisable.

Speakers also clearly feel that they must determine the philosophical grounds on which occult phenomena are to be accepted or rejected. In other words, they take on fundamental epistemological issues. Some speakers object to rationalist dismissals of occult phenomena. (Interestingly, in many conferences on the occult, empiricism functions as a way to undermine too great an emphasis on reason.) Others solidify their definitions (literally) by direct appeals to empiricism. Magnetism, for example, provides an important empirical demonstration of the application of sympathy. But empirical evidence does not necessarily clarify these issues because of the inability of speakers to adjudicate between contradictory claims based on equally probable or improbable empirical evidence. Furthermore, empirical evidence is not universally hailed. One speaker insists that to believe only what we see is to be "too sensual," especially since the evidence from estimable ancient sources, like Aristotle and Plato,[30] confirms that spirits exist. "Too sensual," in this case, connotes too great an insistence on the primacy of one's own experience as opposed to the authority of the opinions of others, especially those of the ancients.

Certain kinds of empirical evidence are harshly castigated. One speaker says about the empirical arguments given in support of the existence of the unicorn: The "marks" given of it are "equivocal, incredible, and ridiculous, " and the

> trials of empirics are even more ridiculous; they boast, that if a circle be described with a piece of this horn upon a table, and an adder or spider laid in the middle of it, they can never come out of it; and, that these animals die, if only held a quarter of an hour under the shadow of this horn.... In brief, these numerous contradictions, impossibilities, and uncertainties make me conclude this story of the unicorn is a mere unicorn.[31]

---

[30]This speaker cites the importance of spirits to Aristotle and Plato: "Although it be an universal doctrine of all sober antiquity that there are spirits and that they appear often times to men in cases of necessity, by which, according to Aristotle himself, the souls of the dead friends are affected ..." and "As Apuleius reports, the Platonists make three sorts of spirits, first, demons or Genii, which are souls while they animate bodies; second, lares, or penates, the souls of those who had lived well and after death were considered tutelary gods of the houses which they had inhabited; third, Demures or Hobgoblins, the souls of the wicked, given to do mischief or folly after death, as they did during their life"; conference 79, part 2, "De l'Apparition des Esprits ou Phantômes," *Deuxième Centurie*, 235.

[31]Conference 248, "De la Licorne," *Quatrième Centurie*, 245–249.

Another speaker criticizes too great a reliance on empirical evidence and suggests that, in maintaining that incubi and succubi exist, he is carving out a moderate position. "As it is too gross to recur to supernatural causes, when natural ones are evident, so it is too sensual to seek the reason of everything in nature and to ascribe to mere phlegm and the distempered fantasy the coitions of demons with men." However, to support his argument with evidence he finds compelling, he cites testimonies of direct confrontations with devils. He is particularly willing to credit accounts from exotic locales, such as Peru and Turkey.[32] Even though he has denounced rationalist arguments against the existence of incubi, he nonetheless offers several arguments about how the propagation of devils might rationally take place. They might well, for instance, "borrow some human seed and transport it almost instantly so as to preserve its spirits from evaporation." Just "as the devil performs the natural actions of animals by supernatural means…so he may make a perfect animal without observing the conditions of ordinary agents."[33] This speaker supports his argument from contradictory perspectives. He denounces excessive reliance on authority and offers empirical evidence in support of his position. He then advances his own rationalistic explanation, enumerating the natural processes which could explain the propagation of incubi by devils. But ultimately, he insists that devils are not bound by natural processes.

This conference highlights just one of the many difficulties involved in defining or categorizing the proceedings as subscribing to a specific philosophical school. These participants use whatever arguments make their case or whatever they conceive as the most persuasive argument or response to another speaker.

UNDERSTANDING NATURE

Despite the obvious confusion on this and other occult topics, the speakers, who firmly believe in phenomena like these, do so in part because they are able to reconcile that belief with an understanding of nature. Often the correspondence between a particular occult phenomenon and their understanding

---

[32]The evidence he provides for accepting coition with demons is drawn from personal testaments, and thus "we cannot deny without giving the lie to infinite of persons of all ages, sexes, and conditions, to whom the same have happened." He also finds accounts from distant places persuasive. "Even at this day, in the Island of Hispaniola, by the relation of Chieza, in his history of Peru, a demon, called by the inhabitants Corocota, who has given women and children horns." And, he points out, "among the Turks, those people whom they call Nephesolians, are believed to be generated by the operation of Demons"; conference 128, "Des Incubes & Succubes & Si les Demons peuvent engendrer," *Troisième Centurie,* 185.

[33]Ibid., 186.

of nature is based on their presuppositions about nature, which we do not necessarily share, such as the presumed existence of the devil and his role in a hierarchy of matter, a commitment to Paracelsian matter theory, a belief in the hierarchy of nature, and so forth. Beliefs such as these do not in any way distinguish participants in these conferences from universally heralded figures of the Scientific Revolution, like Francis Bacon, Robert Boyle, or Isaac Newton. It may be difficult for the modern reader to credit, but it is undeniable on the basis of textual evidence that these views of nature based largely on analogic relationships, like the macrocosm-microcosm, remain persuasive explanatory tools throughout the seventeenth century.

In addressing occult topics, speakers (1) directly confront their presuppositions about things they believe are and are not restricted to operating within natural bounds and (2) insist on uniform and universal operation of nature (although they are not agreed on what those operations are). Thus they circumscribe, to whatever degree possible, the occult within the operations of nature. One speaker integrates the philosophers' stone into a Paracelsian understanding of nature: "salt is its matter, and motion its fire."[34] When discussing sympathy and antipathy, speakers situate the topic within a broader framework of how nature functions. They assume, for example, that all creatures seek self-preservation, using both manifest and occult qualities, by, as one put it, "adhering to what was conductible to it and avoiding the contrary."[35] A speaker dismisses satyrs as fabulous because of his understanding of nature. Although he concedes that extraordinary things make the greatest impression on the mind, nonetheless he insists "those that have most exactly examined the power of nature, find the mixture of these species impossible, not only on the part of the matter...but also in respect of the form, which is indivisible, especially the rational soul." [36]

But some speakers protest these efforts to demystify nature or force it into a mold which conforms to human reason. Another speaker claims that to doubt the existence of the unicorn only on the basis of negative arguments calls into question "the power of nature, to deny such virtue to be found in inanimate bodies, as in the serpentine tongues found in the caves of Malta, sealed earths, and minerals, such as those they call for that reason *unicornu*

---

[34]Conference 43, part 1, "De la Pierre Philosophale," *Récueil Général*, 345–349.

[35]The fourth speaker advocates a Paracelsian understanding of nature: "If their forces and virtues be contrary, they destroy one another: which is called antipathy. If the same be friendly, they unite and join together, the stronger attracting the weaker. Hence, iron does not attract the lodestone, but the lodestone iron"; conference 32, part 1, "De la Sympathie & Antipathie," *Récueil Général*, 259.

[36]Conference 250, "Des Satyres," *Quatrième Centurie*, 258.

minerale."[37] This argument asserts an omnipotent nature which is not susceptible to human reason or standards of evidence.

In a discussion "Of the Mandrake," the first speaker takes the doctrine of
signatures as a given because "Nature has (instead of the instinct bestowed on
other animals to guide them to their good) given man reason, whereby he
may proceed from things known to things unknown; so besides the manifest
and occult qualities of plants, from which their uses may be inferred, she has
marked those which are most useful to us with certain signs and characters."[38]
He accepts the signature theory as a given and the mandrake as the most thor-
oughgoing example. However, the speaker is critical of the overextended
application of signature theory. The mandrake is problematic because, as it
encompasses the whole man, it is such an inclusive signature that it has been
too broadly and too uncritically construed. Because it represents "the figure of
an entire man, and, as the eminent virtues of ancient heroes, being too great
to be comprehended by the wits of these ages, gave occasion to fabulous
Romances, so too, the Wits of Botanists, that have been capable to write the
virtues of other simples, have not been sufficient to speak of these mandrakes."
The mandrake has not been well understood or described by scientists, "leaving the vulgar the liberty to attribute supernatural virtues to them." While this
speaker takes a skeptical stance and assigns belief in the mandrake to the vulgar, he nonetheless relishes telling the tales of the power of the mandrake from
various histories.[39]

The third speaker offers logical reasons why it is possible that a plant like
the mandrake could grow from human sperm on the ground. "Man to whom
niter contributes very much, which as a salt which is not lost by death, nothing hinders, that in a fertile soil, a plant, determined by some form or other,
should arise out of it." However, he is careful to qualify his belief by saying

[37]Conference 248, "De la Licorne," *Quatrième Centurie,* 249.

[38]He points out some of the most striking signatures: "Among these, the mandrake is the
most famous, representing not the eye, as eyebright does; nor the lung, as lungwort; nor the liver
as liverwort"; conference 222, "De la Mandragore," *Quatrième Centurie,* 161.

[39]These are some of the contemporary references: "Our histories report, that in the year of
1420, a certain cordelier named friar Richard, was so persuasive in his sermons, that in two days
the Parisians publicly burnt all the instruments of voluptuousness and debauchery, and particularly, the women their images; and mandrakes which they kept wrapped up in their attires, upon
a belief that as long as they had mandrakes, they should never fail to become rich.... Belleforest,
also relates, that the Maid or Orleans was calumniated for having acquired the valor she testified
against the English by the magical virtue of a mandrake. And Henry Bouquet, a modern author,
affirms, that thieves steal goods out of houses and children from their mother's breasts by its help;
those who behold them being unable to defend themselves, because this plant stupefies their
hands"; conference 222, "De la Mandragore," *Quatrième Centurie,* 162.

that the possibility can be sustained only if the experiments reported are true "that the salts of rosemary, sage, mint, and some other strong-scented herbs, being extracted according to art and frozen in a glass, exhibit the image of those plants, and, if sown in well-prepared earth, produce the plants of same species."[40]

Another speaker insists it is not impossible to fit a creature like the mandrake into an understanding of the organization of nature, "since there are middle natures composed of two extremes, as your zoophytes between plants and animals, to wit, sponges and coral; between brute and man, the ape; between the soul and the body of man, his spirits: why may there not be something of a middle nature between man and plant, to wit, mandrake, a man in external shape, and a plant in effect and internal form."[41] Thus, this speaker suggests that, while creatures which fall between our categories may be difficult to categorize, it is not impossible to reconcile them with the more regular behavior of nature.

Occult subjects also raise other fundamental issues about understanding nature; for example, the appropriate relationship between art and nature.[42] (In these discourses *art* refers to all that is produced by human beings.) One speaker discounts the possibility of the philosophers' stone because its existence would suggest that art could surpass nature, while another responds that drawing out gold from base metals would be but a pale reflection of the vast accomplishments of nature.[43] In other words, this speaker suggests that knowledge of the occult is vouchsafed to man by nature, as a kind of knowledge which demonstrates nature's power without encroaching upon it. Another speaker insists that because nature gives us no desire in vain (another fundamental presupposition about nature), not that the philosophers' stone must exist, but rather that the search for it must be productive. Just as mathematicians, by their quest to square the circle, have arrived at the knowledge of many things which were unknown to them; so too, he argues, though the chemists have not discovered the philosophers' stone, they have, nonetheless, uncovered admirable secrets in vegetables, animals, and minerals.[44] Pursuit of occult knowledge provides a productive research agenda, because nature does

[40]Ibid., 166

[41]Conference 222, "De la Mandragore," *Quatrième Centurie*, 165.

[42]Conference 82, part 1, "Quel est le plus puissant de l'art ou de la nature," *Deuxième Centurie*, 257–262.

[43]But "since art draws so many natural effects out of fitting matter, as worms, serpents, frogs, mice, toads, and bees," he did not consider it absurd that "at least by the extraordinary instruction of good or bad spirits, some knowledge of this operation may be derived to men"; ibid., 160.

[44]Conference 43, part 1, "De la Pierre Philosophale," *Récueil Général,* 345.

not allow man to seek in vain. Once the claim is made that, although man may not find what he is seeking, he will, nonetheless, make discoveries that are useful, productive, and so on, then "science," broadly construed as any systematic investigation, is guaranteed to be productive and utilitarian.

Furthermore, the relationship between nature and the occult works both ways: speakers use their understanding of nature to refute or to corroborate occult phenomena; and, the arguments speakers use for or against a particular occult phenomenon ultimately support their understanding of nature. Despite the difficulties involved in defining and applying these qualities, speakers find such topics particularly engaging and a constructive way to understand and describe natural processes, such as generation, growth, survival, and so forth.

Psychology and the Occult

One particularly interesting facet of their discussion of the occult is that conference participants understand that one way to deal with such topics is to separate the question of whether occult phenomena exist from the question of why people believe they do. Some speakers suggest that the lure of the occult is rooted in human nature. For example, on the question "Whether there be any art of divination," a speaker notes that man alone understands time and "hence his ardent desire of presaging." Other speakers contend that people believe in occult phenomena for various psychological reasons. They believe that they see spirits only because of their fancy, "men being prone to acquiesce in their own imagination though misguided by the passion of fear, hope, love, desire; especially children and women who are more susceptible of all impressions, because their fancies are so weak as to be no less moved with their own fictions than real external representations by the senses." Thus particular individuals, because of the weakness of their minds, are prone to believe in the occult. The criticisms of another speaker are much harder hitting: "Some jugglers pass for sorcerers among the vulgar." Another speaker points out that apparitions are caused when a soul is in pain because of present or future evil, perhaps because of an unfulfilled vow. [45] (This point clearly suggests an understanding of the effect of guilt on the imagination.) Another speaker explains popular credulity as the result of jealousy. For example, "when a private person arrives to great honor or estate suddenly, though it be by his merit, yet the generality of people, the meanest of which account themselves worthy of the

---

[45]"God for his own glory, the ease of his creatures, and conversion of sinners, permits it [an apparition] to manifest itself by ways most convenient"; conference 80, part 2, "S'il y a quelque Art de Déviner," *Deuxième Centurie*, 246.

same fortune, attribute such extraordinary progress to the devil."[46] Interestingly, the gullible, the guilty, and the jealous, identified in these conferences as those most likely to believe in the occult, are also recognized in recent and sophisticated scholarly treatments as the principal players in the drama of the early modern witchcraft trials.[47]

SORCERY AND METEMPSYCHOSIS

Although many speakers approach occult topics from a skeptical perspective, their efforts at demystification, rational clarification, and critical skepticism are frequently undermined if the topic resonates within the Christian tradition. Despite the disclaimer in the preface to the collection which asserts that religion will not be discussed in the conferences, religious arguments are invoked, if infrequently. However, they are more likely to be used in discussing occult topics, particularly those which bear on Christian beliefs. For example, one participant suggests that the cabala should be esteemed especially for "the hieroglyphical and mysterious names of God and angels which it contains." If the cabala can be associated with divine power, how can its powers be questioned? Or, if "black magic can do wonders by the help of malignant spirits,[48] why not the cabala, with more reason, by means of the names of God and the angels of light?"[49] This reverential treatment is quite foreign to the spirit of the conferences. By this statement, this speaker not only casts a religious reverence over the topic; he has effectively cut off subsequent discussion.[50]

---

[46]And yet, this speaker notes it is very rare for one to be enriched by the devil, a phenomenon he explains this way: "either because he reserves his riches for Antichrist so as to seduce the nations; or because God does not allow it, lest men should forsake his service for that of devils, and the good should be too sorely afflicted by the wicked"; conference 80, part 2, "S'il y a quelque Art de Déviner," *Deuxième Centurie*, 246.

[47]See in particular Keith Thomas's *Religion and the Decline of Magic* (Cambridge: Cambridge University Press, 1971).

[48]The tradition of demonic revelation as the source of black magic enters the western tradition through the work of Augustine. For a discussion of this tradition, see Keith Hutchison, "What Happened to Occult Qualities in the Scientific Revolution?" *Isis* 73 (1982): 235–237. For a discussion of the concern with the demonic in the scientific revolution, see Charles Webster, *From Paracelsus to Newton: Magic and the Making of Modern Science* (Cambridge: Cambridge University Press, 1982), 75–100.

[49]Another speaker concurs, noting that the church endorses this notion by using the name of Christ to cast out devils; Conference 37, "De la Cabbale," *Récueil Général*, 297.

[50]Perhaps conscious of the violation of the spirit of the conferences, this speaker then refocuses discussion on more empirical grounds by comparing the cabala to numerology. The sense that he recognizes that he has violated conference norms and retreats to a more acceptable treatment of these topics is simply my conjecture.

On the topic of sorcery, many speakers assume that sorcerers require the cooperation of the devil which further entails God's consent, "without which not one hair falls from our heads." (A scriptural citation is also unusual in these conferences.) Although the actions of the individual sorcerer are grounded in a compact with the devil, speakers insist, his work uses only commonplace items which have no special power in themselves.[51] Other speakers note that many of the effects attributed to sorcery are illusory, produced when the devil "makes use of delusions to cover his impotence, making appearance of what is not, and hindering perception of what really is. Such was Gyges' ring, which rendered him invisible when he pleased."[52]

Despite these criticisms, most speakers are unwilling to deny the existence of sorcerers. To question the power of the devil would implicitly undermine conventional religious beliefs. But some participants try to discount sorcerers by curtailing their influence. For example, one speaker claims "that the power of evil spirits, whose instruments sorcerers are, is so limited that they cannot either create or annihilate a straw, much less produce any substantial form, or cause the real descent of the moon, or hinder the motion of the stars, as heathen antiquity stupidly believed." Despite this rather scathing critique of the credulity of others, he concedes that sorcerers do have power over earthly things; "they are able to move all sublunary things; so they cause earthquakes, the devil either congregating exhalations into its hollowness, or agitating the air included therein."[53]

---

[51]"But the most ordinary means which they use in their witchcrafts are powders, which they mingle with food, or else infect the body, clothes, water, or air…sometimes they perform their witcheries with words, either threats or praises…. Not that these have any virtue in themselves any more than straws, herbs, and other things with which they bewitch people; but because the devil is by covenant able to produce such effects by the presence of these things"; conference 77, part 1, "Des Sorciers," *Deuxième Centurie*, 217. ,

[52]This speaker does allow the devil some real power: "The real are when the devil makes use of natural causes for such an effect, by applying actives to passives, according to them to perfect the knowledge which he has of everything's essence and properties; having lost no gifts of nature by sin, but only those of grace"; conference 77, part 1, "Des Sorciers," *Deuxième Centurie*, 217.

[53]Conference 77, part 1, "Des Sorciers," *Deuxième Centurie*, 222. Although the Christian tradition may predispose some speakers to believe in the occult, the first speaker on the topic of spirits cites many arguments for their existence derived from many kinds of sources within the western tradition. They are based on logic (the perfection of the universe requires the existence of angels), Aristotle ("Aristotle has nine classes of spirits below the level of the First Mover"), and Hermes Trismegistus ("Trismegistus acknowledged only two which hold the Arctic and Antarctic poles"). There are more orthodox arguments for the existence of spirits: some spirits are considered necessary for human preservation like guardian angels; other spirits war with man constantly, like devils; and other spirits animate bodies and separate from them at death. Conference 79, part 2, "De l'Apparition des Esprits ou Phantomes," *Deuxième Centurie*, 235.

Occult topics are treated much more critically when they are not part of the Christian tradition. For example, metempsychosis is described as a "heathen" belief, and speakers are much more explicit in questioning whether such beliefs can be sustained through reason and the "light of nature." Without the constraints of the Christian tradition, participants feel free to assert the necessity of "free and open" inquiry, insisting that "there is nothing which more enriches the field of philosophy than liberty of reasoning." A speaker concludes that "the heathen, guided only by the light of nature," had no reason to "maintain this extravagance." Another speaker refutes metempsychosis as a logical impossibility on several grounds. First, "it is impossible for one and the same thing which has been to be again new." Furthermore, for this speaker, the connection between body and soul, specifically the body as a significant reflection of the soul, would make it impossible for the soul to move to another body which would not reflect it.[54]

This particular conference raises, in a way that is fairly consistent in the treatment of occult topics, questions of what kinds of arguments and evidence are brought to bear to sustain or refute occult phenomena. However, it is significant that metempsychosis is denounced on logical grounds. In light of our understanding of the epistemological evolution of the scientific revolution, it is rather peculiar to note that "new" ways of arguing are used most frequently to bolster the existence of the occult, and conventional arguments are more frequently used to doubt or discredit occult phenomena. In other words, the topics that we and the participants who want to argue against them would consider mystical or bizarre are refuted by syllogism, analogy, or the most traditional kinds of arguments, whereas mystical or occult topics are frequently supported by appeals to historical evidence or medical reports. And, in supporting the occult, speakers are particularly inclined to provide empirical substantiation, which ranges from personal experience to anecdotal evidence to examples from ancient sources. And it is worth noting that citing ancient examples is not considered to be invoking authority but instead is presented as the careful use of evidence drawn from specific cases in ancient sources. These examples, even though derived from ancient sources, are considered credible counters to an excessive reliance on reason.

PARACELSUS AND THE OCCULT

Paracelsian topics are a good place to look for an indication of how participants saw occult topics. Since the conferences treat a fairly inclusive range of

---

[54]Conference 143, "De la Metempsycose," *Quatrième Centurie*, 245–249.

contemporary issues, one would expect Paracelsian topics to be addressed, especially since Renaudot subscribed to iatrochemical medicine and produced chemical remedies. Indeed, one finds a number of topics dedicated to Paracelsian themes, like the power of sympathy, the quintessence, the philosophers' stone, and so forth. In fact, Paracelsus had given many of the occult topics discussed in this article a new currency.

As a final indication of the nature of the treatment of the occult in these conferences, I would like to look at a particularly illuminating conference, "What Paracelsus meant by the *Book of M**," in some depth. By raising questions about the appropriate language for science and issues of secrecy and obfuscation, this conference highlights an important theme of the conferences in general. Both the *avant propos* to the collected discourses and the general statements speakers make about language insist on the value of clear expression and the open dissemination of science. In response to this concern, conference participants indicate both positive and negative assessments of Paracelsus and the Paracelsians. They are generally in sympathy with Paracelsian critiques of existing knowledge, but they disparage the arcane language and the deliberate obfuscation they associate with Paracelsian texts.[55] By and large, they appreciate the reformist endeavors they associate with the new chemical philosophy and are discomfited by the mystical overtones. In general, they put their stamp of approval on a kind of sanitized Paracelsianism.

The first speaker suggests that M stands for *mundus,* "that great book open to all that are minded to read it." Although he criticizes the arcane language of Paracelsus, he is sympathetic to his validation of the book of the world and his claim that the book of nature should replace all other sorts of books. "So remarkable is the difference between the theory and the practice of arts; for almost all books being false copies of that of the world, no wonder if book-doctors are most commonly ignorant of things, whose solid contemplation produces other satisfactions in the informed intellect, than do the empty fancies of those who … never understood what they write." He attacks knowledge which is too theoretical, too remote from nature, too intellectual, as

---

[55]The first speaker points to the fundamental concern. By looking at the frontispiece, he notes, "we may observe how remote this author's manner of writing is from that of the doctors of these times; yes, and of former times too, (if you except the Chemists) who mainly aim to speak clearly, and to render themselves intelligible, many of them professing to wish that things themselves could speak." The author is so committed to secrecy "that he conceals even the name of the Books he studied, by a kind of Plagiarism hiding his theft, lest others should trap him; and the same jealously runs through all his works"; conference 203, "Qu'est-ce qu'a voulu entendre Paracelse par le livre de M*," *Quatrième Centurie,* 73.

"fancies" which cannot be implemented and sees in Paracelsus an important counterweight to these kinds of knowledge.

The next speaker attacks the *Book of M** as an assault on medicine. It must, he insists, stand for magic, which he takes by definition to be diabolical because of the kinds of cures it claims to effect. Paracelsus, by "teaching in many places in his books to cure diseases by words and to produce men by enchantment in a great bottle, with other such abominable proposals, not to be accomplished but by diabolical assistance," must be a practitioner of magic. Anyone, he claims, who would presume to overthrow the art and tradition of medicine, must inevitably act with the help of either God or the devil. For this speaker, the unorthodox treatments Paracelsus suggests can only be the result of diabolical magic.

While speakers are quite critical of claims made for magic, nonetheless, any concerted attack on magic elicits a defense which carves out some acceptable arena for magical practice. For example, a speaker distinguishes between types of magic—natural, which is commendable, and black, which is to be abhorred. He notes "that it may be magic, and yet lawful, to wit, true and natural magic, such as was professed by the Indian Magi; three of them having discovered our savior's Birth, came to worship him; the other black and infamous magic, no more deserving that name, than empirics and mountebanks do that of physicians." He acknowledges magic as a specialized knowledge, available only to the learned.[56]

Another speaker returns to the topic to suggest that "M" is a talismanic figure which Rosicrucians use to recognize one another.[57] The fifth speaker dismisses the "secrets" as mere absurdities and indicts "authors who puzzle their readers minds with such figures." They "are as culpable as those are com-

---

[56]He makes a clear distinction between the kinds of knowledge available: "Now natural magic is the knowledge of the nature and properties of all things hidden to the vulgar, who take notice only of manifest qualities and reduce all to generalities, to avoid the pains of seeking the particular virtues of each thing; and therefore it is no wonder if they see only common effects and successes from them. Thus plants bearing the signature or resemblance of a disease, or the part diseased, such as lungwort, pepperwort, cure by a property independent of the first qualities, though few understand so much. Of this kind are many excellent secrets, whose effects seem miraculous, and much surpass those of ordinary remedies, whose virtues are collected only from their apparent qualities"; conference 203, "Qu'est-ce qu'a voulu entendre Paracelse par le livre de M*,"*Quatrième Centurie*, 74.

[57]He describes the talisman "M", "as a talismanic figure engraved in a seal, and employed by the Rosicrucians to understand one another; and called the Book M, because it represents an M crossed by some other letters, whose combination produces the mystery of the great work, designing its matter, vessel, fire and other circumstances; the first of which is dew, the true menstruum or dissolvers of the red dragon or gold"; ibid., 75.

mendable, who feed them with true and social demonstrations." He ridicules the pretensions and obscurantism of the Paracelsians: "Whereas we thought that this M signified Mons, we now see that it signifies no more than Mus; according to the ancient fable of the laboring mountains, out of which …issued forth nothing but a mouse."

The speaker who most vigorously defends Paracelsus does so, in effect, by defending deliberately obscure language, saying "that high mysteries have always been veiled under contemptible and often ridiculous figures; as if the wisdom of the more sublime spirits meant to mock those of the vulgar, who judge of things only by appearance." Furthermore, because there are many cases of medical treatments which do not reveal any clear affinities between cause and effect, "Why then may not the same reality be admitted between these characters and the effects claimed by those brothers of the Rosie-Cros?"[58]

The very name of Paracelsus flags concern with the occult and provokes sharp division of opinion which sometimes characterizes occult topics. Since the topic is so open-ended, that is to say, what did Paracelsus mean by "M" in the *Book of M**, it leaves speakers full range to insert whatever word beginning with the letter M they associate with Paracelsus. Obviously, they must first decide whether M should carry a positive or negative association. Then, if the word is one like magic, it raises the further questions about what magic is, the relationship between claims to magical knowledge and the practice of magic, and whether it has positive or negative connotations. This conference also vividly demonstrates the division between proponents of clear public expression of knowledge and proponents of knowledge as the hidden and deliberately obscured realm of the special practitioner. This conference also returns to the starting point of this paper by raising the question once again of talismans and the efficacy of symbolic representations.

Conclusion

Examining the treatment of the occult in these discourses is revealing. First, and perhaps most striking, the discussion is quite deliberately restrained. There are no gory details and almost no reveling in the bizarre. They do not look to occult phenomena as signs of demonic magic or use them to predict the future or the second coming. Instead, participants want to address these

---

[58]Conference 203, "Qu'est-ce qu'a voulu entendre Paracelse par le livre de M*," *Quatrième Centurie*, 76.

phenomena from the highest possible intellectual level. They are, in effect, engaged in an effort to sanitize and rationalize the occult. Second, speakers are acutely aware of the difficulties involved in treating these issues: they require definition, a restraining of the topic within appropriate parameters. As a result, such discussions illuminate standards of argumentation and evidence in cases that are frequently undemonstrable. Discussions of occult topics also provoke skeptical responses.

Occult topics consistently address epistemological issues, particularly questions of what standards of evidence should be argued for and how far one should go in insisting on the value of one kind of evidence over another. (Occult qualities, like many of the claims of the new mechanical science, contravene sensory evidence.) They offer oblique recognition of the damper religion put on scientific discussion. Perhaps because these are occult or hidden topics, they, ironically, offer a clearer indication of what counts as evidence than do discussions of more conventional topics.

Participants approach occult topics from a number of different scientific traditions. Interestingly, although they invoke traditions, the conferences do not offer set pieces—for example, the speech of an Aristotelian challenged by a Paracelsian, and so forth, as more orthodox scientific topics sometimes do. Instead (and this has proven to be exceedingly frustrating for those who have worked on the science in Renaudot's conferences), these speakers invoke tradition as they see fit, borrowing freely without regard for theoretical consistency or any notion that they would be expected by subsequent historians to evince a consistent theoretical position! Because these speakers meld together pieces of various traditions irrespective of the internal logic of the theory and because they use whatever pieces of the theory seem persuasive, they suggest a much more complicated and diverse evolution of scientific opinion in the Scientific Revolution than the replacement of an Aristotelian understanding of science with a new mechanical worldview.

Ultimately these documents are particularly good to think with. They allow one to explore the early seventeenth century from a great variety of perspectives. Occult topics, in particular, challenged participants to reconcile a number of contradictory elements in their worldview—demonstrable evidence and traditional beliefs, the scientific and the religious, experience and reason or logic, nature and the devil. They also challenge modern historians to expand notions of "science" to include such discussions and to reappraise the Scientific Revolution by acknowledging the fundamental significance of the occult within groups like the one which met at the *Bureau d'adresse*. However unorthodox its form and conclusions might appear in the positivist story of the Scientific Revolution, these conferences, like the proceedings of other gatherings committed to the diffusion of knowledge, demonstrate a quest to evaluate traditional knowledge in light of science.

Ursula Klein

NATURE AND ART IN SEVENTEENTH-CENTURY FRENCH CHEMICAL TEXTBOOKS

PARACELSIAN PHILOSOPHY HAD A STRONG INFLUENCE on seventeenth-century chemists, even on those not Paracelsians strictly speaking. Besides chemical philosophers, like Daniel Sennert, Joachim Jungius, or Robert Boyle, who often remained negatively conditioned by Paracelsianism while criticizing it, there was also a group of more craft-oriented educated chemists who were somewhat influenced by Paracelsian philosophy. Chemical producers like Rudolf Glauber (1604–1670) and chemical practitioners engaged in teaching like Jean Beguin (ca. 1550–ca. 1620), William Davisson (1593–1669), Estienne de Clave, Nicaise Le Febvre (1610–1669), Christopher Glaser (1621–1679), and Nicolas Lemery (1645–1715), who practiced and taught chemistry in France, mostly at the Jardin Royal des Plantes, belonged to this group of chemists. These educated chemical practitioners were authors of a specific kind of chemical book. The bulk of their books consisted of recipes for the preparation of medicines. These books depict in detail and at length the technical procedures of manufacturing drugs, often enlarged by the description of metallurgical operations and enriched by drawings of chemical instruments and vessels.[1]

---

[1] See Jean Beguin, *Les Elemens de Chymie* (Paris, 1615), originally published as *Tyrocinium Chymicum* (Paris, 1610); William Davisson, *Les Elemens de la Philosophie de l'Art du Feu ou Chimie* (Paris, 1651); Estienne de Clave, *Cours de Chimie* (Paris, 1646); Christopher Glaser, *Traité de la Chymie* (Paris, 1663); Nicaise Le Febvre, *A Compendious Body of Chymistry: Teaching the whole Practice Thereof by the most exact Preparation of Animals, Vegetables and Minerals, preserving their essential Vertues* (London, 1664), originally published as *Traicté de la Chymie*, 2 vols. (Paris, 1660); Nicolas

Detailed and unconcealed description of chemical operations distinguishes these books from sixteenth-century Paracelsian texts. Overall, they were chemical-technological manuals rather than philosophical texts,[2] although containing philosophical parts. However, the philosophical parts which use the basic conceptions and images of the Paracelsian philosophy were restricted, and confined to an introduction.[3]

In this paper I study the image of chemistry of these chemists and their understanding of the relationship between chemical art and nature. Since the authors of the chemical recipe books knew well contemporary chemical craft, and had been educated in Paracelsian natural philosophy, their conception of the relationship between chemical art and nature is particularly revealing.[4] It is well known that in Aristotelianism a distinction was made between mechanical art (mechanice techne) and nature. The Paracelsians and their followers revised Aristotelianism profoundly and supplemented it by alchemical and neoplatonic ideas, yet they also used some Aristotelian conceptions. This is the background against which my analysis of the nature-art relationship in the chemical recipe books should be seen. Although my examples come from the chemical textbook of Nicaise Le Febvre, my analysis is not confined to Le Febvre's image of chemistry.[5] Few authors discussed the nature-art relationship in chemistry as explicitly as Le Febvre. His textbook *Traicté de la Chymie* (1660) was translated into English and German, ran through various editions, and signified a culminating point of French chemical textbooks influenced by Paracelsianism.[6] As with many authors of the chemical recipe books, Le

---

Lemery, *Cours de Chymie* (Paris, 1675). On these books see Allen G. Debus, *The French Paracelsians—The Chemical Challenge to Medicine and Scientific Tradition in Early Modern France* (New York: Cambridge University Press, 1991), 123 ff.; Ursula Klein, *Verbindung und Affinität: Die Grundlegung der neuzeitlichen Chemie an der Wende vom 17. zum 18. Jahrhundert* (Basel, Boston: Birkhauser, 1994); idem, "Origin of the Concept of Chemical Compound," *Science in Context* 7, no. 2 (1994): 163–204; Hélène Metzger, *Les doctrines chimiques en France du début du XVIIe à la fin du XVIIIe Siècle* (Paris: PUF, 1923); James Riddick Partington, *A History of Chemistry*, 4 vols. (London: Macmillan, 1961–1970), 1:32 ff., and 2:2 ff.

[2] This portrayal differs from Metzger's; see Hélène Metzger, *Les doctrines chimiques en France.*

[3] An exception is Nicolas Lemery's textbook, which was strongly influenced by the mechanical corpuscular philosophy.

[4] For a much more encompassing study on the Paracelsian commitments of the authors of the French chemical textbooks, see Debus, *The French Paracelsians*, 123 ff.

[5] My analysis is based on a detailed examination of a series of the French chemical textbooks. See Klein, *Verbindung und Affinität.*

[6] It was followed by the textbooks of Nicolas Lemery's *Cours de Chimie* in which Paracelsian influences are still present but considerably weaker than in Le Febvre's book and those before it. Besides his textbook, Le Febvre published only a description of a specific pharmaceutical preparation entitled *A Discourse upon Sir Walter Rawleigh's Great Cordial,* English trans. Peter Belon (London, 1664).

Febvre had finished an apothecary apprenticeship. He became demonstrator in chemistry at the Paris Jardin des Plantes in 1652, professor of chemistry and apothecary in ordinary to King Charles II in 1660, and was elected a fellow of the Royal Society in 1663.[7]

Artificial and Natural Separation of Natural Mixts into Their Principles

Le Febvre defined the chemical art as follows:

> You see by the enumeration of these Mixts, of what vast extent is the Empire of Chymistry, since her operation is based upon these so different Compounds: for she may choose any of these bodies, *either to divide and resolve it into its Principles,* by making a separation of the Substances which do compound it; or she uses them, *to extract the mystery of nature out of them,* which contains the Arcanum, Magistery, Quintessence, Extract and Specifick, in a much more eminent degree, than the body from whence it is extracted.[8]

According to this definition, the chemical art had two goals, namely the separation of natural mixts into their principles and the extraction of substances like arcana, magisteries, and so forth, in general referred to as "essences" or the body's "mystery." Similar definitions of the art of chemistry can be found in other contemporary French chemical textbooks. The conceptions of principles and of the separation of principles within these textbooks was influenced by the Paracelsian philosophy.

The exact meaning of the term *principle* varied according to the theoretical context in which it was applied.[9] Within the Paracelsian theory of the constitution of natural mixts, principles were viewed as constituents of natural bodies, but not in the sense of corporeal parts but as carriers of sets of qualities which invested natural bodies with sensible properties and virtues. Thus, all natural mixts were seen as completely homogeneous, the same in all their parts.[10] Homogeneous natural bodies were called "mixts" not because they consisted of different corporeal parts but because they were constituted from

---

[7]For biographical details on Le Febvre, see Owen Hannaway, "Le Febvre, Nicaise," *Dictionary of Scientific Biography,* and Partington, *History of Chemistry,* 3:17ff.

[8]Le Febvre, *A Compendious Body of Chymistry,* 70–71. Parenthetical references are to this work; emphases added.

[9]On the Paracelsian conception of principles and natural mixts, see also Walter Pagel, *Paracelsus: An Introduction to Philosophical Medicine in the Era of the Renaissance* (Basel: Karger, 1958), 86ff.

[10]The speech of an outer shell and inner spirits had a metaphorical rather than a physical meaning. The criterion of this distinction was sensual perception. The outer corporeal shell was tangible and visible, whereas the inner spiritual essence was not sensible but could only be experienced through its effects.

different spiritual entities. Whereas in the theory of the constitution of natural mixts, the terms *principle* and *element* were synonymous,[11] their meaning differed slightly in the theory of the generation of natural mixts.[12] The Paracelsian theory of the generation of natural mixts assumed that natural mixts were created from one element and three principles. The element—either earth or water—was seen as the "matrix" or "womb," and the principles as "semina" that invested natural bodies with different qualities.[13] Although elements were understood as imprinting their "signature" on their fruits, the element-principle distinction in the Paracelsian theory of generation was largely based on the Aristotelian matter-form dualism.

According to Paracelsus' theory of generation the three principles were potentially contained in the elemental matrix.[14] Le Febvre's theory of generation differs in this respect. According to Le Febvre the principles originate in the universal or seminal spirit, which was "divested of all Corporeity" (13). The three principles—sulphur, mercury, and salt—are potentially contained in the universal spirit which was "one, simple and homogeneous."[15] In the generation of natural bodies, the universal spirit descends from heaven to earth, where it is corporified by the specific matrixes or wombs either of the element water or earth. At the same time, the three seminal principles of the universal spirit are actualized (16ff., 29–30, 39, 41–42). Whereas the elemental matrix invests natural bodies with corporeal qualities, like consistency, continuity, hardness, viscosity, and so on—in other words, creates corporeality itself—all other qualities of the bodies are derived from the three seminal principles. In particular, the principles carry all virtues and activities of natural bodies (16, 18).

---

[11]See, e.g., Le Febvre, *A Compendious Body of Chymistry*, 19–20.

[12]On the relation between elements and principles, see also Pagel, *Paracelsus*, 83, and R. Hooykaas, "Die Elementenlehre des Paracelsus," *Janus* 39 (1935): 175–187, here 184.

[13]See Paracelsus, "Philosophie and die Athener," in *Paracelsus' Sämtliche Werke*, transl. into modern German, Bernhard Aschner, from the ten-vol. Huser edition (1589–1591) (Jena: G. Fisher, 1930), 3; Paracelsus, "Das Buch über die Minerale," *Paracelsus' Sämtliche Werke*, 3.

[14]Paracelsus applies formulations like "contained in a subtle way" or "contained like a picture in wood"; see Paracelsus, *Paracelsus' Sämtliche Werke*, 3:778–779

[15]Le Febvre does not use the term *potential* but distinguishes between "distinct but not differing substances" and between the homogeneity of the universal spirit and its "threefold denomination": "This spiritual substance, which is the primary and sole substance of all things, contains in it self three distinct, but not differing substances: For they are homogeneous, as we have already said.... Nature is one, simple and homogeneous; if the seminal principles were heterogeneous, nothing would be found in nature one, simple, and homogeneous.... Let us then conclude, that this radical and fundamental substance of all things [the universal spirit], is truely and really one in its essence, but hath a threefold denomination"; see Le Febvre, *A Compendious Body of Chymistry*, 15.

Another difference between Paracelsus' conception of principles and that of Le Febvre and most other authors of French chemical textbooks concerned the number of principles (three, as opposed to five). This difference was based on the different empirical evidence available to these theories. Paracelsus referred to combustion as an operation that gave empirical evidence of his three-principle theory,[16] whereas the authors of the French textbooks referred to the distillation of plants. Plant distilling was a central operation for the preparation of medicines in the seventeenth century. If plants were distilled, one could obtain three kinds of volatile substances (water, spirit, and oil) and a residue which could be separated into a component soluble in water (salt) and an insoluble one (earth):

> After that the Artist hath performed the Chymical resolution of bodies, he doth finde last of all five kinde of substances, which Chymistry admits for the Principles and Elements of natural bodies…; [T]hese are, the Phlegmatick or waterish part, the Spirit or Mercury, the Sulphur or Oyl, the Salt, and the Earth. (19–20)

The term *principle* had a third meaning when it referred to substances separated by distillation. The separated principles of the Paracelsians were viewed as both corporeal and spiritual. They shared this ontological ambiguity with the arcana, elixirs, and other chemically processed substances called essences. Speaking of essences, Le Febvre emphasizes their intermediate state between the corporeal and the spiritual by suggesting a possible misreading of Paracelsus: "But it is here be noted, that when Paracelsus saith, that this mystery must be devested of its body, he means only that it must be freed from that gross body whererin it is imprisoned…"(55). Le Febvre made a similar statement discussing the separation of the five principles:

> But after these Principles are separated one from the other, and from the terrestreity and corporeity which they draw from their Matrixes, they make it plain enough by their powerful effects, that it is in this state they ought to be reduced, before they can work with efficacy, though they retain yet still their character and internal Idea. Thus some few drops of the true spirit of Wine will be more powerfull, then a whole glasse of this coporeal liquor wherein it was enclosed. (18)

---

[16]See Paracelsus, "Opus Paramirum," *Paracelsus' Sämtliche Werke*, 1:64 ff. See also Allen G. Debus, "Fire Analysis and the Elements in the Sixteenth and Seventeenth Centuries,"*Annals of Science* 23 (1967): 127–147, and idem, *The Chemical Philosophy: Paracelsian Science and Medicine in the Sixteenth and Seventeenth Centuries*, 2 vols. (New York: Science History Publications, 1977), 81 ff.

Thus, the separation of the five principles was a purification of the rough corporeal qualities of a body while the principles retained their specificity and the more subtle corporeal qualities. This conception of separation differs remarkably from the modern conception of chemical analysis. In contrast to modern views, it did not mean a separation into preexisting physical parts of a body, since natural mixts were seen as completely homogeneous. The conception of homogeneity entailed that separation was at the same time a creation of distinct physical constituents, or the re-creation of the constituent principles of the natural body. The original constituent principles and the chemically separated ones differed insofar as the former were purely spiritual whereas the latter still retained some corporeal qualities of the natural body. Hence the chemically separated principles were visible and tangible bodies despite their subtlety and purity. According to a familiar idea in the seventeenth century—that of the great chain of being[17]—they occupied an intermediary position between the universal spirit and the raw natural mixts.

If chemistry was largely the art of separating principles united together in the natural generation of the mixts, did this imply an image of chemical artificial separation violating nature? Nothing was farther from the truth, since Le Febvre as well as Paracelsians complemented the theory of generation by a theory of natural corruption according to which all natural mixts eventually undergo a natural destruction or putrefaction. In Le Febvre's version of natural corruption, bodies were separated into their constituent principles, the principles being gradually spiritualized, thus reverting to the universal spirit (45, 57 ff.). The Paracelsians and their followers had an image of an active nature, of one that was "never idle, but perpetually in action" (35). Corporification of the universal spirit and respiritualization of the corporified principles constituted a perpetual natural cycle. The separation of chemical principles in chemical art was part of this natural cycle. Hence, artificial separation was nothing else than an imitation and enforcement of natural corruption. Referring to the chemists' separation of natural mixts into principles, Le Febvre states that the "Chymical Artist, [is] fetching his instruction from nature itself" (19). He emphasizes that chemical art only contributes the chemical instrument fire which enforces natural processes, and vessels receiving the products of separation (21). Not only were the products themselves "merely and purely Natural," but the chemical process itself was "a mere natu-

[17]Arthur O. Lovejoy, *The Great Chain of Being: A Study of the History of an Idea* (Cambridge: Harvard University Press, 1936).

ral separation, assisted by the heat of the Vessels and the hand of the Artist" (21–22).

ENHANCEMENT AND EXTRACTION OF ESSENCES

The extraction of essences (also known as arcana, magisteries, balsams, flowers, and so on) was the main goal of the chemical practice to which Le Febvre refers, namely drug manufacturing. Two chemical operations were dominant in sixteenth- and seventeenth-century chemical drug preparations, distillation,[18] and slow extraction by means of a solvent called menstruum. Most of the distillations and extractions were interpreted by the authors of the seventeenth-century chemical-pharmaceutical books of recipes as the separations or extractions of "essences."

Why was it possible both to extract essences from natural bodies and to separate them into principles. How did essences differ from principles? Le Febvre writes:

> Therefore it cannot be thought strange, that other substances then the fore-mentioned five [the five principles], should be extracted from Mixt Bodyes by Chymical Operations, when the way of operating is altered, and proceeds by another way, then by separation of Principles, such as are the Quintessences, Arcana, Magisteries, Specificks, Tinctures, Extracts, Facula, Balsams, Flowers, Panacea's, and Elixirs, whereof Paracelsus treats at large, in his Books of Archidoxa; since all these several preparations take their vertues from the various mixture of the Principles.... (22)

Since all natural mixts were viewed as homogeneous, and separation as well as extraction accompanied the creation of distinct physical bodies, it depended on the chemical operation in question how the sets of qualities carried by the different principles were reorganized during the creation and separation of a substance from the natural body. Different reorganizations of qualities, or different mixtures of principles yielded different products of extraction.

Terms like "spirits," "essences," and so forth that were given to the extracted substances had both a technological and an interpretational meaning. Distilled "essences" were characterized as "subtle" and "pure," since they were more volatile compared with the basic substances and more effective as

---

[18]On the chemical operations done in seventeenth-century chemical-pharmaceutical practice and their interpretation by the authors of the French chemical textbooks, see Ursula Klein, *Verbindung und Affinität*; and idem, "Origin of the Concept of Chemical Compound" *Science in Context* 7 (2) (1994), 163–204.

medicine. Simultaneously essences were conceived of as pure and enhanced substances, nobler than unprocessed bodies:

> Besides the five Substances or Principles, which we have formerly said may be extracted out of natural Compounds, by the ministery of fire, there may be yet some Essences drawn, by diversifying the Operations of Art, which *exalts, and do ennoble the Principles of these Mixts, and raise it to their purity*. These Essences do not only differ in body, from that of the Compound whence they were extracted, but are *advanced also to nobler and more efficacious qualities and vertues*, than those which during it's intireness did adorn their bodies…." (55; empahsis added)

The conception of enhancement was closely related to the conception of purity. Le Febvre had at least four different notions of purity. First, substances referred to as pure were homogeneous, i.e. not mixed with other substances (49, 54). Second, pure substances were useful to "Man's Nature" (49). Third, pure substances were deprived of their corporeality, thus being spiritual. Fourth, they had one gender and species. When essences were interpreted as enhanced substances only the two latter meanings of purity were important: spirituality and an identical gender and species.

Exaltation was a purification whereby extracted essences were less corporeal and more spiritual than raw natural bodies. Extracted essences were not absolutely pure or spiritual, since they were still visible and tangible things applied in chemical operations. This ontological ambiguity of chemical essences as substances occupying an intermediary position between raw bodies and genuine spirits is emphasized by Le Febvre:

> Paracelsus in his first Book of Archidoxa's, saith, that the six following Preparations, viz. Essences, Arcana's, Elixirs, Specificks, Tinctures, Extracts, are contained in the mystery of Nature, which he calls Purity…thereby insinuating, that these Essences are brought neer and assimilated to their first Principle, which is of the nature of Fire, since Light it self, which is but Fire, is the first Principle of all things: In the same place, he calleth also the Body Impurity, which keepeth in Prison this mystery; and therefore saith, that he that will enjoy this mystery, must devest it of all Corporeity…. But it is here to be noted, that when Paracelsus saith, that this mystery must be devested of its body, he means only that it must be freed of that gross body wherein it is imprisoned, to impart him a more subtle one, which he may shake off with ease, and spiritualize himself, to be the more capable thereby to penetrate into our last digestions, and there correct all those defects which impurity might have caused." (55–56)

Now I come to the question of the relationship between chemical or artificial extraction and natural processes. In analogy to the separation of the principles of natural bodies, the chemical art of extracting and enhancing essences was seen as enforcing natural processes, namely the natural tendency of bodies to return to the universal spirit. Extractions not merely enforced natural processes, but were also a "correction" of nature (53). The idea of a correction of nature had its basis in Le Febvre's cosmographical ideas. Impurity could interrupt the natural perfection of bodies as a consequence of the deluge. The deluge yielded a mixture of the two elements water and earth—the former generating minerals and the latter vegetables and animals—and of their spiritual seeds. Hence, all Mixts came "under several genders, and different species," "as when Minerals become by some way or other, united to Vegetables or Animals" (52–53). Chemical Art had to "conduct the Mixt to the end of its natural predestination"; it had to free the natural body from its "domestick enemy, which insensibly doth creep into the Compounds" (53).

ARTIFICIAL MIXTURES

Le Febvre's image of nature compared nature's activity with human "workmanship" (60). Both kinds of workmanship—the natural and the human—were seen to a large degree as complementary. Hence, artificial chemical separation and extraction was conceived of as an imitation and enforcement of natural processes.[19] Did this imply there was no distinction at all between the chemical art and nature? Could chemistry imitate all actions of nature?

Le Febvre specifies nature's activities as follows:

> Nature which is still in action and busie about productions, makes use of the said substances [the separated principles], and applyes them to the generation of several other existencies, as Aristotle hath very well observed, when he saith that, Corruptio unium est generatio alterium. (21–22)

Thus, nature's activity comprised the production or regeneration of bodies. Did this image of chemistry also entail that chemical art could imitate natural generation? Le Febvre's theory of generation which incorporated the basic ideas of the Paracelsian theory of generation included the assumption that the generated natural mixts are homogeneous, the same in all their parts. Did Le

---

[19]Le Febvre does not mention transmutations in his definitions of chemistry, but he makes a few remarks on the transmutation of metals in the chapter on metals. There he states that "the power of Art" is able to transmute imperfect metals into noble ones, and that "both Art and Nature" are acting in this case in the same way. Thus, the conception of transmutation fits largely into the image of chemical art as imitating and enforcing natural processes. See Le Febvre, *A Compendious Body of Chymistry*, 65ff.

Febvre therefore believe that chemistry could create homogeneous artificial mixts analogous to natural mixts?

Le Febvre repeatedly emphasized that the goal of chemical art was the separation of natural bodies and the separation of impurity from purity during the extraction of essences. However, he never claimed that chemistry could imitate natural generation or create new homogeneous mixts from heterogeneous ingredients.[20] In the chapter on natural generation, chemical art is not mentioned at all (56ff.). This is somewhat paradoxical, since the practical part of Le Febvre's textbook as well as other French textbooks indicate that, for example, artificially created salts were quite familiar in the second half of the seventeenth century.[21] Some of these homogeneous products of chemical transformation were seen as being analogous to natural salts, and, for example, called "sal marinus regeneratus," "artificial saltpetre," and so forth. However, Le Febvre did not discuss such homogeneous chemical artifacts in the theoretical part of his textbook. On the contrary, when it comes to generation, alteration, and the creation of new mixts, he made a sharp distinction between nature and art. Referring to these transformations, he maintained the Aristotelian distinction between artificial and natural mixtures. In "artificial mixtures" the parts were seen as "really mixt together, but without change or alteration of the whole substance..." (58). Examples from mechanical mixtures provided the necessary evidence. When "particles of Wheat and Barley mixt in a heap, are mingled in the same mass of Flower," the product was heterogeneous and the parcels were still perceptible to the eye (59). This kind of

[20]Besides the definition of chemistry quoted above, Le Febvre, *A Compendious Body of Chymistry*, 19, 34–35, 70, and 74, gives the following additional definitions: "For as the Anatomist doth make use of Rasors and other sharp Tools in his Dissections, to separate the better the several parts of the human body, which is his chief object: The same doth the Chymical Artist, fetching his instruction from Nature it self, to attain his end, which is nothing but to join homogeneal and separate heterogeneal things by the means of Heat." "For as Nature cannot communicate its Treasures unto us, but under the shade of Bodies, so can we do no more then to devest them by the help of Art from the grossest and most material part of that Body, to apply to our uses: for if we urge them, and spiritualize too much, so as they should fly from our sight and contact, then do they lose their bodily Idea and character, and return again to ther Universal Spirit..." "Chymistry worketh upon all these Mixts, to extract what is pure in them; and rejects their impurity." "Though Chymistry takes for its object all natural Bodies, yet properly and particularly she confines her Operations upon Mixt Bodies, which she teacheth how to exalt by the help of Solution and Coagulation, who do contain under them several kinds of Operations, tending all eithr to spiritualize or corporifie, Minerals, Vegtables, and Animals: so that the exaltation of any Mixt or Compound, is nothing else but the purest part of the same, by the help of several Solutions and coagulations often reiterated, brought to its highest prfection."

[21]For a detailed examination of the chemical practice of the creation of salts and their interpretation by the authors of the French chemical textbooks, see Klein, *Verbindung und Affinität*.

artificial mixture was called an "apposition" of the mixed parts. In the case of the mixture of wine and water and the apothecaries' mixtures of drugs the product was called a "confusion." Although in the artificial confusion, the parts of the mixed substances were imperceptible, it was heterogeneous, too, since there was no alteration of the whole substance. In contrast to the heterogeneous artificial mixture, the "natural mixture properly so said" was "strict union of the substances, whence some things substantial doth result, and yet different from the other Substances which constitute it, by the help of Alteration" (58–59). Once more, there is no hint in the theoretical part of the textbook, that chemical art could perform this kind of transformation.

Why was the chemical art not able to imitate natural generation? Le Febvre does not explicitly answer this question, but the answer is provided by his theory of generation and his statements on the constraints of chemical operations. Generation was a process that started with the universal spirit which was deprived of corporeality (i.e., that which was intangible, invisible, insensible). Natural mixts and their corporeality were only constituted in generation. Their constituents created corporeality, but were themselves not corporeal, and hence not sensible. However, chemistry was a "sensual philosophy" and art (72). Le Febvre's description of chemistry as an art and science that "takes for its object all natural Bodies, yet properly and particularly she confines her Operations upon Mixt Bodies" (74), also defines the constraints of chemical art. Chemical art could only manipulate visible and tangible natural things, but it could not act on pure spirits. Le Febvre even emphasizes that for practical ends chemists should refrain from spiritualizing bodies too much, since thus they would become unavailable to chemical operations:

> For as Nature cannot communicate its Treasures unto us, but under the shade of Bodies, so can we do no more then to devest them by the help of Art from the grossest and most material part of the Body, to apply to our uses: for if we urge them, and spiritualize too much, so as that they should fly from our sight and contact, then do they lose their bodily Idea and character, and return again to the Universal Spirit...." (34–35)

Conclusion

Le Febvre's Paracelsian image of chemistry restricted chemical transformations to the separation of principles and the extraction and enhancement of essences, and to transmutations of metals as marginal transformations. As to these kinds of chemical transformations chemical art was conceived of as imitating and enforcing nature. The artificial separation of principles was seen as imitation and enforcement of the natural corruption of mixts, and the exaltation of essences during their extraction as a process that brings natural substances to their natural predestination. Le Febvre distinguished sharply between artificial mixtures and natural mixts, in contrast to what was the case for separation and extraction. Natural mixts were understood as completely homogeneous bodies that could only be created by nature. Chemical art could merely produce mechanical or artificial mixtures, i.e. mixtures which were heterogeneous, since the mixed substances were not altered.

Le Febvre had two notions of the artificial, one as imitating and enforcing nature, the other as opposing nature. The latter continued the Aristotelian distinction between mechanice techne or mechanical art and nature. The true art of chemistry did, however, not resemble mechanical art but the art of the gardener.

Vera Cecília Machline

THE CONTRIBUTION OF LAURENT JOUBERT'S *TRAITÉ DU RIS* TO SIXTEENH-CENTURY PHYSIOLOGY OF LAUGHTER

TODAY'S INTEREST in the sixteenth-century Montpellier physician Laurent Joubert (1529–1582) springs from two vernacular works whose study has led in two separate directions.[1] However, as this paper suggests, these writings have in common certain traits worth exploring.

Since the mid-1970s, owing to Natalie Zemon Davis' *Society and Culture in Early Modern France,* Joubert's *Erreurs populaires* has been well known.[2] Furthermore, beginning in the late1980s, thanks to Gregory D. de Rocher's

---

[1] Besides a successful career both in Montpellier and in the French Court, a biographical sketch of Laurent Joubert includes a sizable list of Latin and vernacular writings on assorted medical subjects. Fashionable at his time, they include paradoxical demonstrations, arquebus wounds, various diseases, and mineral waters. Apart from the two works focused in this article, also noteworthy are *Pharmacopée,* and a revised edition of the *Chirurgia magna* written by Guy de Chauliac (c. 1300–1368). Joubert reached the highest point of his career in 1579. In that year, on top of already being first physician of Catherine de Médicis (1519–1589) and chancellor of the school of medicine of Montpellier, he was titled Ordinary Physician of the King of France, Henry III (1551–1589). Biographical sources of Joubert include Pierre-Joseph Amoreux, *Notice historique et bibliographique sur la vie et les ouvrages de Laurent Joubert, Chancelier en l'Université de médecine de Montpellier, au XVIe siècle* (Montpellier: J. G. Tournel, 1814; facs. reprint, Geneva: Slatkine, 1971); Louis Dulieu, "Laurent Joubert, Chancelier de Montpellier," *Bibliothèque d'Humanisme et Renaissance: Travaux et Documents* 31 (1969): 139–167; and idem, *La Médecine à Montpellier,* vol.2 (Avignon: Les Presses Universelles, 1979), 105–108, 340–343.

[2] This article relies on the Brazilian translation of Davis' study, originally published by Stanford University Press in 1975; it is entitled *Culturas do Povo: Sociedade e cultura no início da França Moderna, oito ensaios* (Rio de Janeiro: Paz e Terra, 1990); Joubert's *Erreurs populaires* is discussed 182–185, 210–217.

endeavors, both of its parts have become available to English readers.[3] Reputed earlier this century by Ernest Wickersheimer as a valuable document of Renaissance medical scholarship,[4] the *Erreurs populaires* was credited by Davis with the merit of inaugurating a novel strand of popular medical literature, namely, amendments to vulgar misconceptions. According to Davis, this stratagem allowed Joubert not only to profess the authority of university-trained physicians over competing medical "empirics," but also to control popular opinion.[5]

In addition to the *Erreurs populaires,* Joubert has also been in the public eye owing to his *Traité du ris.* This work was brought to light in the late 1960s by Mikhail M. Bakhtin's study of *Rabelais and His World,* which argues that laughter had a "positive, regenerating, creative meaning" in the age of the medical humanist François Rabelais (c. 1494–1553). Yet, for reasons left unclear by Bakhtin, this understanding soon gave way to a narrower view. From the seventeenth century onwards, besides pertaining only to low literary genres, laughter has been deemed "[either] a light amusement or a form of salutary punishment of corrupt and low persons."[6]

Thanks to Bakhtin, the *Traité du ris* received some attention in the 1970s. For one thing, dating from 1579 and consisting of three books, its complete version became available in facsimile reprint in 1973.[7] For another, it was subject to three relevant reviews by scholars curious about Rabelais's ideas on

---

[3]Joubert, *Popular Errors,* English trans., Gregory D. de Rocher (Tuscaloosa: University of Alabama Press, 1989); idem, *The Second Part of the Popular Errors,* English trans. Gregory D. de Rocher (Tuscaloosa: University of Alabama Press, 1995).

[4]Ernest Wickersheimer, "Un brave homme et un bon livre: Laurent Joubert et les *Erreurs populaires* au fait de la médecine et du régime de santé," in *La Médecine et les Médecins en France à l'époque de la Renaissance* (Paris: A. Maloine, 1905; facsimile reprint, Geneva: Slatkine, 1970), 497–542.

[5]Davis, *Culturas,* 184; see also Alison K. Lingo, "Empirics and Charlatans in Early Modern France: The Genesis of the Classification of the 'Other' in Medical Practice," *Journal of Social History* 19 (1986): 583–603. Joubert explains his concept of "empiric" medical practitioners in *Popular Errors,* 93.

[6]Bakhtin, *Rabelais,* English trans. (Bloomington: Indiana University Press, 1984), 67, 71; the *Traité du ris* is mentioned on 68. The edition used here succeeded the publication, in 1968, by the Massachusetts Institute of Technology, which in turn preceded the French translation by Gallimard in 1970. Earlier this century, the French literary scholar Jean Plattard, *La Vie de François Rabelais* (Paris: Van Oest, 1928), alluded to Joubert's *Traité du ris*; this reference occurs on p. 99 of the British translation *(The Life of François Rabelais,* London: Frank Cass, 1968); yet, Joubert's treatise on laughter received no real attention until Bakhtin's dissertation on Rabelais, already penned in the 1940s, was eventually published in the 1960s.

[7]Joubert, *Traité du ris, contenant son essance, ses causes, et mervelheus effais, curieusemant recerchés, raisonnés & observés* in *Traité du ris suivi d'un dialogue sur la Cacographie Française* (Paris: Nicolas Chesneau, 1579; facsimile reprint, Geneva: Slatkine Reprints, 1973).

laughter, as well as his claims that his amusing chronicles *Gargantua and Pantagruel* had therapeutic value.[8]

Indeed, it was quite a meager outcome, considering that "Rabelais does not go into much detail over the physiology of laughter," as remarked by Michael A. Screech and Ruth Calder in their survey on "Some Renaissance Attitudes to Laughter."[9] Screech and Calder noticed that man's risible disposition had been "a major concern" in early modern times. Overwhelmed by the "various opinions" held by Rabelais's contemporaries, they ventured only one generalization. According to them, "the classical authors…are rather weak on laughter, and this was recognized by Renaissance scholars." To substantiate their conclusion that these men "simply could not build up a satisfactory theory from the bric-à-brac of classical notions alone," Screech and Calder quoted a brief passage from the *Traité du ris* which actually bears witness to Joubert's vindication of his medical skills: "The subject of laughter is so elevated and profound, that few philosophers have attempted it, and none has won the prize of treating it properly."[10] Otherwise, this statement is even nowadays a fashionable commonplace.[11]

While Screech and Calder contend that there barely was a Renaissance revival of the classical physiology of laughter, Roland Antonioli asserts in *Rabelais et la Médecine* the continuance of a long-standing "tradition of medical laughter," embracing both a scholarly and a popular version. Thus, according to Antonioli, however playful, Rabelais' claims were not preposterous, as expounded in detail in the *Traité du ris*.[12]

---

[8]This claim occurs in practically all the prologues of *Gargantua and Pantagruel;* they are best interwoven in Rabelais' dedicatory letter to Odet de Coligny, Cardinal of Chastillon, which opens the *Fourth Book;* it comprises 517–521 in Rabelais, *Oeuvres complètes,* ed. Mireille Huchon (Paris: Gallimard, 1994).

[9]Michael A. Screech and Ruth Calder, "Some Renaissance Attitudes to Laughter," in *Humanism in France at the end of the Middle Ages and in the Early Renaissance,* ed. Antony H. T. Levi (Manchester: Manchester University Press/Barnes & Noble, 1970), 216–228; at 220.

[10]Screech and Calder, "Some Renaissance Attitudes to Laughter," 216–218. Based on the facsimile reprint of the *Traité du ris,* one finds that the passage borrowed by Screech and Calder from Joubert is in the thirteenth, unnumbered page of the dedicatory letter opening the *Traité du ris.* This letter was addressed to Marguerite de Valois (1553–1615), daughter of Henry II and Catherine de Médicis and wife of Henry of Navarre (the future Henry IV of France).

[11]See for instance Charles R. Gruner, *Understanding Laughter: The Workings of Wit & Humor* (Chicago: Nelson-Hall, 1978), 23, as well as the 1995 "Preface" to *Humor and Laughter: Theory, Research, and Applications,* ed. Antony J. Chapman and Hugh C. Foot (New Brunswick: Transaction Publishers, 1996), xxvii–xxviii.

[12]Roland Antonioli, *Rabelais et la Médecine* (Geneva: Droz, 1976), 356–364.

Before publishing his translation of this work,[13] Rocher applied it to classify the outbursts of laughter exhibited by characters in *Gargantua and Pantagruel*.[14] Rocher resorted to Joubert's laughing theory in view of the possibility that he perhaps "began composing his treatise as early as 1552—the year in which Rabelais ended...his four unquestionably authentic books."[15]

Yet, the actual date when Joubert penned the *Traité du ris* remains obscure. On the one hand, he himself claims that this work was the first one he composed in his life. Originally written in Latin, it languished in his private library for years. He was brought to recognize its worth much later, when a student of his showed him the French translation he had secretly made of this Latin manuscript, after chancing upon it by accident.[16] On the other hand, the publication in 1560 of the first book of the *Traité du ris*, which was nineteen years later avowed "unauthorized," encourages speculation. For instance, it raises the possibility that the two subsequent books could have been written as late as 1578, the year when the first part of the *Erreurs populaires* was initially printed.[17]

It is far more certain that, because Wickersheimer preferred to dwell upon the *Erreurs populaires*, Alexis Bertrand's short overview in 1904 ended up being the last time the *Traité du ris* was appraised in the realm of history of medicine.[18] Since then, this treatise has only concerned scholars pursuing Rabelais' fusion of medicine and literature in *Gargantua and Pantagruel*. For that matter, carrying out a study foreseen in the late 1920s,[19] Rocher proposed that these chronicles are a prose enactment of the Renaissance notion that laughter

---

[13]Joubert, *Treatise on Laughter*, English trans., Gregory D. de Rocher (Tuscaloosa: University of Alabama Press, 1980).

[14]Rocher, *Rabelais's Laughers and Joubert's Traité du ris* (Tuscaloosa: University of Alabama Press, 1979).

[15]Rocher, *Rabelais's Laughter*, 3.

[16] This claim is in the dedicatory letter described in n. 10 above; it occurs in the seventeenth, unnumbered page in the facsimile reprint of the *Traité du ris*.

[17]The possibility that Joubert wrote the first book of his *Traité du ris* in 1559, from the very beginning in French, is investigated by Claude Longeon, "Loys Papon, Laurent Joubert et le *Traicté du Ris*," *Réforme Humanisme Renaissance* 7 (1978): 9–11. The "unauthorized" publication of Joubert's treatise on laughter is entitled *Traicté du Ris*, French translation by Loys Papon (Lyon: Jean de Tournes, 1560). Rocher included a detailed account of the editions of the first part of the *Erreurs populaires* in his translation of the *Popular Errors*, xix–xxv; by the way, this work eventually incorporated references to the complete version of the *Traité du ris*.

[18]Bertrand, "Une théorie du rire: Laurent Joubert" in his *Mes Vieux Médecins* (Lyon/Paris: A. Storck & Cie., 1904), 65–98; see also Wickersheimer, "Un brave homme," 501, in which this historian of medicine estimates Bertrand's overview sufficient.

[19]About the origins of this scheme see n. 6 above, and Rocher, *Rabelais's Laughter*, 3.

was "paradox made flesh."[20] As explained by him, his conclusion was conditioned by the fact that the intellectual arena of laughter in Rabelais' time was medicine, and its underpinning, physiology.[21]

This much said by way of introduction, the present paper shall be arguing that the *Traité du ris* was also intended to manipulate popular opinion. It is true that this work conveys a far less patronizing Joubert than the *Erreurs populaires,* in which the excellence of physicians is trumpeted to the full. However, in light of sixteenth-century physiology of laughter, the *Traité du ris* betrays the same intent. Furthermore, except for being centered upon laughter, it seeks also to amend common knowledge just as well. Thus, to afford a better appreciation of fundamental subtleties underlying the *Traité du ris,* instead of focusing on it immediately, this paper will initially discuss why the Cinquecento was a turning point in European ideas about laughter.

A significant factor that fostered such change was the "civilizing process" described by Norbert Elias. Coupled with the Renaissance revival of Epicurean and Stoic ideas, it brought forth an earnest concern about man's risible disposition.[22] It is true that, regardless of its relaxing virtue, laughter had also been a vexing question in classical times, having busied thinkers such as Plato (c. 428–c. 348 B.C.), Aristotle (284–322 B.C.), Cicero (106–43 B.C.), and Quintilian (c. 25–c. 96).[23] Nevertheless, the guidelines of social decorum, initially fashioned in courtly households and soon extended to bourgeois homes, gave rise to an intense contempt for boisterous laughter and abusive deriding in early modern times. A good example is the book of manners written by Baldassare Castiglione (1478–1529), originally published by the Aldine press in 1528. Titled *Il cortegiano,* one fourth of its pages are dedicated entirely to laugh-

[20]Rocher, *Rabelais's Laughter,* 141; this passage alludes not only to Joubert's theory, but also to Barbara C. Bowen, *The Age of Bluff: Paradox & Ambiguity in Rabelais & Montaigne* (Urbana: University of Illinois Press, 1972).

[21]Rocher, *Rabelais's Laughter,* 140.

[22]Elias, *The Civilizing Process,* English trans. (Oxford/: Blackwell, 1994); see esp. part 2 of "The History of Manners,"pp. 42–215; among other articles in *Atoms, Pneuma and Tranquility: Epicurean and Stoic Themes in European Thought,* ed. Margaret J. Osler (Cambridge: Cambridge University Press, 1991), see Letizia A. Panizza, "Stoic Psychotherapy in the Middle Ages and Renaissance: Petrarch's *De remediis,*" 39–65, and Louise Fothergill-Payne, "Seneca's role in popularizing Epicurus in the Sixteenth Century," 115–133.

[23]See for instance Plato, *Philebus* (esp. 30–67) in *The Dialogues of Plato,* English transl. (Chicago: Encyclopædia Britannica, 1978), 619–639; Aristotle, *Nichomachean Ethics,* book 2, chap. 7 (esp. 1108a.20–30) in *The Works of Aristotle,* ed. W. David Ross, English trans. (Chicago: Encyclopædia Britannica, 1978), 2:353; Cicero, *De oratore,* book 2, chaps. 54–71, of vol. 1, English trans. (Cambridge, Mass.: Harvard University Press/William Heinemann, 1988), 356–419; and chapter 3, book 6, of Quintilian', *The Institutio oratoria of Quintilian,* book 6, chap. 3 in vol. 2, English transl. (Cambridge, Mass.: Harvard University Press/William Heinemann, 1985), 439–501.

ter as well as to formalizing socially acceptable forms of witticism, that is to say, jokes not relying on ridiculing infirmities and misfortunes of fellow-men.[24]

A flagrant symptom of this nonreligious sensibility to exorbitant laughing was the progressive restriction of Carnival-like festivities, which were far more numerous and longer than today. Until the early days of the sixteenth century, they had been tolerated by the Catholic Church—notwithstanding their burlesque jibes, notable for an irreverence nowadays unthinkable.[25] In other words, amidst Reformation and its countermovement, nonclerical scruples about laughter prompted a diligent effort to understand this easily inconvenient human trait.[26] A clue to the changing mainstream thought is outlined in the work on human emotions written by the Spanish-born humanist Juan Luis Vives (c. 1492–1540). Published in 1538, Vives' *De Anima et Vita* maintains that, even though laughter

> is always natural rather than willed... it can be controlled by habit and reason to prevent excessive outbursts that shake the entire body. Such are the convulsions of the ignorant, the peasants, children, and women, when they lose their self-control as they are overcome by laughter of this kind.[27]

Closer to the original meaning of natural philosophy speculating about the workings of a world made up of both a macro- and a microcosm,[28] sixteenth-century physiology tended to consider laughter as one of about thirty

---

[24]*The Book of the Courtier* is available to English readers in more than one translation; the second book here referred to comprises pp. 89–197 in Charles S. Singleton's English translation (Garden City: Doubleday, 1959); see also Peter Burke, *The Fortunes of the Courtier: The European Reception of Castiglione's Cortegiano* (University Park: Pennsylvania State University Press, 1995), esp. 8–18, where Elias' "civilizing process" is interwoven with the revival of Cicero's *urbanitas* and kindred concepts.

[25]Peter Burke, *Cultura Popular na Idade Moderna,* Brazilian trans. of *Popular Culture in Early Modern Europe* (São Paulo: Companhia das Letras, 1989); see esp. 202–265, and John H. Towsen, *Clowns* (New York: Hawthorn Books, 1976), 16–48.

[26]The same applies to our modern concept of humor, namely, an amusing stimulus sometimes stirring up laughter. As rightly remarked by William F. Fry, "Humor and Paradox," *American Behavioral Scientist* 30 (1982): 42–71, no "one has yet been able to provide an understanding or recognition that makes it possible to reconcile humor's powerfully pleasurable, recreational, creative, and constructive nature with its potential for hostility and destruction....This is paradoxical"; "Humor and Paradox," *Americn Behavioral Scientist* 30 (1982): 42–71.

[27]Vives, *The Passions of the Soul: The Third Book of De Anima et Vita,* trans. Carlos G. Noeña (Lewiston: Mellen, 1990), 58; for further details of Vives' *De Anima et Vita,* see Carlos G. Noreña, *Juan Luis Vives and the Emotions* (Carbondale: Southern Illinois University Press, 1989).

[28]Since its origins in Presocratic times, physiology has varied considerably its range of scientific inquiry, along with changes in philosophical and cosmological views regarding vital phenomena; see e.g. Karl E. Rothschuh, *History of Physiology,* English trans. (Huntington: Krieger Publishing, 1973).

passions of the soul or the mind.[29] Currently known as emotions, the passions were seen in very distinct terms before the nineteenth century, as part of the doctrine of reflex action as an explanation of muscular movement,[30] which is the basis of today's understanding of laughter.[31] Also known as perturbations, affections, or affects, they were regarded in Joubert's time as sensual "movements" of the soul or mind, aroused by the imagination of some good or ill thing. While on the one hand they were "acts," or "operations" of the appetitive faculty of the soul (or mind), on the other hand, they were thought capable of causing "passive" alterations on the body.[32]

Before the rise of seventeenth-century mechanical philosophy, which turned the soul (or mind) into little more than a passive observer of bodily changes, the passions had a corporeal instrument. According to Aristotelian physiology, the heart as seat of all vital and mental powers, expanded or contracted, depending on the heating or cooling nature of the ongoing affection. For example, joy and pleasure dilated the heart and warmed the body, whereas grief and fear were responsible for its constriction and the ensuing feeling of coldness.[33] As pointed out by Owsei Temkin in his study on Galenism, the heart remained the center of life with Galen (129–c. 199) in spite of his Platonic view, which gave the liver, heart, and brain their respective share of the soul.[34] Thus, unless reason intervened, the heart continued subservient to the passions, whose somatic effects on the body went beyond cardiac commo-

---

[29]This estimate is based on the total number of passions analyzed by Vives in *Passions*. Interestingly, Vives himself did not consider laughter an emotion, but "an external action proceeding from within ... caused by joy and pleasure"; for further details, see chap. 10, pp. 57–59, which covers of most of Vives' ideas on laughter. Throughout time, the passions have been ascribed either to the soul or to the mind; the roots of this long-standing divergence are briefly discussed in Aristotle, *On the Soul*, book 1, chaps. 1–2, (esp. 403a.1–404b.7) in *The Works of Aristotle*, 1:632–633, and in Thomas S. Hall, *History of General Physiology, 600 B.C. to A D. 1900*, vol. 1 (Chicago/London: University of Chicago Press, 1975), 38, 142.

[30]See for instance Georges Canguilhem, *La formation du concept de réflexe aux XVIIe et XVIIIe siècles* (Paris: PUF, 1955), 3.

[31]William F. Fry, "The Respiratory Components of Mirthful Laughter," *Journal of Biological Psychology* 19 (1977): 39–50; Arthur Koestler, *The Act of Creation* (Harmondsworth: Penguin, 1989), 27–32.

[32]Lelland J. Rather, "Old and New Views of the Emotions and Bodily Changes: Wright and Harvey versus Descartes, James, and Cannon," *Clio Medica* 1 (1965): 1–25.

[33]Ibid., 1–3; Thomas S. Hall, "Greek Medical and Philosophical Interpretations of Fear," *Bulletin of the New York Academy of Medicine*, 2d series, 50 (1974): 821–832.

[34]Owsei Temkin, *Galenism: Rise and Decline of a Medical Philosophy* (Ithaca: Cornell University Press, 1973), 121.

tions and included possible changes in the qualitative mixture, or the mutual balance, of bodily humors.[35]

This physiological understanding explains why emotions had long been taken into consideration by medical theory.[36] Formally speaking, however, they were incorporated into medicine in the wake of twelfth-century Galenism,[37] either by the author or the translator of the primer known as the *Isagoge*.[38] Henceforth, practically until the last century, together with ambient air, food and drink, sleep and watch, motion and rest, evacuation and repletion, the passions became one of the six "non-natural" sets of factors that, despite being exogenous, could either promote or undermine health.[39]

Recognized since biblical times, mirth was often stressed in late medieval *consilia* and *regimina sanitatis*.[40] For that matter, well known among historians of medicine is the recommendation given by the *Regimen Sanitatis Salernitanum* of resorting to "Doctor Merry-Man" to assure good health.[41] By the same token, as told by Glending Olson in his study on *Literature as Recreation in the Later Middle Ages,* listening to cheerful stories was a customary medical

[35]Ibid., 88–89, 181; see also Luis García-Ballester, *Alma y Enfermedad de la obra de Galeno* (Granada: Secretariado de Publicaciones de la Universidad de Granada, 1972), 113–152.

[36]For instance, in book 2, sec. 4 of the Hippocratic work *On Epidemics,* there is the following advice: either "to regain color, or to reanimate [somebody], one should provoke an intense choler—and joy, fear, and the like." This passage is quoted from *Tratados Hipocráticos,* Spanish trans., vol. 5 (Madrid: Editorial Gredos, 1989), 171.

[37]Temkin, *Galenism,* 97–114; and Michael R. McVaugh, "The Nature and Limits of Medical Certitude at Early Fourteenth-Century Montpellier," *Osiris,* 2d series, 6 (1990): 64–84, esp. 62–65.

[38]For further details about the *Isagoge,* a Latin adaptation of c. 1100 of an Arabic work attributed to the Nestorian physician Joannitius, or Hunayn ibn Ishaq al-'Ibodi (809–c. 877), see Temkin, *Galenism,* 105–107; also, Jerome J. Bylebyl, "The Medical Meaning of Physica," *Osiris,* 2d series, 6 (1990): 16–41, esp.y 32; an English translation of the *Isagoge* constitutes appendix 4 of Edward T. Withington, *Medical History from the Earliest Times: A Popular History of the Healing Art* (London: Scientific Press, 1894), 386–396.

[39]Besides the "six non-naturals," there were seven endogenous "natural" agents as well as an infinite number of pathological "contra-natural" causes. The few discussions on these three sets of factors include: Jerome J. Bylebyl, "Galen on the Non-Natural Causes of Variation in the Pulse," *Bulletin of the History of Medicine* 45 (1971): 482–485; Luis García-Ballester, "On the Origins of the 'Six Non-Natural Things' in Galen," in *Galen und das hellenistische Erbe,* ed. Jutta Kollesch and Diethard Nickel (Stuttgart: Steiner, 1993), 105–115; Peter J. Niebyl, "The Non-Naturals," *Bulletin of the History of Medicine* 45 (1971): 486–492; and Lelland J. Rather, "The 'Six Things Non-Natural': A Note on the Origins and Fate of a Doctrine and a Phrase," *Clio Medica* 3 (1968): 337–347.

[40]E.g., Prov. 17:22 advises: "A cheerful heart is a good medicine, but a downcast spirit dries up the bones." As for the subtleties distinguishing *consilia* from *regimina sanitatis,* see Jole Agrimi and Chiara Crisciani, *Les Consilia Médicaux,* French trans. (Turnhout: Brepols, 1994), esp. 18–24.

[41]See, e.g., David Riesman, *The Story of Medicine in the Middle Ages* (New York: Paul B. Hoeber, 1936), 45.

advice in those times,[42] a fact that makes clear why, just like Rabelais, Renaissance comic authors often boasted about mitigating the sufferings of their readers with their funny stories.[43] Another source of amusement still prevalent in Joubert's age was the entertainment provided by itinerant healers. As surveyed by Alison K. Lingo in her research about "Empirics and Charlatans in Early Modern France," these healers lured customers in many different ways, including magical tricks and comic antics.[44]

While gaiety was encouraged, there was much reticence about laughing carelessly.[45] This was because, akin to strokes of excessive joy, the explosive outbursts of laughter seemed to challenge the doctrine of the mean, that is to say, *sophrosyne*.[46] Dating back to Pythagorean cosmology, this all-embracing physiological canon, holding weighty ethical and medical implications, was consecrated by Galenism as mediocrity.[47] Better known as the principle of moderation, it postulated that any intemperate action was an infringement of rational and virtuous conduct. This was particularly true of inordinate passions.[48] Likely to bring about widespread misfortune such as warfare, they could cause death to individuals if they reached paroxysmal proportions amounting to a fatal expansion or contraction of the heart.

It goes without saying that, aware of ancient reports of casualties from excessive joy,[49] the sixteenth-century intelligentsia were eager to determine

[42]Glending Olson, *Literature as Recreation in the Later Middle Ages* (Ithaca/London: Cornell University Press, 1986), 39–89.

[43]Deborah N. Losse, *Sampling the Book: Renaissance Prologues and French Conteurs* (Lewisburg : Bucknell University Press, 1994), 57–78.

[44]Lingo, "Empirics and Charlatans," 583–587.

[45]Olson, *Literature as Recreation,* 11.

[46]About this golden rule, see Whitney J. Oates, "The Doctrine of the Mean," *The Philosophical Review* 45 (1936): 382–398; F. la T. Godfrey, "The Idea of the Mean," *Hermathena* 81 (1953): 14–28; Theodore J. Tracy, *Physiological Theory and the Doctrine of the Mean in Plato and Aristotle* (Chicago: Loyola University Press, 1969).

[47]Galen, *A Translation of Galen's Hygiene (De Sanitate Tuenda)* (Springfield, Illinois: Charles C. Thomas, 1951), 20–21.

[48]E.g., see Galen, *On the passions and errors of the soul,* English trans. (Columbus: Ohio State University Press, 1963); James Hankinson, "Actions and Passions: Affection, Emotion, and Moral Self-Management in Galen's Philosophical Psychology" in *Passions and Perceptions: Studies in Hellenistic Philosophy of Mind*, Proceedings of the 5th Symposium Hellenisticum, ed. Jacques Brunschwig and Martha C. Nussbaum (Cambridge: Cambridge University Press, 1993), 184–222; Norenā, *Vives*, 213–218; Anthony Levi, *French Moralists: The Theory of the Passions 1585 to 1649* (Oxford: Clarendon Press, 1964), 234–256.

[49]Obviously, one source was Pliny the Elder (A.D. 29–79); see book 7 of his *Natural History,* vol. 2, English trans. (Cambridge, Mass.: Harvard University Press, 1989), 584–585, 626–627. Although possibly not entirely trustworthy, a comprehensive list of ancient and medieval sources is given by Rabelais in chapter 10 of *Gargantua;* see his *Oeuvres complètes,* 32–33. Bakhtin, *Rabelais,* 408–410, also deals with fatal cases of laughter.

whether laughter complied with the doctrine of the mean. Far from easy, this appraisal stumbled upon a long-standing puzzle, seldom discussed by classical thinkers. As pointed out by Joubert in the opening of his *Traité du ris,* being conversant with the propositions of earlier authorities who had dwelt on the subject, it had come to his notice that none of them had arrived at a satisfactory explanation of "all the effects and the sudden convulsions" accompanying laughter. According to him, they all lacked determining at what we laugh.[50] In other words, Joubert was pointing out that almost nothing had been written about "the ridiculous,"[51] or, strictly speaking, the actual cause giving rise to bursts of laughter.[52]

Due to the relevance of this topic in the Cinquecento, even physicians were pondering over a matter possibly postulated for the first time in the Aristotelian *Poetics.* According to this work, the ridiculous was "a species of the Ugly.… a mistake or deformity not productive of pain or harm to others; the mask, for instance, that excites laughter, is something ugly and distorted without causing pain."[53]

Rather vague outside classical Greek thought, this definition was known by most Renaissance scholars through borrowings or paraphrases of second-hand sources, due to the late recovery of the *Poetics.* Even though officially inaugurated in 1498, its rebirth only warmed up in the 1550s, when there was an upsurge, particularly in the Italian peninsula, of several translations. Usually in Latin but occasionally in vernacular, these renderings sometimes included glosses on the ridiculous, penned by industrious translators.[54]

Similarly to contemporary attempts to reconstruct the Aristotelian theory of comic catharsis,[55] these sixteenth-century commentaries tried to make up for the inherent laconism of the *Poetics,* even more prominent when dealing

---

[50]Joubert, *Traité du ris,* 14, which pertains to the prologue of the first book.

[51]Mary E. Grant, "The Ancient Rhetorical Theories of the Laughable: The Greek Rhetoricians and Cicero," *University of Wisconsin Studies in Language and Literature* 21 (1924): 1–166;; for instance, Castiglione, *Courtier,* 145, practically repeats the difficulty in grasping the ridiculous already recognized in Cicero, *De Oratore,* 1:372–373, and later seconded in Quintilian, *Institutio,* 2:440–443.

[52]For further details about the causes of passions according to Aristotle, see W. W. Fortenbaugh, *Aristotle on Emotion: A Contribution to Philosophical Psychology, Rhetoric, Poetics, Politics and Ethics* (New York: Harper & Row, 1975), 15.

[53]Aristotele, *On Poetics* (1449a.32–35), in *Works of Aristotle,* 2:683.

[54]For further details, see Marvin T. Herrick, *Comic Theory in the Sixteenth Century* (Urbana: University of Illinois Press, 1950), 37–52.

[55]Apart from Umberto Eco's playful *The Name of the Rose,* recent speculations include Richard Janko, *Aristotle on Comedy: Towards a Reconstruction of Poetics II* (Berkeley: University of California Press, 1984); or Dana F. Sutton, *The Catharsis of Comedy* (Lanham: Rowman & Littlefield, 1994).

with laughing matters.[56] Thus, the Paduan humanist Antonio Riccoboni (1541–1599) suggested in *Ex Aristotele ars comica* that laughter sprung from both joy and pleasure,[57] while the Brescian commentator Vincenzo Maggi (c. 1500–1564) proposed in his *De ridiculis* that laughing was a double movement of expansion and contraction of the heart, caused by turpitude and wonder.[58]

Usually relying on hearsay sources of the *Poetics, Cinquecento* physicians exhibited the same lack of consensus. For instance, according to the Paduan doctor Girolamo Fracastoro (c. 1478–1553), laughter was a twofold movement made up of wonder and joy, which accounted for it conveying an intrinsic contradiction. While wonder kept the soul in suspense, joy promoted its expansion. Consequently, as warned his *De sympathia et antipathia liber unus*, laughing became difficult after the heart reached its maximum limit of normal expansion. This problem, however, only concerned people who were easily surprised. Apart from morbid cases, they included immature youngsters and simpleminded people.[59]

Differently from Fracastoro, the Turin professor of medicine François Valeriole (1504–1580) seems to have suggested in his *Énarrationes medicimales* that man's "risible affection" was a hazardous fit of intense joy.[60] Explicitly wishing to rebut Valeriole's extreme position and to improve Fracastoro's hint of a halfway alternative, Laurent Joubert came up with a third proposition to an old-time dilemma in his *Traité du ris*.[61]

Making the most of the doctrine of the mean, Joubert defined laughter as practically "the middle ground between joy and sadness, each of which in their extremities [could] cause loss of life." As explained in the first book, what accounted for laughter being a compound passion made up of opposite emotions, and for happiness exceeding grief by just a little, was the nature of ridic-

---

[56]David W. Ross, *Aristotle* (London: Methuen, 1964), 16–19, 290.

[57]Antonio Riccoboni, *Ex Aristotele ars comica* in Riccoboni, *Poetica Aristotelis Latine Conversa* (Padua: Apud Paulum Meietum, 1587; facs. reprint, Munich: Wilhelm Fink Verlag, 1970), 139–172; dealing with the ridiculous, chap. 20 comprises 164–168; Riccoboni uses the words *leticia* and *voluptas*.

[58]Vincenzo Maggi, *De ridiculis* in Vincenzo Maggi and Bartolomeo Lombardi, *In Aristotelis librum de poetica communes explanationes* (Venice: Officina Erasmiana Vicentii Valgrisii, 1550; facsimile reprint, Munich: Wilhelm Fink Verlag, 1969), 301–317; Maggi uses the words *admiratio* and *turpitude*.

[59]Fracastoro, *De sympathia*, German trans. (Zurich: Juris Druck/Verlag, 1979); Fracastoro's ideas on laughter are in chap. 20, pp. 199–203. Considering that this work was originally published in 1546, according to the posthumous edition *Opera omnia, in unum proxime post illius mortem collecta: Quorum nomina sequens pagina plenius indicat* (Venice: Apud Iuntas, 1574), 74.a, Fracastoro's words were *admiratione* and *laetitia*.

[60]Joubert, *Traité du ris*, 163–164, which pertains to chap. 1 of the second book.

[61]Ibid., 13–15, 163–170.

ulous things. Based on Cicero's sketch of the ridiculous, Joubert presumed that everything laughable was "ugly or improper, yet unworthy of pity or compassion." Consequently, sadness derived from its ugliness and impropriety, while joy resulted from the awareness that, in everything that is ridiculous, "there is nothing to pity (other than a false appearance)." The reason why happiness always outweighed sorrow was that there never was any serious harm or evil in laughable matters. Succeeding one another rapidly, joy and grief protected man from the danger of an acute heart expansion or contraction caused by a plethoric fit of either passion.[62]

The possibility that laughter would prompt a wholesome mean applied only to the variant Joubert considered "genuine," or natural. This type sprang from the heart of healthy individuals after they apprehended a ridiculous deed or word.[63] Conversely, the kind of laughter he named "bastard," or illegitimate, often was a sign of ill health. As detailed at length by Joubert, such laughter stemmed from an infinite number of maleficent causes, the most common being humoral imbalance, tickling, rupture of the diaphragm or certain nerves, an ill-functioning spleen, the poison of the spider popularly called tarantula, excessive intake of wine or saffron, and the plants called gelotophyllis and sardomia.[64]

Usually bearing all the ordinary physical signs of true laughter such as the jostling of the chest and the broken voice, a false mode could nevertheless be distinguished from its genuine counterpart by symptomatic facial evidences of intemperance. As explained by Joubert, when laughter "is dissolute or of long duration the throat opens wide and the lips draw back to an extreme.... And because of this, laughter becomes ugly, improper, and lascivious." According to the Montpellier physician, immoderate laughter tired "the muscles, which are then unable to draw up the mouth and put it back in its right position, due to which it remains indecently open." Another effect of dissolute laughing was the appearance of wrinkles in the face and round the eyes. As stated by Joubert, that is why "young girls are warned not to laugh foolishly, and threatened that they will become old sooner."[65]

Talking about paroxysm, a plethoric state characterized nearly all the ancient epithets minutely reviewed by Joubert in the second book. Among many more, these included Ajax, Ionic, Megaric, Cynic, Sardonian, Canine,

---

[62]Joubert, *Traité du ris*; these passages are from 88, 16, and again 88.

[63]For further details about the traditional distinction between the comic as it is witnessed and as it is recounted, see Rocher, *Rabelais's Laughers,* 11–14.

[64]Joubert, *Traité du ris;* these explanations extend from the first to the third book, 133–318.

[65]Ibid., 103–115.

and Homeric laughs. Together with cachinnation, they were variations of inordinate laughing caused by an unhealthy state that, if not duly treated, was bound to be fatal, either as a consequence of the original ailment or as a result of the exhaustion ensuing from excessive laughing.[66]

Modest laughter was the only type that matched Joubert's concept of legitimate laughter. Nevertheless, one should be sparing even of it. Actually, like all "non-naturals," depending on the physical disposition of each individual, even a nonindulgent laugh could be harmful, as readers are warned in the final chapters of the third book of the *Traité du ris*.[67]

Although much more could be said about this treatise, the time has come to draw some conclusions. Having initially pointed out the present existence of both a medical and a literary interest in Laurent Joubert, this article has attempted to suggest that there may exist a strong link between the *Popular Errors* and the *Treatise on Laughter*. Apart from the possibility that they could have been partly written just a year apart, these works appear to share the same twofold goal: advocating the status of the physician while correcting popular misconceptions. Such resemblance, however, only reveals itself once there is an acquaintance with sixteenth-century physiology of laughter. Ushered by the Ciceronian ideal of urbanity, this chapter of the history of ideas regarding laughter seems to foretell later developments, including the Romantic concept of humor, namely, "the happy compound of pathos and playfulness."[68] In early modern times, as discussed here, the physiology of laughter busied scholars such as Joubert, who took pains to grasp the elusive nature of "the ridiculous" and to decry boisterous laughing.

In light of this background, Joubert's contribution to sixteenth-century physiology of laughter is at least bifold. First, considering his concept of a moderate, genuine mode of laughter, he should be credited for having arrived at a proposition that complied with both the standards of decorum and the physiological premises of his time. Secondly, in view of his initiative to disclose in French his ideas on the subject, he may also be acknowledged for having fashioned a popular medical work that disseminated among commoners both a physician's expertise in the complexities of laughter, and the notion

---

[66]Ibid., 170–219.

[67]Joubert, *Traité du ris*, 330–352; the expression "modest laughter" occurs in the first book, 114, and is repeated in book 2, p. 213.

[68]Louis Cazamian, *The Development of English Humor*, parts 1 and 2 (Durham: Duke University Press, 1952; facsimile reprint, New York: AMS, 1965), 411; see also Raymond Klibansky, Erwin Panofsky, and Fritz Saxl, *Saturn and Melancholy: Studies in the History of Natural Philosophy, Religion, and Art* (London: Thomas Nelson & Sons, 1964), 233–235.

that there is only one kind of laugh truly wholesome and socially acceptable. An indication of Joubert's design, perhaps derived from a good use of Castiglione's *Il cortegiano*,[69] is the fact that he chose to comment on the giggling disposition of young girls rather than on the fits of laughter of simpletons, objected to in Latin by Vives and Fracastoro.

Joubert's *Traité du ris* raises the question as to the actual extension, and success, of an early modern popular literature dealing with the appropriate nature of moderate laughing. But this is only a minor point since there are abundant grounds for the future investigation of laughter—today proclaimed "the best medicine" owing to its beneficial impact upon the physiology of the body and the psychological disposition of our minds.[70]

We will probably never fully understand what makes us laugh, and why a good-humored disposition is wholesome. At any rate, the future does not immediately concern historians of science. Still, it is worth considering that, nowadays, hospitals are welcoming clowns incarnating the "Doctor Merry-Man," metaphorically envisaged in the late Middle Ages and virtually enacted in early modern times by anonymous itinerant healers as well as men of letters such as François Rabelais.

[69]Rocher, *Treatise on Laughter,* 136 n. 20, raises the possibility that Joubert was acquainted with Castiglione's *The Book of the Courtier.*

[70]Fry, "Laughter: Is It the Best Medicine?" *Stanford Medical Alumni Association* 10 (1971): 16–20; idem, "The Biology of Humor," *Humor* 7 (1994): 111–126; see also Joseph D. Dunn, "New Discoveries in Psychoneuroimmunology: An Interview with Dr. Lee S. Berk," *Humor & Health Letter* 3 (1994): 1–8.

ACKNOWLEDGMENTS

This article was possible thanks to two Brazilian funding institutions and two research facilities of The Johns Hopkins University. The Coordenação de Aperfeiçoamento de Pessoal de Nível Superior (CAPES) has provided for my doctoral research into sixteenth-century physiology of laughter, between 1992 and 1996, under the direction of Professor Ana Maria Alfonso-Goldfarb; the Conselho Nacional de Desenvolvimento Científico e Tecnológico, CNPq, has enabled me to pursue my studies in Baltimore, Maryland, in 1994; last but not least, The Johns Hopkins University Institute of the History of Medicine and the Milton S. Eisenhower Library generously shared with me their bibliographical resources.

CONTRIBUTORS

ANA MARIA ALFONSO-GOLDFARB chairs the Centro Simão Mathias de Estudos em História da Ciência, as well as the newly founded Graduate Program on History of Science, both linked to the Pontifícia Universidade Católica de São Paulo in Brazil. Her research is centered mainly on the history of chemistry, particularly on issues related to hermeticism, including its transition to modern science.

MARTHA BALDWIN is an assistant professor in the Department of the History of Science,Stonehill College, North Easton, Massachusetts. Her research interests include early modern medicine, folk medicine, and medical experiments. Her scholarly articles on such matters have appeared in *Isis*, *The Bulletin for the History of Medicine*, and *Ambix*.

NICHOLAS H. CLULEE received his Ph.D. from the University of Chicago and is professor of history at Frostburg State University, Frostburg, Maryland, where he teaches medieval, Renaissance, and early modern European history. He is the author of *John Dee's Natural Philosophy* (1988) and his current research focuses on early modern natural philosophy, alchemy, and magic.

ALLEN G. DEBUS is the Morris Fishbein Professor Emeritus of the History of Science and Medicine at the University of Chicago. He has published extensively on Renaissance and early modern science and medicine including *The English Paracelsians* (1965), *The Chemical Philosophy: Paracelsian Science and Medicine in the Sixteenth and Seventeenth Centuries*, 2 vols. (1977), *Man and Nature in the Renaissance* (1978), and *The French Paracelsians: The Chemical Challenge to Medical and Scientific Tradition in Early Modern France* (1991). In addition, he has published new editions of works by John Dee, Elias Ashmole, Robert Fludd, and John Webster as well as many research papers. He has achieved the Sarton Medal and the Pfizer Award of the History of Science Society, the Dexter Award of the American Chemical Society, the Edward Kremers Award of the American Institute of the History of Pharmacy, and an honorary degree from the Catholic University of Louvain.

CHARLES D. GUNNOE, JR., Department of History, Calvin College, Grand Rapids, Michigan, is completing his dissertation at the University of Virginia under H. C. Erik Midelfort entitled "Thomas Erastus: A Renaissance Physician in Reformation Heidelberg." He has written articles and reviews on Reformed Protestantism, the Palatinate, and Paracelsianism.

265

URSULA KLEIN is a research fellow at the Max Plank Institute for the History of Science, Berlin. She was a visiting scholar at Harvard University, 1996–1997. She is author of *Verbindung und Affinitat: Die Grundlegung der neuzeitlichen Chemie an der Wende vom 17 zum 18. Jahrhundert* (1994).

VERA CECÍLIA MACHLINE participates in the faculty of the recently founded graduate program on history of science at the Pontifícia Universidade Católica de São Paulo. Centered in the history of medicine, her research is presently focused on early modern concepts of laughter, particularly those concerned with its psychological and humoral aspects.

STEPHEN A. MCKNIGHT is professor of European intellectual and cultural history at the University of Florida. His publications include *International and Interdisciplinary Perspectives on Eric Voegelin* (1997), *Science, Pseudo-science and Utopianism in Early Modern Thought* (1992), *The Modern Age and the Recovery of Ancient Wisdom: Historical Consciousness, 1400–1650* (1991), *Sacralizing the Secular: The Renaissance Origins of Modernity* (1989), and *Eric Voegelin's Search for Order in History* (1978). He is also recipient of the Mahon Undergraduate Teaching Award (1992), the College of Arts and Sciences Teaching Award (1994), and the University Teaching Excellence Award (1994).

BRUCE T. MORAN is professor of history at the University of Nevada, Reno, where he teaches the history of science and early modern Europe. He is the author of *The Alchemical World of the German Court: Occult Philosophy and Chemical Medicine in the Circle of Moritz of Hessen (1572–1632)* and has edited *Patronage and Institutions: Science, Technology and Medicine at the European Court, 1500–1750*, both published in 1991. Currently, he is preparing a cultural study of the works of Andreas Libavius, entitled *Chemists and Cultures in Early Modern Germany: Andreas Libavius and His War of Words*.

WILLIAM R. NEWMAN received his Ph.D. in history of science from Harvard University in 1986. He has published two books on the history of alchemy: *The Summa perfectionis of pseudo-Geber* (1991) and *Gehennical Fire: The Lives of George Starkey, an American Alchemist in the Scientific Revolution* (1994). He is associate professor of the history and philosophy of science at Indiana University, Bloomington.

LAWRENCE M. PRINCIPE holds a Ph.D. in chemistry from Indiana University and a Ph.D. in the history of science from The Johns Hopkins University, and he is currently a senior lecturer at Johns Hopkins. He has recently completed his first book, *The Aspiring Adept: Robert Boyle and His Alchemical Quest* (in press).

JOLE SHACKELFORD recent publications include "Rosicrucianism, Lutheran Orthodox, and the rejection of Paracelsianism in Early Seventeenth-Century Denmark," *Bulletin of the History of Medicine* 70 (1996), and "Early Reception of Paracelsian Theory: Severinus and Erastus," *Sixteenth Century Journal* (26 (1995); and a chapter entitled ""Unification and the Chemistry of the Reformation" in *Infinite Boundaries: Order, Disorder, and Reorder in Early Modern German Culture*, edited by Max Reinhart (1998). He is currently assistant professor at the University of Minnesota, teaching in the history of science and technology program.

MICHAEL T. WALTON's most recent works are "Should Genetic Health Care Providers Attempt to Influence Reproductive Outcome Using Directive Counseling Techniques," in *Genetic Services Proceedings*, ed. Freeman, Hinton, and Elsas (1996;with Robert M. Fineman) and "Witches, Jews and Spagyrists: Blood Remedies and Blood Transfusion in the Sixteenth Century," *Cauda Pavonis*, (Spring 1996; with Phyllis J.Walton). He is completing a study of law and medicine in fifteenth-century London.

KATHLEEN WELLMAN is an associate professor of history at Southern Methodist University and the author of *La Mettrie: Medicine, Philosophy and Enlightenment* (1992). Her article in this book is part of a larger study of the content of Renaudot's conferences which places them in a broad seventeenth-century context and conceives of them as a crucial link between Renaissance humanism and Enlightenment social science.

THOMAS WILLARD has edited the alchemical tracts of Jean D'Espagnet for the English Renaissance Hermeticism Series (1997). He serves as review editor of *Cauda Pavonis Studies in Hermeticism* and teaches English at the University of Arizona.

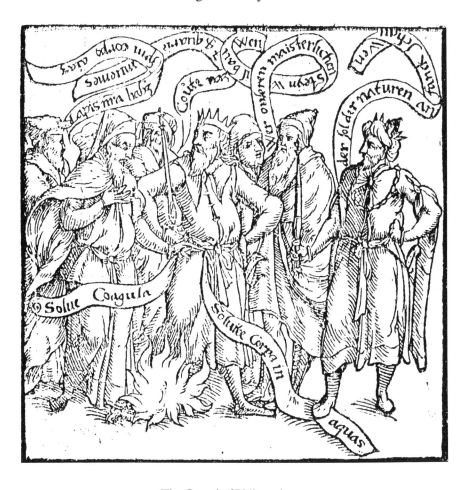

The Crowd of Philosophers,
Auriferae artis, quam chemiam vocant antiquissimi authores sive Turba philosophorum,
P. Perna (Basle, 1572)

INDEX